Infections in Bones and Joints

Infections in Bones and Joints

Carl Norden, MD
American Cyanamid Company
Medical Research Division
Lederle Laboratories
Pearl River, New York

Formerly of
Department of Medicine
University of Pittsburgh School of Medicine
Pittsburgh, Pennsylvania

William J. Gillespie, FRCSEd, FRACS
Clinical Research Unit
Princess Margaret Rose Orthopedic Hospital
Edinburgh, Scotland

Sydney Nade, DSc, MD
Department of Surgery
Westmead Hospital
Westmead, Sydney, Australia

Boston
BLACKWELL SCIENTIFIC PUBLICATIONS
Oxford • London • Edinburgh • Melbourne
Paris • Berlin • Vienna

Blackwell Scientific Publications

EDITORIAL OFFICES:

238 Main Street, Cambridge, Massachusetts 02142, USA
Osney Mead, Oxford OX2 0EL, England
25 John Street, London WC1N 2BL, England
23 Ainslie Place, Edinburgh EH3 6AJ, Scotland
54 University Street, Carlton, Victoria 3053, Australia
Arnette SA, 1 rue de Lille, 75007 Paris, France
Blackwell-Wissenschaft, Kurfürstendamm 57, D-10707 Berlin, Germany
Blackwell MZV, Feldgasse 13, A-1238 Vienna, Austria

DISTRIBUTORS:

USA
Blackwell Scientific Publications
238 Main Street
Cambridge, Massachusetts 02142
(Telephone orders: 800-215-1000 or 617-876-7000)

Canada
Times Mirror Professional Publishing
130 Flaska Drive
Markham, Ontario L6G 1B8
(Telephone orders: 800-268-4178 or 905-470-6739)

Australia
Blackwell Scientific Publications (Australia) Pty Ltd
54 University Street
Carlton, Victoria 3053
(Telephone orders: 03-347-5552)

Outside North America and Australia
Blackwell Scientific Publications, Ltd.
c/o Marston Book Services, Ltd.
P.O. Box 87
Oxford OX2 0DT, England
(Telephone orders: 44-865-791155)

Typeset by Huron Valley Graphics
Printed and bound by Braun-Brumfield, Inc., Ann Arbor, MI
Designed by Joyce C. Weston

Printed in the United States of America
94 95 96 97 5 4 3 2 1

Library of Congress Cataloging in Publication Data

Norden, Carl.
Infections in bones and joints / Carl Norden. William J. Gillespie, Sydney Nade.
p. cm.
Includes bibliographical references and index.
ISBN 0-86542-273-7
1. Musculoskeletal system—Infections. I. Gillespie, William J. (William John) II. Nade, Sydney. III. Title.
[DNLM: 1. Bone Diseases—microbiology. 2. Bone Diseases—diagnosis. 3. Joint Diseases—microbiology. 4. Joint Diseases—diagnosis. WE 251 N8291 1994]
RC925.5.N67 1994
616.7—dc20
DNLM/DLC
for Library of Congress 94-12123
CIP

Contents

Notice: The indications and dosages of all drugs in this book have been recommended in the medical literature and conform to the practices of the general medical community. The medications described do not necessarily have specific approval by the Food and Drug Administration for use in the diseases and dosages for which they are recommended. The package insert for each drug should be consulted for use and dosage as approved by the FDA. Because standards of usage change, it is advisable to keep abreast of revised recommendations, particularly those concerning new drugs.

Preface

The basic terminology of musculoskeletal infections (e.g., septic arthritis or osteomyelitis) is well established and clinically useful. It identifies the tissue or space to which the infection is at least initially confined, or whose structure and function are most obviously affected. The infections that primarily affect soft tissues, with the exception of a few, such as clostridial myonecrosis and the various manifestations of necrotizing fasciitis, have a reputation of easier resolution, which has persisted since before the introduction of antimicrobial agents. Osteomyelitis, in contrast, conjures in many minds an image of a chronic disabling disease for which surgery, often difficult, is always required.

Antimicrobial agents, when readily available, have profoundly changed the incidence and outcome of musculoskeletal infections. Contrary to the hopes and expectations of many, they have not, however, abolished the need for surgical drainage or surgical debridement in chronic bone infection. In the developed world, diagnosis and treatment are generally early. Antibiotics are readily available and widely prescribed. Specialist attitudes to management tend to reflect training; surgeons operate, internists prescribe and aspirate, and the imaging department has techniques that compete for a role in diagnosis and increasingly allow effective minimal interventions that might replace surgical procedures. In the developing world, diagnosis is often late, antibiotics are scarce, and medical services are poorly resourced.

Although some good comparative studies are emerging in the field of prevention, they are scarce in the management of musculoskeletal infections. As better methods for such studies have been defined, so has hematogenous osteomyelitis, for example, declined significantly in incidence in the developed world. A difficulty that remains to be overcome is the development of generally accepted staging protocols for both acute and chronic bone and joint infections.

In this book, we attempt to review the range of musculoskeletal infection to provide a synthesis of current views from the perspective of clinical management and an entrée for interested readers to the history of how these views have emerged, as well as to some aspects of contemporary research that seem to explain old problems or clarify the value of traditional clinical approaches.

In the first section, some general aspects of pathogenesis are discussed, including the strengths and weaknesses of current classification schema, microbial and host factors, and an issue of potential importance in outcome, structural degradation and repair of bone and cartilage. Experimental models have contributed substantially to contemporary knowledge; these models are reviewed in some detail.

The second section covers diagnostic strategy in evaluating potential musculoskeletal infection. If some aspects appear self-evident to experienced clinicians, they will no doubt move on; but we make no apology for stressing the critical importance of clinical evaluation in different contexts, and the inherent waste and occasional danger in relying on investigations that, although well described and readily available, contribute little or nothing to an optimal management algorithm.

The various clinical syndromes are covered from two directions. After an introduction to the principles of management, osteomyelitis, infectious arthritis, and soft-tissue infections are covered systematically. The problem of the infected joint replacement, although conceptually a special case of chronic osteomyelitis, is important enough to deserve its own chapter. Prevention and management of infection following fractures have become increasingly important with the increased use of internal fixation techniques. Discussion follows of the special features of infections caused by a number of organisms, including spirochaetes and mycobacteria, which are re-emerging as important pathogens in the developed world and have continued to provide major problems elsewhere. Finally, a number of conditions that mimic infection in bone are briefly considered.

Throughout, we tried not only to indicate the uncertainties that make decision-making difficult, but also to suggest a recommended course of action for contemporary practice. Particularly, but not exclusively, in the field of antibiotic prophylaxis and treatment, we believe that many of these recommendations could change over the next number of years as new agents and comparative studies become available. The need for continuing research in the area of bone and joint infections is critical and has increased, rather than diminished, in an era of exciting new diagnostic modalities, antimicrobial agents, and surgical techniques. The ability to incorporate these methods in a cost-effective manner into the management of bone and joint infections will determine our success. Answers to the questions posed in this book must come from data obtained from carefully conducted research that can be appropriately integrated into clinical practice.

Carl Norden
William J. Gillespie
Sydney Nade

Acknowledgments

Each author owes a major debt to an individual who stimulated a deep interest in musculoskeletal infection. We acknowledge the late Dr. Edward H. Kass, former Professor of Medicine of Harvard University School of Medicine, the late Mr. J. D. Morgan, Nuffield Orthopaedic Centre, Oxford, England, and his mentor Professor Josep Trueta, and the late Dr. K. M. Mayo, formerly Director of Radiology, Middlemore Hospital, Otahuhu, Auckland, New Zealand.

Our secretaries, Mrs. Gloria Zoda, Mrs. Miriam Messick, Mrs. Lyndie Barrkman, and Mrs. Cheryl Dineen, patiently handled the many revisions required to bring the manuscript to its final form.

We are grateful to Victoria Reeders and Coleen Traynor for their professional and patient advice and editorial assistance.

Our wives, Joyce, Lesley and Sally, provided support and encouragement to complete this work; we owe them a major debt for this and much more.

We also acknowledge assistance from the following for the provision of text figures: Dr. Alex Norman, Dr. Gary Wormser, Dr. Jack Lawson, Dr. Martin McHenry, Dr. Benjamin Lipsky, Dr. Peter Rissing, Dr. Thomas Berquist, Dr. Robert Klein, Dr. Denise Leslie, Dr. Arnold Jacobson, Dr. Kenneth Sherbon, Dr. Roger Uren, Dr. Kazimir Kozlowski, Dr. George Chapman and Dr. Ian Beggs. The Radiological Libraries of Princess Margaret Hospital for Children, Perth, Western Australia, and Westmead Hospital, Sydney, NSW, Australia were also a source of radiographs.

PART ONE

Pathogenesis

CHAPTER 1

Nomenclature and Classification Systems

Comparability between outcomes reported in bone and joint infections is dictated by the limitations of nomenclature and the available classification and staging systems. Problems are experienced particularly in the many presentations of osteomyelitis and in some of the extensive soft-tissue infections considered in Chapter 20. The increasing sophistication of available imaging modalities allows a much more detailed assessment of both soft-tissue involvement and changes within bone than was historically possible; their availability is likely to determine the scope of future comparative studies.

The term *osteomyelitis* is now widely used in the English language to describe any infection involving bone. It appeared first in the French literature in the mid-nineteenth century (1), prior to which a range of other terms, notably *necrosis,* was employed (2). The term *osteomyelitis* applies to medullary infections involving trabecular bone and marrow. Some prefer *osteitis,* which is more logical, but on the whole convention has prevailed, and we use *osteomyelitis* in that wide context.

A number of classification systems, of varying degrees of formality, have been devised for osteomyelitis. Broadly, they are anatomical, etiological, or clinical in context and claim utility as guides to clinical diagnosis and management or as predictors of outcome (3–9). None has so far proved universally applicable as a basis for outlining management strategy or for comparative studies, as have some staging systems used in oncology.

The etiological classification of Waldvogel and colleagues (3) has been widely used and is the basis of the manner in which osteomyelitis is approached in this book. Trueta (4) proposed a system that he applied to acute hematogenous osteomyelitis; however, because it considers primarily the extent of soft-tissue involvement, it could also be usefully applied to chronic disease with established radiological signs in bone. The classifications of Cierny and Mader (5), Roberts and associates (6), and Gledhill (7) describe the anatomy of the bone lesion and, in some cases, the quality of the skeletal response to infection. Kelly (8) distinguished between post-traumatic cases with fracture union and nonunion. Petersen (9) noted that the diagnosis of osteomyelitis made without confirmation of the organism involved can only be considered "possible" or "probable." Although inability to culture a pathogen may indicate technical failure, it may also reflect the paucity of organisms present and the nature of the balance between bacteria and host.

Each of these classifications identifies features of importance in planning management and thus in evaluating outcome. Ideally, therefore, their essential elements should be incorporated into a staging system that would allow more detailed comparison between patients and between series. Such a system would detail the route by which the infecting organisms accessed the bone, identification of the organism or organisms, host status with respect to nutrition, immune competence, and comorbidity, disease activity at the onset of treatment, and anatomical involvement of bone and soft tissue, as determined by well-defined imaging strategies.

After some debate, we decided not to attempt a synthesis of all these elements in this book. That it can be done, albeit with some difficulty, we have little doubt. However, it would be best achieved by the consensus of a much larger group of interested individuals and should be designed with a view to a subsequent program of validation and utility assessment. We expect that this task will be undertaken in the next few years, and that from it will follow more rigorous multicenter comparative studies addressing some of the unanswered questions posed in later chapters.

References

1. Nelaton A. Elements de pathologie surgicale. Paris: Bailliere, 1844.
2. Smith N. Observations on the pathology and treatment of necrosis. Phil J Med Surg 1827;1:11–19;66–75.

3. Waldvogel FA, Medoff G, Swartz MN. Osteomyelitis: a review of clinical features, therapeutic considerations and unusual aspects. N Engl J Med 1970;282:198–206.
4. Trueta J. The three types of acute haematogenous osteomyelitis. A clinical and vascular study. J Bone Joint Surg [Br] 1959;41:671–680.
5. Cierny G, Mader JT. Adult chronic osteomyelitis: an overview. In: D'Ambrosia RD, Marier RL, eds. Orthopaedic infections. Thorofare, NJ: Slack, Inc., 1989:31–48.
6. Roberts JM, Drummond DS, Breed AL. Subacute haematogenous osteomyelitis in children. J Pediatr Orthop 1982;2:249–254.
7. Gledhill RB. Subacute osteomyelitis in children. Clin Orthop 1973;96:57–69.
8. Kelly PJ. Infections of bones and joints in adult patients. Instr Course Lect 1977;26:3–13.
9. Peterson HA. Musculoskeletal infections in children. Instr Course Lect 1984;33:33–37.

CHAPTER 2

Microbial and Host Factors

The difficult reputation of osteomyelitis arises from the tendency toward chronic, recurrent infection. Before the introduction of antimicrobial drugs, it was observed that previous infection with *Staphylococcus aureus* was associated with an increased risk of infection at subsequent surgery (1). In some hosts, clinical infection is more or less constant, with continuing fistulous discharge; in others, episodes of inflammation occur unpredictably at variable intervals. Although most recurrent infections are recognized within one year of the primary episode (2), delays of up to 80 years have been reported (3). Thus, it is clear that colonies of some pathogenic organisms are capable of long-term symbiotic existence in bone. Until the last decade, the mechanisms were poorly understood. There is now a plausible description of the events that surround establishment of bacterial colonies in bone, although as yet only limited understanding of the dynamics of recurrent infection exists.

Microbial Factors

The initial event in localization of infection appears to be adhesion (4–7). The presence of a solid phase, whether encountered by chance or on a chemotactic gradient, encourages initial loose adhesion, which is potentially reversible (8). If at its surface the solid phase offers a configuration for which the micro-organism possesses a receptor, or if it is coated by one of a number of matrix glycoprotein molecules, a highly specific molecular adhesion occurs (9). For example, *S. aureus* strains have been shown to possess receptors for types I (10,11) and II collagen (12), fibrinogen, laminin, fibronectin, thrombospondin, bone sialoprotein, and heparin sulphate (13–17). A collagen receptor gene from a strain of *S. aureus* has been cloned (18).

The conservation of expression of these receptors between strains is not known, nor is the localization of different matrix proteins mapped out clearly throughout skeletal development and growth. However, it is clear that regional variation in matrix protein distribution does exist in the growing skeleton. Bone sialoprotein is expressed particularly in fetal growth plate chondrocytes, particularly in the hypertrophic zone: It appears to be expressed at later stages of differentiation to an osteoblast phenotype (19). The adjuvant role of injury in experimental models and perhaps in clinical practice may be explained by exposure of binding sites for strains of *S. aureus*. Strong morphological evidence for the importance of collagen binding has been demonstrated (20). Variable expression of bacterial surface ligands could account for the failure of some strains to produce infection in otherwise standardized experimental situations.

Following adhesion, firm attachment occurs. In the case of *S. aureus*, this process involves elements of the polysaccharide pseudocapsule, which form strong links between the bacterial cell and the solid surface. Polysaccharide production is essential for the development of surface films on solid surfaces but not for initial adhesion (21), although it may be triggered by some adhesion-associated factor. Such surface films have been demonstrated in human and experimental osteomyelitis, on both bone and implant surfaces (22). The synthesis of capsular polysaccharide 8 (CP8) has been studied in an experimental model of foreign body infection (23). Synthesis begins shortly after adherence and increases over one week, after which the rate stabilizes. It appears likely that these extracapsular polysaccharides offer substantial protection against antibiotic activity. Agents such as rifampicin, clindamycin, and some of the fluoroquinolones have a degradative effect on biofilms (24–27). Polysaccharide biofilms may also inhibit elements of both specific and nonspecific immunity in experimental preparations (28). In mice, T- and B-cell blastogenesis, chemotaxis, and opsonization appear inhibited, and virulence is increased. Leukocyte locomotion may also be disturbed (29). Adherence of *S. aureus* to fibronectin-coated surfaces can be inhibited by immunoglobulin (30).

The mode of growth of bacterial pathogens and the factors that allow them to infect human bone have become increasingly elucidated within the past several years. In vitro incubation of *S. aureus* with bone chips, when interrupted at approximately 48 hours, produces glycocalyx formation (Figures 2-1A, B). Electron microscopic studies of bacterial growth, from two patients with chronic osteomyelitis (31), showed a "biofilm" mode of growth. It was noted that this method of growth resembles that seen on surfaces of medical biomaterials and in infections of prostheses in humans. Within the biofilm, the bacteria tended to form microcolonies, and cells within these microcolonies were connected to the surrounding environment and to each other by a fibrous exopolysaccharide matrix of glycocalyx material. It was postulated that this mode of growth may allow the bacterial population to interact with the colonized tissue (bone) and may also allow protection of the organisms from host defense mechanisms. In addition, it was noted that strains of *S. aureus,* which produced osteomyelitis in experimental animals, strongly bound to

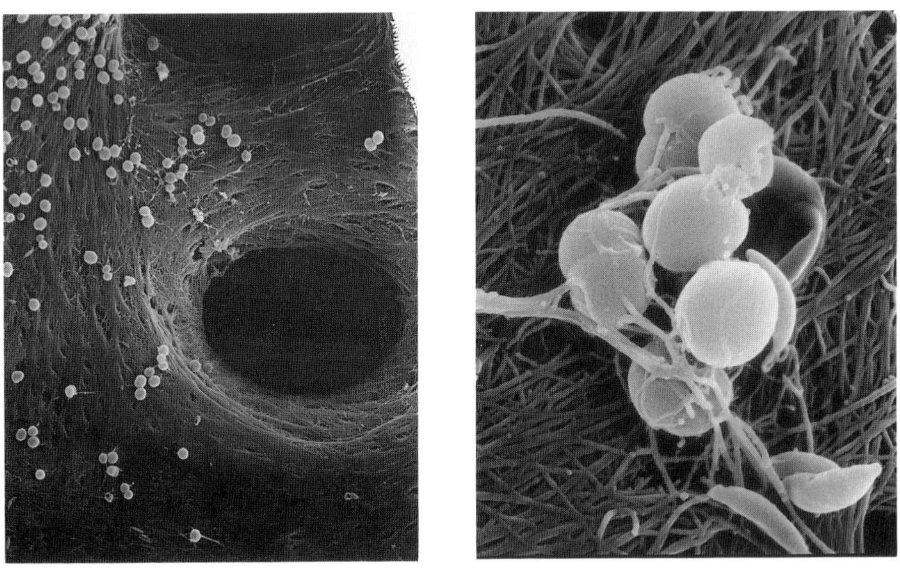

Figure 2-1. *In vitro incubation of bone chips with* Staphylococcus aureus *interrupted at 48 hours. (A) Endosteum of bone showing staphylococcus near the endosteal Haversian canal (×2,000). (B) Staphylococci enmeshed in glycocalyx near the Haversian osteum (×20,000).* (Courtesy of Dr. Peter Rissing.)

type I collagen; the authors suggested that this binding is a likely early event in acute osteomyelitis (32).

Changes have been noted in the patterns of cell wall development in staphylococci growing in situ in models of experimental osteomyelitis (33). When cells of *S. aureus* and *S. epidermidis* are grown in culture in nutrient-rich media, cell walls are regular in thickness, cell size is normal, and the patterns of septation are orderly. In contrast, when either species is examined in infected rabbit bone, the cell wall thickness is often greater and is more irregular, the size of the organisms is increased, and their septation patterns are abnormal. All these alterations occurred in the absence of antibiotics and suggested that they may be a response to alternate environmental conditions as well as growth of the organisms on hard surfaces.

Bacterial adherence and glycocalyx formation were studied in an experimental model of osteomyelitis caused by *S. aureus* in rabbits (34). Both transmission and scanning electron microscopy of the infected bone revealed bacteria embedded in a very extensive matrix of glycocalyx adhering to the bone and the surgically implanted catheter. Masses of gram-positive cocci were observed and it was postulated that if such large numbers of organisms, encased in glycocalyx, were typical of the disease, then the organisms could be protected from antibiotics and from phagocytosis by macrophages. Glycocalyx might serve a protective function for bacteria by interfering with phagocytosis (35,36); by covering the teichoic acid, which enhances opsonization (37); and by consuming or covering and altering the configuration of complement (37,38). Similar findings were noted in a rat model of experimental staphylococcal osteomyelitis, thus showing that formation of glycocalyx occurs in more than one animal species (39) (Figure 2-2). An apparent reduction in glycocalyx has been observed after treatment with clindamycin in animal models (40); clindamycin was found to be the most effective single agent in the treatment of experimental *S. aureus* osteomyelitis in rabbits (41). It is tempting to conclude that the ability of antibiotics, such as clindamycin, to reduce glycocalyx production is in some way associated with efficacy of the antimicrobial agent.

Others have further examined bacterial adherence in the problem of biomaterial-centered infection. Observations regarding the growth of organisms in biofilms in osteomyelitic bone (42) have been extrapolated to a sophisticated analysis of bacterial adhesion to biomaterials.

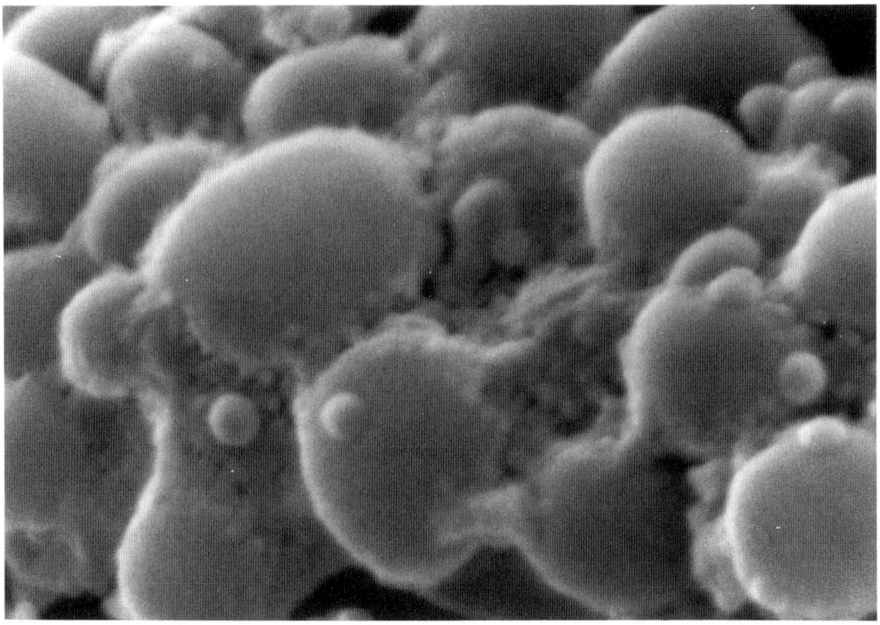

Figure 2-2. *Experimental osteomyelitis in the rat caused by* Staphylococcus aureus. *A high magnification of the coccoid-studded biofilm. Note the tendency for glycocalyx to form globular-shaped microspheres.* (Reproduced by permission from Buxton T, Horner J, Hinton A, Rissing J. In vitro glycocalyx expression by *Staphylococcus aureus* phage type 52/52A/80 in *S. aureus* osteomyelitis. J Infect Dis 1987;156:942.)

The following sequence has been postulated (43). (a) Invading bacteria introduced into the operative field or reach biomaterial by the hematogenous route are usually phagocytized by tissue macrophages, but the effect of biomaterial on phagocytic cells may impede that function and allow the organisms to adhere and multiply. (b) Even when the host responds to the presence of invading bacteria, it is not a totally effective response because bactericidal antibodies may not reach the bacterial cell surface (due to glycocalyx) and because leukocytes may not be able to phagocytize the large adherent masses of bacteria even if specific opsonizing antibodies are present. (c) The ion exchange function of the glycocalyx may protect the bacteria from antibiotics. (d) If all these steps occur, the bacteria will continue to grow and produce more glycocalyx and the infection will become well established. These processes call attention to the importance of biomaterials, which can block initial adherence of bacterial organisms, but also promote phagocytosis and bactericidal activity at their surfaces (44,45).

In a review of infections in prosthetic devices, bacterial adherence and slime production are discussed, and the importance of bacterial glycocalyx or extracellular slime substance as one mechanism of bacterial attachment is noted (46). Strains not producing slime appear less likely to adhere to plastic surfaces and are less likely to produce infection (47,48). It is unclear whether slime is necessarily involved in the intial phase of attachment (49) or if it is mainly produced after adherence takes place (50). The structure of extracellular slime substance is not totally clear; it is known to be water-soluble and to contain 40% sugar and 27% protein (51) and probably varies for different organisms. In culture, its production is markedly affected by the growth media used (51). All the following properties have been observed with slime obtained from coagulase-negative staphylococci: (a) inhibition of phagocytosis (52,53); (b) inhibition of chemotaxis and oxidative metabolism (54,55); and (c) suppression of mononuclear cell lymphoproliferative response, killer cell cytotoxicity, T helper suppressor cell ratio, and immunoglobulin synthesis (56,57).

Taken in conjunction with the adverse effects of tissue hypoxia in established osteomyelitis on host defenses, particularly on leukocyte function (58,59), this emerging picture of adhesion and biofilm production offers a plausible basis for the ability of bone infections to remain dormant for long periods. It could also account for the failure of antibiotics, in general, to achieve long-term cure in chronic osteomyelitis; for the lowering of the effective challenge dose of organisms (ID50) in the presence of implanted materials (60); and for the pathogenicity of biofilm-formers of low virulence, such as *S. epidermidis.*

Bone Resorption: Structural Effects of Osteoarticular Infection

The osteoclast is responsible for bone resorption in normal growth and remodeling and in pathological states, such as hyperparathyroidism. Cytokines capable of osteoclast stimulation, which appear to be involved in bone resorption in infection, include tumor necrosis factor (TNF)-alpha, TNF-beta, interleukin-1 (IL-1)-alpha and -beta, and prostaglandin E_2 (PGE_2) (61–63). Careful examination of the histology of recent models of osteomyelitis indicates that osteoclasts may be observed resorbing bone in acute bacterial infections (64). However, it is not clear that this process is entirely osteoclast-mediated. Release of calcium from devitalized bone in vitro by both macrophages (65,66) and polymorphonuclear leukocytes (PMNs) (67) has been demonstrated. Provided that the bone is stripped of its periosteum, it may also be demonstrated when mouse calvaria in tissue culture are exposed to PMNs in high concentrations (67). Although this latter effect might be indirect (mediated through the activation of osteoclasts), the results from devitalized bone indicate that direct bone degradation by inflammatory cells also occurs. These observations are supported by the morphological evidence that inflammatory cells derived from the joint capsule around prosthetic hip joints resorb devitalized bone slices (68).

Aspects of the biochemistry of resorption have been studied in a number of in vivo and in vitro models. Prostaglandin release from explants of normal and osteomyelitic human bone has recently been measured (69). The activity in osteomyelitic bone is 5 to 30 times that in normal bone. Administration of cyclo-oxygenase inhibitors reduces radiographic changes and prostaglandin production in the rabbit (70) and the rat (71). Injection of the prostaglandin precursor arachidonic acid augments bone degradation (72). Synergy between aerobes and anaerobic pathogens, which enhance prostaglandin production through phospholipase activity, also reduces the size of inoculum of *S. aureus* required to produce experimental osteomyelitis in the rat (73).

In summary, bone degradation in infection appears to involve both stimulation—by cytokine products of inflammation of resident cell populations normally involved in bone turnover—and direct resorptive effects produced by inflammatory cells of both monocyte/macrophage and granulocyte families. Although aspects of the kinetics have been studied, the relative importance of these mechanisms at different stages of the process has yet to be established.

Destruction of Articular Cartilage

There has been a strong association observed between pus and gross cartilage destruction in septic arthritis. The precise mechanisms of joint destruction remain unknown, although many chondrolytic enzymes and the factors involved in their elaboration have been identified in recent years. The major components of extracellular cartilage matrix are water (65%–80%), collagens (10%–30%), and proteoglycans (5%–10%). The balance of extracellular matrix is composed of noncollagenous matrix proteins and small amounts of lipids. Chondrocytes occupy only 2% to 10% of the tissue volume (74).

S. aureus is a frequent pathogen in septic arthritis. Strains isolated from patients with septic arthritis possess a collagen receptor that contains either two or three copies of an 187 amino acid repeat motif (75). Collagen receptor positive strains adhere to both collagen substrate and cartilage in a time-dependent process. It is believed that the collagen receptor is both necessary and sufficient to mediate bacterial adherence to cartilage and is an important part of the pathogenesis of septic arthritis (75).

Cartilage degradation appears to result from two principal degradative pathways: (a) direct invasion of synovium with local release of destructive enzymes, and (b) an indirect pathway that requires participation by chondrocytes activated by informational factors from synovium (76). Infection is not the only cause of articular cartilage degradation, and the specific mechanisms due to the presence of bacteria in a joint remain unclear. To try and answer some of these questions, several animal models for septic arthritis have been utilized. Despite these studies, there is still controversy about the initial events leading to erosion of the articular surface and the method of spread to the epiphysis and the growth plate (77,78).

The bacteriology and histopathology of an avian model of acute septic arthritis have been described (79). The first histopathological changes in the joints of chickens were detected 60 minutes after injection with *S. aureus*. At this time, there was slight inflammation of the synovium and intracapillary accumulation of polymorphonuclear neutrophils. Inflammation of the synovium was more extensive after 90 minutes, and by 3 hours, an exudate of neutrophils was observed in the joint lumen.

Bacteria were first detected histologically 6 hours after injection, when a small focus of staphylococci was located along the surface of the articular cartilage. After 12 hours, the bacteria had invaded the articular surface and occluded blood vessels within the cartilage. Twenty-four hours after intra-articular injection, invasion of articular cartilage by bacteria was quite obvious. Multiple abscesses were seen in the articular cartilage, and many blood vessels were occluded with bacteria. Adjacent vessels contained many inflammatory cells. The synovium was markedly inflamed and areas of necrosis were seen.

Destruction of articular cartilage had progressed by 48 hours, and several abscesses were surrounded by inflammatory cells. Loss of cartilage glycosaminoglycans was far more extensive. Masses of neutrophils were seen in the joint lumen as well as in the synovial and subsynovial tissues.

Four days after inoculation, clusters of staphylococci lined large areas of the joint, on both synovial and cartilage surfaces. Articular cartilage showed loss of staining for glycosaminoglycans through its entire thickness. Bacterial abscesses invaded into the deep zones of the articular cartilage, often adjacent to the secondary epiphyseal ossification center. A pannus had formed on the cartilage surface, and necrotic debris was found in the joint lumen.

By the eighth day after injection, the cartilage had further degenerated. Inflammation had spread into the secondary (epiphyseal) ossification center and occasionally deeper, into the growth plate. Articular cartilage vessels were occluded with either bacteria or inflammatory cells. Polymorphonuclear leukocytes were seen clumped together against exposed cartilage matrix and adjacent to necrotic chondrocytes. Damage to the whole joint was very extensive by 14 days.

Previous studies (80,81) demonstrated that the first histological evidence of degenerative changes in articular cartilage appeared 3 days after bacterial injection. The first changes were superficial erosion and loss of glycosaminoglycan staining at 3 days, followed by chondrocyte degeneration and finally mild loss of collagen at 7 days. Gross damage to articular cartilage only occurred after loss of collagen. In contrast, authors of another study (82) found bacteria congregated along the surface of the articular cartilage at 6 hours, followed by invasion of cartilage matrix and cartilage blood vessels at 12 hours and loss of uptake of glycosaminoglycan stain and cartilage erosion as early as 24 hours after injection.

These observations do not support the view that purulent fluid is the sole cause of cartilage destruction, in which case uniform cartilage destruction might be expected. It is postulated that the focal adherence of bacteria to the cartilage surface permits destruction of the cartilage matrix to occur first in those regions.

Antibiotics can prevent the adhesion of bacteria to the articular surface, but unless adequate doses are given, cartilage destruction is not entirely prevented.

Metalloendopeptidases, also known as matrixins, are a family of protein-degrading enzymes, which includes collagenase, proteoglycanase, and stromelysin (83). They are found universally among mesenchymal cells of all types. The catalytic activity of matrixins depends on the presence of zinc. They are secreted in an inactive zymogen form and can be activated by a variety of proteases as well as physical agents and chemical compounds. Activation by either method is usually accompanied by a decrease in molecular weight of approximately 10 kd. This family of endopeptidases cleaves, with rather a broad specificity, components of the extracellular matrix. All the enzymes of this family are inhibited by another family of proteins, the tissue inhibitors of metalloproteinases (TIMPs). Chondrocytes express and secrete all three major classes of metalloproteinases (i.e., collagenases, stromelysin, gelatinase). Collagenase is also found in chondrocytes. Platelet-derived growth factor (PDGF) initially released by degranulating platelets has chemotactic properties attracting inflammatory cells and acts as a strong stimulator of mesenchymal cell proliferation.

Cytokines are a family of polypeptide hormones produced by a wide variety of cell types, including chondrocytes. Among the cytokines are IL-1 and IL-6, which have a major role in extracellular matrix regulation. IL-1 stimulates production of collagenase and proteoglycanase in articular cartilage (84). IL-1 acts as a differentiation facilitator by suppressing the cellular proliferation of chondrocytes and down-regulating the expression of cartilage-specific type II and IX collagens, as well as proteoglycans. IL-1 has been detected in synovial fluids of patients with various arthritides. IL-1 is presumed to act through a specific receptor on cartilage cells about which little is currently known (85). IL-6 induces the synthesis of TIMPs. IL-1, IL-6, and probably other cytokines actively participate in the regulation of matrix degradation. In addition to IL-1, several other chondrocyte active agents are now known and include bacterial products, bacterial lipopolysaccharides (endotoxin), prostaglandins, and cyclic adenosine monophosphate (AMP) (76). Bacterial endotoxin can promote rapid cartilage breakdown, but requires living chondrocytes. Prostaglandins E_2, $F_{1\alpha}$, and $F_{2\alpha}$ are stimulated at such times. Although synthesis of prostaglandins is an important aspect of the inflammatory response, it seems unlikely that they have a significant role in the cartilage degradative process (76). Cyclic AMP-dependent mechanisms may be important in modifying the chondrocyte degradative response, and hence in determining the outcome at active resorption sites in inflammatory arthritides. It is probable that cytokines in synovial fluid can only act on human cartilage synergistically with some other components of synovial fluid, such as cartilage-degrading proteases (86).

Host Factors

It is unclear whether there is innate susceptibility to bone or joint infections in individuals in whom osteomyelitis or suppurative arthritis develop. A characteristic of defective host resistance is a tendency to recurrent and severe infection. In the preantibiotic era, osteomyelitis fit into this pattern; however, with the advent of antibiotics, the incidence of recurrent infectious episodes has dramatically decreased.

S. aureus is one of the major pathogens in bone and joint infection. The major reservoir for coagulase-positive staphylococci is the anterior nares (87). Although 30% of the population are carriers (87), the actual incidence of staphylococcal invasive disease is small (88). This finding suggests that normal defense mechanisms are relatively effective against *S. aureus;* among known factors that may decrease host resistance to *S. aureus* are viral infections, such as influenza (89,90). Authors of one study (91) set out to identify factors that might increase susceptibility to invasion by staphylococci in individuals with a proven diagnosis of staphylococcal osteomyelitis. Among 20 children with a proven episode of hematogenous osteomyelitis caused by *S. aureus* one year or more previously, the following observations were made in 18 index patients, 34 first-degree relatives, and 52 age- and sex-matched controls subjects. (a) The only significant differences, in a series of determinations that included histocompatibility antigen profile, leukocyte phagocytosis and killing, leukocyte locomotion and chemotaxis, peripheral leukocyte migration inhibition, immunoglobulin levels, myeloperoxidase activity, and NBT test, were found in total immunoglobulin G (IgG) levels, which were lower in both patients and relatives than in control subjects. However, the total levels were still in a normally expected range. IgG subclasses were not measured. (b) One other significant difference noted was that the incidence of nasal carriage of *S. aureus* in the index patients was 65% and was significantly higher than in the control group. Among first-degree relatives, the incidence was 38%, which was higher than control subjects, but not significantly so. There was no association of risk of nasal carriage with any human leukocyte antigen (HLA) group. The authors concluded that after acute osteomyelitis due to *S. aureus,* they could demonstrate an increase in nasal carriage rate of this organism and decreased IgG levels. They were unable to attach significance to these observations. Another study (92) noted that there was a greater affinity of *S. aureus* for the nasal mucosal cells of carriers rather than noncarriers and suggested that this was a property of the mucosal cells rather than the bacteria. In a study of patients with multiple diseases and laboratory workers, certain HLA groups were found to be associated with carriage of *S. aureus* in the nares (93). These observations were not confirmed in the smaller sample cited earlier (91).

Another intriguing but not easily explored phenomenon is the immune response of the host to chronic staphylococcal osteomyelitis. Of 20 patients, 13 of whom had osteomyelitis caused by *S. aureus* (the remainder by miscellaneous organisms, mostly gram-negative), most had chronic infections present for months or years, none was acutely ill, and most had high titers of antibacterial agglutinating antibodies in the face of weak gamma G opsonic capacity (94). This observation contrasted with that made in patients with subacute bacterial endocarditis in which both high agglutinin and high opsonic titers were the general rule. It was speculated that a relative gamma G opsonin deficiency could develop from the relative isolation of dead bone and a weak antigenic stimulus by invading bacteria, but concluded that there was no easy explanation for these observations, nor did they suggest that the weak opsonic activity could be a prime cause of the chronicity.

In our opinion, the precise role of the immune response of the host to staphylococcal infections of bone remains to be determined.

References

1. Davis JB. Recurrence of infection after elective operations in cases of healed suppuration in bones and joints. Arch Surg 1940;41:1426–1436.

2. Gillespie WJ, Mayo KM. The management of acute haematogenous osteomyelitis in the antibiotic era: a study of the outcome. J Bone Joint Surg [Br] 1981;63:126–131.
3. Gallie WF. First recurrence of osteomyelitis eighty years after infection. J Bone Joint Surg [Br] 1951;33:110–111.
4. Gristina AG, Oga M, Webb LX, Hobgood CD. Adherent bacterial colonization in the pathogenesis of osteomyelitis. Science 1985;228:990–993.
5. Gristina AG, Costerton JW. Bacterial adherence to biomaterials and tissue. The significance of its role in clinical sepsis. J Bone Joint Surg [Am] 1985;67:264–273.
6. Gristina AG, Naylor PT, Myrvik QN. Musculoskeletal infection, microbial adhesion, and antibiotic resistance. Infect Dis Clin North Am 1990;4: 391–408.
7. Gristina AG, Naylor PT, Myrvik QN. Mechanisms of musculoskeletal sepsis. Orthop Clin North Am 1991;22:363–371.
8. van Loosdrecht MCM, Lyklema J, Norde W, Zehnder AJB. Influence of interfaces on microbial activity. Microb Rev 1990;54:75–87.
9. Wadstrom T. Molecular aspects of bacterial adhesion, colonization and development of infections associated with biomaterials. J Invest Surg 1989; 2:353–360.
10. Buxton TB, Rissing JP, Horner JA, et al. Binding of a Staphylococcus aureus bone pathogen to type I collagen. Microb Pathog 1990;8:441–448.
11. Speziale P, Raucci G, Visai L, Switakski LM, Trimpl R, Hook M. Binding of collagen to Staphylococcus aureus Cowan 1. J Bacteriol 1986;167:77–81.
12. Speziale P, Hook M, Wadstrom T. Binding of type II collagen to Staphylococcus aureus. Zentralbl Bakteriol Parasitenkd Infektionskr Hyg 1985;14 (suppl):191–196.
13. Herrmann M, Vaudaux PE, Pittet D, et al. Fibronectin, fibrinogen and laminin act as mediators of adherence of clinical staphylococcal isolates to foreign material. J Infect Dis 1988;158:693–701.
14. Herrmann M, Suchard SJ, Boxer LA, Waldvogel FA, Lew PD. Thrombospondin binds to Staphylococcus aureus and promotes staphylococcal adherence to surfaces. Infect Immun 1991;59:279–288.
15. Liang OD, Ascencio F, Frannson LA, Wadstrom T. Binding of heparin sulphate to Staphylococcus aureus. Infect Immun 1992;60:899–906.
16. Ryder C, Yacoub AI, Maxe I, et al. Specific binding of bone sialoprotein to Staphylococcus aureus isolated from patients with osteomyelitis. Eur J Biochem 1989;184:331–336.
17. Vercelloti GM, Lussenhop D, Peterson PK, et al. Bacterial adherence to fibronectin and endothelial cells: a possible mechanism for bacterial tissue tropism. J Lab Clin Med 1984;103:34–43.
18. Patti JM, Jonsson H, Guss B, et al. Molecular characterization and expression of a gene encoding a Staphylococcus aureus collagen adhesion. J Biol Chem 1992;267:4766–4772.
19. Bianco P, Fisher LW, Young MF, Termine JD, Robey PG. Expression of

bone sialoprotein (BSP) in developing human tissues. Calcif Tissue Int 1991;49:421–426.

20. Speers DJ, Nade SML. Ultrastructural studies of adherence of Staphylococcus aureus in experimental acute haematogenous osteomyelitis. Infect Immun 1985;49:443–446.
21. Falcieri E, Vaudaux P, Huggler E, Lew D, Waldvogel F. Role of bacterial exopolymers and host factors on adherence and phagocytosis of Staphylococcus aureus in foreign body infections. J Infect Dis 1987;155:524–531.
22. Mayberry-Carson KJ, Tober-Meyer B, Smith JK, Lambe DW, Costerton JW. Bacterial adherence and glycocalyx formation in osteomyelitis experimentally induced with Staphylococcus aureus. Infect Immun 1984;43: 825–833.
23. Arbeit RD, Dunn RM. Expression of capsular polysaccharide during experimental focal infection with Staphylococcus aureus. J Infect Dis 1987;156: 947–952.
24. Mayberry-Carson KJ, Tober-Meyer B, Lambe DW, Costerton JW. An electron microscopic study of the effect of clindamycin therapy on bacterial adherence and glycocalyx formation in experimental Staphylococcus aureus osteomyelitis. Microbios 1986;48:189–206.
25. Nichols WW, Evans MJ, Slack MPE, Walmsley HL. The penetration of antibiotics into aggregates of mucoid and non-mucoid Pseudomonas aeruginosa. J Gen Microbiol 1989;135:1291–1303.
26. Desnottes JF, Diallo N, Loubeyre C, Moreau N. Effect of pefloxacin on microorganism-host cell interaction. J Antimicrob Chemother 1990;26(suppl B):17–26.
27. Gagnon RF, Harris AD, Prentis J, Richards GK. The effects of heparin on rifampin activity against Staphylococcus aureus. Adv Perit Dial 1992;5: 138–142.
28. Wilkinson BJ, Sisson SP, Kim Y, Peterson PK. Localisation of the third component of complement on the cell wall of encapsulated Staphylococcus aureus M: implications for the mechanism of resistance to phagocytosis. Infect Immun 1979;26:1159–1163.
29. Muller C, Zielinski CC, Passl R, Eibl MM. Divergent patterns of leukocyte locomotion in experimental post-traumatic osteomyelitis. Br J Exp Pathol 1984;65:299–303.
30. Vaudaux PE, Huggler E, Lerch PG, et al. Inhibition by immunoglobulins of Staphylococcus aureus adherence to fibronectin-coated foreign surfaces. J Invest Surg 1989;2:397–408.
31. Marrie T, Costerton J. Mode of growth of bacterial pathogens in chronic polymicrobial human osteomyelitis. J Clin Microbiol 1985;22:924–933.
32. Buxton TB, Rissing JP, Horner JA, et al. Binding of a Staphylococcus aureus bone pathogen to type I collagen. Microb Pathol (Engl) 1990;8:441–448.
33. Costerton J, Lambe D, Mayberry-Carson K, Tober-Meyer B. Cell wall alterations in staphylococci growing in situ in experimental osteomyelitis. Can J Microbiol 1987;33:142–150.

34. Mayberry-Carson K, Tober-Meyer B, Smith J, Lambe D, Costerton J. Bacterial adherence and glycocalyx formation in osteomyelitis experimentally induced with Staphylococcus aureus. Infect Immun 1984;43:825–833.
35. Peterson P, Kim Y, Wilkinson B, et al. Dichotomy between opsonization and serum complement activation by encapsulated staphylococci. Infect Immun 1978;20:770–775.
36. Peterson P, Wilkinson B, Kim Y, et al. Influence of encapsulation on staphylococcal opsonization and phagocytosis by human polymorphonuclear leukocytes. Infect Immun 1978;19:943–949.
37. Wilkinson B, Kim Y, Peterson P, et al. Activation of complement by cell surface components of Staphylococcus aureus. Infect Immun 1978;20:388–392.
38. Wilkinson B, Peterson P, Quie P. Cryptic peptidoglycan and the antiphagocytic effect of the Staphylococcus aureus capsule: model for the antiphagocytic effect of bacterial cell surface polymers. Infect Immun 1979; 23:502–508.
39. Buxton T, Horner J, Hinton A, Rissing J. In vitro glycocalyx expression by Staphylococcus aureus phage type 52/52A/80 in S. aureus osteomyelitis. J Infect Dis 1987;156:942–946.
40. Mayberry-Carson K, Tober-Meyer B, Lambe D, Costerton J. An electron microscopic study of the effect of clindamycin therapy on bacterial adherence and glycocalyx formation in experimental Staphylococcus aureus osteomyelitis. Microbios 1986;48:189–206.
41. Norden C, Shinners E, Niederriter K. Clindamycin treatment of experimental chronic osteomyelitis due to Staphylococcus aureus. J Infect Dis 1986; 153:956–959.
42. Gristina A, Oga M, Webb L, Hobgood C. Adherent bacterial colonization in the pathogenesis of osteomyelitis. Science 1985;228:990–993.
43. Gristina A, Costerton J. Bacterial adherence and the glycocalyx and their role in musculoskeletal infection. Orthop Clin North Am 1984;15:517–535.
44. Gristina A. Biomaterial-centered infection: microbial adhesion versus tissue integration. Science 1987;237:1588–1595.
45. Beachey E. Bacterial adherence: adhesion-receptor interactions mediating the attachment of bacteria to mucosal surfaces. J Infect Dis 1981;143: 325–345.
46. Dougherty S. Pathobiology of infection in prosthetic devices. Rev Infect Dis 1988;10:1102–1117.
47. Christensen G, Baddeur L, Simpson W. Phenotypic variation of Staphylococcus epidermidis slime production in vitro and in vivo. Infect Immun 1987;55:2870–2877.
48. Christensen G, Simpson W, Bisno A, Beachey E. Experimental foreign body infections in mice challenged with slime-producing Staphylococcus epidermidis. Infect Immun 1983;40:407–410.
49. Peters G, Locci R, Pulveror G. Adherence and growth of coagulase-negative staphylococci on surfaces of intravenous catheters. J Infect Dis 1982;146: 479–482.

50. Hogt A, Dankert J, Hulstaert C, Feijen J. Cell surface characteristics of coagulase-negative staphylococci and their adherence to fluorinated poly (ethylenepropylene). Infect Immun 1986;51:294–301.
51. Ludwicka A, Uhlenbruck G, Peters G, et al. Investigation on extracellular slime substance produced by Staphylococcus epidermidis. Zentrabl Bakteriol Mikrobiol Hyg [A] 1984;258:256–267.
52. Vandaux PE, Zulian G, Huggler E, Waldvogel FA. Attachment of staphylococcus aureus to polymethylmethacrylate increases its resistance to phagocytosis in foreign body infection. Infect Immun 1985;50:472–477.
53. Johnson GM, Lee DA, Regelmann WE, Gray ED, Peters G, Quie PG. Interference with granulocyte function by staphylococcus epidermidis slime. Infect Immun 1986;54:13–20.
54. Johnson GM, Regelmann WE, Gray ED, Quie PG. Effects of staphylococcus epidermidis slime on PMN chemotaxis and degranulation (abstract no. 55). Program and abstracts of the 24th Interscience Conference on Antimicrobial Agents and Chemotherapy, Washington, DC, American Society for Microbiology, 1984.
55. Schumacher-Perdreau F, Peters G, Pulverer G, Quie PG. Effect of cell wall components and extracellular slime substance of S. epidermidis on the chemiluminescence of human polymorphonuclear granulocytes (abstract no. 61). Abstracts of the Third European Congress of Clinical Microbiology, The Hague, 1987.
56. Gray ED, Peters G, Verstegen M, Regelmann WE. Effect of extracellular slime substance from staphylococcus epidermidis on the human cellular immune response. Lancet 1984;1:365–367.
57. Gray ED, Regelmann WE, Peters G. Staphylococcal slime and host defenses: effects on lymphocytes and immune function. In: Pulverer G, Quie PG, Peters G, eds. Pathogenicity and clinical significance of coagulase-negative staphylococci. Stuttgart: Gustave Fischer Verlag, 1987:45–54.
58. Niinikoski J, Hunt TK. Oxygen tensions in healing bone. Surg Gynecol Obstet 1972;134:746–750.
59. Hohn DC. Host resistance to infection: established and emerging concepts. In: Hunt TK, ed. Wound healing and wound infection: theory and surgical practice. New York: Appleton Century Crofts, 1980:264–279.
60. Nelson DR, Buston TB, Luu QN, Rissing JP. The promotional effect of bone wax on experimental Staphylococcus aureus osteomyelitis. J Thorac Cardiovasc Surg 1990;99:977–980.
61. Stashenko P, Wang CY. Characterization of bone resorptive mediators in active periapical lesions. Proc Finn Dent Soc 1992;882(suppl 1):427–432.
62. Bataille R, Cahppard D, Klein B. The critical role of interleukin-6, interleukin-1B and macrophage colony-stimulating factor in the pathogenesis of bone lesions in multiple myeloma. Int J Clin Lab Res 1992;21:283–287.
63. Wang CY, Stashenko P. Kinetics of bone-resorbing activity in developing periapical lesions. J Dent Res 1991;70:1362–1366.
64. Whalen JL, Fitzgerald RH, Morrissy RT. A histological study of acute

haematogenous osteomyelitis following physeal injuries in rabbits. J Bone Joint Surg [Am] 1988;70:1383–1392.
65. Mundy GR, Altman AL, Gondek MD, Bandelin JG. Direct resorption of bone by human monocytes. Science 1977;196:1109–1112.
66. Gray TK, Amico CD, Kaplan R, Dodd RC, Mesler D, Cohen MS. Mononuclear phagocytes secrete a protein that directly resorbs devitalized bone particles. Bone Miner 1986;1:235–245.
67. Wang JH, Rogers GR, Allardyce RA, Gillespie WJ. Soluble products of Staphylococcus aureus stimulated blood mononuclear cells in enhancing polymorphonuclear leukocyte degradation of bone. Chin Med J [Engl] 1990;103:326–330.
68. Athanasou NA, Quinn J, Bulstrode CJ. Resorption of bone by inflammatory cells derived from the joint capsule of hip arthroplasties. J Bone Joint Surg [Br] 1992;74:57–62.
69. Plotquin D, Dekel S, Katz S, Danon A. Prostaglandin release by normal and osteomyelitic human bones. Prostaglandins Leukotrienes Essent Fatty Acids 1991;43:13–15.
70. Dekel S, Francis MJO. Treatment of osteomyelitis of the tibia with sodium salicylate. J Bone Joint Surg [Br] 1981;63:178–184.
71. Rissing JP, Buxton TB. Effect of ibuprofen on gross pathology, bacterial count, and levels of prostaglandin E_2 in experimental staphylococcal osteomyelitis. J Infect Dis 1986;154:627–630.
72. Rissing JP, Buxton TB, Fisher J, Harris R, Shockley RK. Arachidonic acid facilitates experimental chronic osteomyelitis in rats. Infect Immun 1985; 49:141–144.
73. Rissing JP, Buxton TB, Horner JA, Shockley RK, Fisher JF, Harris R. Synergism between Bacteroides fragiliss and Staphylococcus aureus in experimental tibial osteomyelitis. J Lab Clin Med 1987;110:433–438.
74. Kuettner KE, Aydelotte MB, Thonar EJ-MA. Articular cartilage matrix and structure: a minireview. J Rheumatol 1991;18(suppl 27):46–48.
75. Switalski L, Patti J, Butcher W, Gristina A, Speziale P, Hook M. A collagen receptor on Staphylococcus aureus strains isolated from patients with septic arthritis mediates adhesion to cartilage. Molec Microbiol 1993;7:99–107.
76. Steinberg JJ, Hubbard JR, Sledge CB. Chondrocyte-mediated breakdown of cartilage. J Rheumatol 1987;14(suppl 14):55–58.
77. Curtiss PH, Klein L. Destruction of articular cartilage in septic arthritis. I. In vitro studies. J Bone Joint Surg [Am] 1963;45:797–806.
78. Roy S, Bhawan J. Ultrastructure of articular cartilage in pyogenic arthritis. Arch Pathol 1975;99:44–47.
79. Alderson MR, Nade SML. Natural history of acute septic arthritis in an avian model. J Orthop Res 1987;5:261–273.
80. Bhawan J, Roy S. Pathology of experimental pyogenic arthritis. Indian J Med Res 1973;61:1604–1613.
81. Goldenberg DL, Chisolm PL, Rice PA. Experimental models of bacterial arthritis: a microbiologic and histopathologic characterization of the arthritis after

the intra-articular injections of Neisseria gonorrhoeae, Staphylococcus aureus, group A streptococci and Escherichia coli. J Rheumatol 1983;10:5–11.
82. Patel H, Nade S. Acute staphylococcal septic arthritis: the effect of cloxacillin therapy in an avian model. J Orthop Res 1987;6:63–72.
83. Woessner FJ. Matrix metallopeptidases and their inhibitors in connective tissue remodelling. FASEB 1991;5:2145–2154.
84. Gowen M, Wood DD, Ihrie EJ, Meats JE, Russell GG. Stimulation by human interleukin-1 of cartilage breakdown and production of collagenase and proteoglycanase by human chondrocytes but not human osteoblasts in vitro. Biochem Biophys Acta 1984;797:186–193.
85. Steinberg JJ, Sledge CB. Chondrocyte-mediated cartilage degradation: regulation by prostaglandin E_2, cyclic AMP and interferon a. J Rheumatol 1991;18(suppl 27):63–65.
86. Hollander AP, Atkins RM, Eastwood DM, Dieppe PA, Elson CJ. Degradation of human cartilage by synovial fluid but not cytokines in vitro. Ann Rheum Dis 1991;50:57–58.
87. Solberg C. A study of carriers of Staphylococcus aureus with special regard to quantitative bacterial estimations. Acta Med Scand 1965;178(suppl 436):1–96.
88. McCarthy P, Grundy G, Spiegel S, Dolan T. Bacteremia in children: an outpatient clinical review. Pediatrics 1976;27:861–868.
89. Fainstein V, Musher D. Bacterial adherence to pharyngeal cells during viral infection. J Infect Dis 1980;141:172–176.
90. Kleinerman E, Synderman R, Daniels C. Depressed monocyte chemotaxis during acute influenza infection. Lancet 1975;2:1062–1066.
91. Gillespie W, Haywood-Farmer M, Fong R, Harding S. Some aspects of the microbe-host relationship in staphylococcal haematogenous osteomyelitis. Orthopedics 1987;10:475–480.
92. Aly R, Shinefield H, Strauss W, Mailbach H. Bacterial adherence to nasal mucosal cells. Infect Immun 1977;17:546–549.
93. Kinsman O, McKenna R, Noble W. Association between histocompatibility antigens (HLA) and nasal carriage of Staphylococcus aureus. J Med Microbial 1983;16:215–220.
94. Williams R, Dossett J, Quie P. Comparative studies of immunoglobulin opsonins in osteomyelitis and other established infections. Immunology 1969;17:245–265.

CHAPTER 3

Experimental Studies of Osteoarticular Infection

The realization in the late 1870s and early 1880s that it was usually possible to culture a micro-organism from the local lesion in osteomyelitis encouraged the development of experimental animal models designed to examine hypotheses of the pathophysiology of the human disease. Since the introduction of antibiotics and sophisticated imaging technology, animal models have also been extensively used to study treatment and outcomes and to validate imaging techniques.

The complexity of evaluating the host–organism interaction in whole animals has also led naturally to many in vitro experiments, which have directly examined various aspects of osteoarticular infection. Data on the mechanisms of inflammation in general, and of the molecular biology of host–bacterial interactions, are accumulating rapidly. We discuss the experimental approaches to three separate groups of infection: (a) hematogenous osteomyelitis, (b) septic arthritis, and (c) chronic post-traumatic osteomyelitis. Experimental models of some other infections are briefly considered with the relevant clinical syndromes in later chapters.

Hematogenous Osteomyelitis

Pathogenesis

For much of the nineteenth century, the characteristic metaphyseal lesion of hematogenous osteomyelitis of childhood was known as "necrosis." Early experiments concentrated on the production of necrotic metaphyseal lesions by physical means. Rosenbach (1) damaged metaphyseal bone in rabbits and guinea pigs using a range of physical and chemical irritants; in some experiments, he locally introduced bacteria. As reports of the discovery of micro-organisms in clinical cases of osteomyelitis accumulated (2,3), attempts were made to reproduce the disease by the induction of septicemia. Kocher (4) and Becker (5) reported production of suppurative osteomyelitis at the site of closed contusion or fracture in rabbit long bones. In a more rigorous experimental program, Krause (6) established that both osteoarticular and muscular abscesses could follow the intravenous injection of micrococcus (*Staphylococcus aureus*), provided the animal survived the initial septicemic episode. Such abscesses occurred both at the site of experimental trauma and in uninjured bones. Using rabbits and guinea pigs, Rodet (7) established osteomyelitic lesions in 8 of 14 animals injected with micrococcus without limb trauma. Lexer (8) was able to repeat this result in immature rabbits.

Despite these successes, the concept of the "locus minoris resistantiae" as a necessary adjuvant to the establishment of experimental osteomyelitis has persisted in experimental studies and in clinical practice, and the difficulty in establishing reliable mammalian models based on the induction of septicemia alone has been repeatedly emphasized. Recent experiments have confirmed that adjuvant local tissue damage using mechanical trauma (9) or implantation of prosthetic materials (10) facilitates the induction of hematogenous osteomyelitis (HO) following bacteremia. It is also clear that, in some models and in the hands of some experimenters, osteomyelitis has followed induction of septicemia alone (11–16). These data are compatible with variations between and within animal and bacterial populations and are an indication of the probability that, for a given strain, a nonfatal *S. aureus* bacteremia may initiate an osteoarticular infection.

A reliable avian model has allowed careful description of the natural history (17–19). The earliest abnormality identified after injection is deposition of bacteria within metaphyseal vascular tunnels in the hypertrophic region of the growth plate. By 12 hours, local inflammatory response and changes in the molecular configuration of the cartilage matrix, as evidenced by histochemical staining, have occurred. By 24 hours, abscesses are visible to the naked eye on careful dissection. Necrosis of bone and cartilage extend over the following eight days, by which time repair is beginning in both growth plate and the adjacent metaphysis.

In the rabbit model described by Whalen and colleagues (9), carefully controlled experimental injury of the growth plate was followed by intravenous injection of *S. aureus*. In contrast to the findings in the avian model, bacterial aggregation was greatest in the spongiosa of the metaphysis or in the epiphyseal nucleus, although organisms were occasionally seen in the damaged growth plate itself. Loss of normal staining of the physeal cartilage was again observed. The time course of the inflammatory response and the onset of repair was similar to that in the chicken. The rapid resorption of bone appeared to be osteoclast-mediated in this model, in which the possible role of inflammatory cells in the resorptive process was not examined.

A model of hematogenous osteomyelitis in the dog has been described (20,21). Although somewhat contrived (using intra-arterial injection of both micro-organisms and barium sulphate), it does produce a progressive, chronic, hematogenous diaphyseal osteomyelitis. A hematogenous model in the mouse has also been reported (22).

A main research question with regard to experimental HO is "what determines localization?" Various hypotheses proposed over the last 100 years are reviewed briefly in Chapter 2. The studies of Nade and colleagues (17–19,23) using the avian model suggest that endothelial gaps in the growing metaphyseal vessels allow access of organisms to binding sites on cartilaginous matrix. It has not been determined which of the known potential ligand/receptor interactions of *S. aureus* with mammalian tissue are critical in the establishment of HO. Ultrastructural studies in the chicken suggest binding directly to cartilage matrix (24); some strains of staphylococci express receptors for collagen II (25). *S. aureus* may also bind to a number of other matrix proteins and to human endothelial cells (26,27). Concentrations of bone sialoprotein, for which the ligand/receptor interaction has been characterized, are highest in areas of endochondral bone formation and in cartilage cells of the transitional and hypertrophic zones in fetal rat long bones (28).

Management

Most studies of management have been carried out in models of osteomyelitis with direct implantation of micro-organisms. These studies are discussed in detail later in this chapter. However, aspects of the management of HO have been examined experimentally in the avian model (18,19,23). Delay in the commencement of antibiotic therapy of four days instead of one resulted in halving the number of chickens in which bone sterilization was achieved, as well as a large increase in the number and size of abscesses detected. Surgical drilling of abscesses performed within four days of onset of the infection was associated with extension of the zone of metaphyseal necrosis. These studies support the importance of early antibiotic therapy and suggest that the traditional and still widely held view that acutely infected bone should be "decompressed" is questionably based.

Spinal Infections

Two models of hematogenous vertebral osteomyelitis have been described, both based on observations of naturally occurring disease. In chickens (29), localization was in the thoracic spine and appeared to be associated with pre-existing degenerative disease. In a more recent mouse model, osteomyelitis occurred in the tail in 5% of mice given an intravenous injection of a strain of *S. aureus* from a spontaneous joint infection in laboratory mice (30).

Reactive Osteitis

Although the bacterial etiology of HO is not seriously in doubt, changes that resemble bacterial osteomyelitis both histologically and radiologically may be produced in experimental animals by exposure to repeated challenges of foreign protein administered locally, intramuscularly, or intravenously. In Russia in the 1930s, a rabbit model was developed (31) in which the animals were sensitized with a subcutaneous injection of horse serum; some days later, local injection of serum into the tibial diaphysis was carried out. Changes characteristic of HO occurred in prechallenged animals who survived anaphylaxis, but were not seen in those who had not been previously sensitized. The changes were largely preventable by administration of ganglion blocking drugs. Later, similar experiments were carried out in Japan (32). Microvascular changes were prominent. Endothelial gaps resembling those observed in the avian model of HO developed in the sinusoidal capillaries.

Prechallenge with foreign serum has been used as a prelude to induction of osteomyelitis by injection of *S. aureus* (33). This approach raises questions about the role of previous sensitization in the localization of osteomyelitis and in the severity of the lesion produced. In an experimental situation, repeated challenge with staphylococci may produce delayed hypersensitivity without increased resistance (34).

Post-traumatic Osteomyelitis

The majority of models of osteomyelitis have employed local injection of micro-organisms into bone and are therefore strictly analogous to post-traumatic osteomyelitis, because the skin and bone have been locally breached. Furthermore, most also use adjuvant mechanical or chemical trauma, or prosthetic implantation, to increase reliability. Most are well documented, reliable, and have been thoroughly evaluated in many laboratories over the last two decades. Their impact on contemporary understanding of pathogenesis, diagnostic strategies, and management has been substantial.

Rabbit Models

Rabbit models involving local injection of micro-organisms were described by a number of groups more than 50 years ago (35,36). Norden and Kennedy (37,38) developed a modified protocol that has been widely used with minor variations to study natural history (39–42), radiological and scintigraphic diagnosis (43–46), antibiotic management programs (47–58), and use of adjuvant therapy, such as hyperbaric oxygen (59–61). Briefly, the proximal tibial metaphysis is injected with a suspension of bacteria, along with a fish-oil–derived irritant, sodium morrhuate. Over the ensuing weeks, a progressive osteomyelitis ensues in almost all infected animals. Modifications of this model have been described with the additional insertion of a silicone implant (62), petroleum jelly (63), demineralized bone preparations (64), mass spectrometer probes for tissue blood flow and gas analysis measurement (61), and implantable antibiotic delivery systems (49).

Other rabbit models have been described. Andriole and co-workers (65,66) employed local injection of organisms into the rabbit tibia, along with insertion of a metal intramedullary rod, with or without associated fracture. No chemical adjuvant was used. The model of Worlock and colleagues (67,68) is similar. These models have allowed experimental evaluation of protocols in prevention and treatment of implant- and fracture-associated infections. A slightly different model system using the femoral metaphysis of the rabbit has been used for studies of local antibiotic administration in polymethylmethacrylate cement (PMMA) (69). Mandibular infections, both with and without fracture, have also been described (70,71). The guinea pig has been used occasionally as an alternative to the rabbit in experimental osteomyelitis. An infected femoral fracture model was described by Passl and colleagues (72) to study aspects of nonspecific immune response.

Other Animal Models

Considerations of cost and convenience have encouraged the development of programs using rat models of osteomyelitis. Apparently first described in 1945 (73) and subsequently used in early studies of hyperbaric oxygen therapy (74), the increased popularity of rat models followed a description (75) in 1982. They have been used extensively by a number of groups (76–80) over the last decade and are now reliable and well characterized with respect to natural history and response to treatment. A mouse model using injection of a coagulase-negative staphylococcus and ornithosis virus has also been described (81).

Dog models, although expensive, offer (because of their size) a significantly better opportunity to evaluate pathology and management programs involving surgical procedures (82), including implant infections. Fitzgerald's model (83) creates a cortical window in the canine tibial diaphysis, through which organisms are introduced; the defect is sealed with a PMMA plug. The natural history of this model is well established. A second canine model described by Petty and associates (84) allowed implantation of cylinders of different prosthetic materials in the femoral canal to evaluate their effect on the size of bacterial inoculum required to initiate infection and on host defense mechanisms. A model of infected fracture of the canine ulna has been used to study the effect of antibiotic impregnated bone graft (85).

In the spine, models of spinal epidural abscess (86) and autoimmune spondylodiskitis (87) are also available. A model of iatrogenic diskitis has been used to study the utility of antibiotics in prevention and treatment of infection following disk surgery or diskography (88).

Models of Infectious (Septic) Arthritis

Models of infectious arthritis have been described in rabbit (89–101), mouse (30,102) chicken (17,24,103), and hamster (104). Most have used intra-articular injection of organisms to resemble the arthritis that may follow penetrating injury, wounding, or surgery. In the recently described mouse model (30), a sialoprotein-binding strain of *S. aureus* injected intravenously caused arthritis in 75% of treated animals. A rat model of reactive *Streptococcus pyogenes* arthritis is also available (105).

The rabbit models have varied widely in the susceptibility of the animals to death from septicemia as a result of the inoculation. They have been used to study the pathogenesis of the arthritis and the efficacy of antibiotic management. Two distinct processes have been observed developing concurrently in the infected rabbit knee joint. The first is inflammation and hypertrophy of synovium, which begin within minutes and progressively erodes and lifts cartilage from the underlying bone in an advancing front of pannus (95). At the same time, loss of the normal staining of glycosaminoglycan of the articular cartilage is seen, which is similar to the changes seen in physeal cartilage in osteomyelitis. This polysaccharide-depleted cartilage is destroyed over a period of approximately two weeks by leukocyte collagenase (106,107) and destruction of underlying metaphyseal bone begins. Irreversible changes appear to supervene if the joint is not sterilized within five days of the onset of infection.

In animals with infection introduced into a previously established adjuvant arthritis, joint destruction is particularly florid and rapid (108); the reason for this finding is not known. Alderson and colleagues (17,24) described the early natural history of septic arthritis in the hock joint of chickens. From one to 24 hours after inoculation, bacterial numbers increased rapidly, remaining steady thereafter until approximately eight days and then decreasing slowly. Subsequent events resembled those in the rabbit model in distribution and time course. Antibiotic administered early reduced the destructive effect on cartilage (98).

Absorption of systemically administered antibiotics into inflamed joints is good (98,99). Although high antibiotic levels and rapid joint sterilization were demonstrated in experiments using intra-articular agents (89), clinical reports of chemical synovitis have restricted their use. Surgical lavage of infected joints has been examined in the rabbit model (109). No effect on proteoglycan loss was seen. The breakdown of articular cartilage collagen was slowed but not abolished. It is concluded that early intervention with both systemic antibiotic and thorough joint lavage is important in the management of infectious arthritis; antibiotic treatment alone is insufficient (94). Antibiotics administered prophylactically before experimental infection are preventive (98).

Imaging Techniques

Diagnostic imaging techniques have been studied in both rabbit and dog models. Briefly, these studies (43–46,110–113) suggest the following. (a) Radionuclide imaging is a sensitive technique for the detection of infection in its early stages, but discrimination between bone and soft-tissue infections is poor. In soft tissue, drainable abscesses are poorly demonstrated by scintigraphy, but readily distinguished by magnetic resonance imaging (MRI) and ultrasound. (b) Indium 111-chloride is superior to ^{99m}Tc-MDP in differentiating infected from noninfected sites. (c) Detection of infection in bone with MRI may be technique-dependent; axial imaging is superior to coronal.

Antibiotic Therapy

Studies of antibiotic management of experimental osteomyelitis have confirmed its resistance to cure (114). As a corollary, it has not been possible to identify minimum effective dosage schedules. Briefly, the published studies suggest the following in *S. aureus* osteomyelitis:

1. Of the agents tested thus far, only rifampicin and clindamycin are predictably capable of sterilizing rabbit experimental osteomyelitis. Rifampicin must be used in combination with other agents (51,55). Clindamycin, which is also effective in dogs, appears to inhibit the formation of bacterial glycocalyx in rabbits and in in vitro models (115,116).
2. Other agents—including beta-lactams, vancomycin, and fluoroquinolones—are ineffective, either alone or in combinations with each other, despite in vitro sensitivities (42,50–55).
3. In multiple resistant *S. aureus* (MRSA), ciprofloxacin and rifampicin combinations and vancomycin have been examined but are not particularly reliable (117–119).

In *Pseudomonas aeruginosa* infections, fluoroquinolones are capable of sterilizing experimental osteomyelitis, although resistance may occur (56,57).

The effect of systemic antimicrobial prophylaxis against implant infection has been examined in rabbit and canine models (10,120), confirming the validity of the general principle laid down by Burke (121): the presence of antibiotic in the wound at the time of contamination offers protection against infection (122).

Reduced perfusion and a low PAO_2 are features of the osteomyelitic lesion (60,61,123). Oxygen tension in the capillary circulation and the diffusion distance of oxygen in the tissues are both increased by hyperbaric oxygen treatment (60), and it is probable that this effect accounts for its beneficial effects as an adjunctive therapy in antibiotic-treated experimental osteomyelitis.

Conclusion

Experimental models of osteoarticular infection have clarified many aspects of pathogenesis and management and elaborated perspectives gained from the observation of human and veterinary infections.

Current progress in molecular biology suggests that the probability of resolving a number of outstanding problems in the next decade is good. These include the bacterial mechanisms of localization, and colonization within a protective biofilm; the host immune response and methods for its augmentation; and the elaboration of antimicrobial agents effective against protective biofilms. The range of experimental models available should contribute to the solution of these problems.

References

1. Rosenbach J. Beitrage zur Kenntniss der Osteomyelitis. Dtsch Z Chir 1878;10:369–393.
2. Garre C. Zur aetiologie acut eitriger Entzundungen (Osteomyelitis, Furunkel, und Panaritum). Fortschr Med Berlin 1885;3:165–173.
3. Ogston A. Micrococcus poisoning. J Anat Physiol 1882;17:24–58.
4. Benaroyo L. The research of Theodor Kocher on the etiology of osteomyelitis and acute struma. Gesnerus 1992;49:151–160.
5. Becker PF. Le microcoque specifique de l'osteomyelite aigue. Semin Med 1883;3:374.
6. Krause F. Uber einen bei der akuten infektiosen osteomyelitis des messchen vorkommenden mikrokokkus. Fortschr Med Berlin 1884;2:222–261.

7. Rodet A-J. De la nature de l'osteomyelite infectieuse. Rev Chir 1885;5: 273–287.
8. Lexer E. Zur experimentellen Erzeugung osteomylitischer Herde. Arch Klin Chir 1894;48:181–200.
9. Whalen JL, Fitzgerald RH, Morrissy RT. A histological study of acute haematogenous osteomyelitis following physeal injuries in rabbits. J Bone Joint Surg [Am] 1988;70:1383–1392.
10. Blomgren G. Hematogenous infection of total joint replacement. Acta Orthop Scand 1982;52(suppl 187):7–64.
11. Baudet G, Cahuzac M. Recherches experimentales sur l'infection osteomyelitique. Rev Chir 1935;73:801–813.
12. Joyner AL, Smith DT. Acute staphylococcus osteomyelitis. The use of staphylococcus antitoxin as aid to management of toxemia and staphylococcemia. Surg Gynecol Obstet 1936;63:1–6.
13. Shioda T. Experimentelle Beitrage zur Frage der akuten eitrigen Osteomyelitis. Arch Klin Chir 1936;185:141–163.
14. Takahashi R. Zur Frage der Infektion bei Vitaminmangel, inbesondere der Enstehung der akuten infektiosen Osteomyelitis. Arch Klin Chir 1934; 181:103–128.
15. Thompson RHS, Dubos RJ. Production of experimental osteomyelitis in rabbits by intravenous injection of Staphylococcus aureus. J Exp Med 1938;68:191–206.
16. Weaver JB, Tyler MW. Experimental staphylococcaemia and hematogenous osteomyelitis. J Bone Joint Surg [Am] 1943;25:791–802.
17. Alderson M, Speers D, Emslie K, Nade SML. Acute haematogenous osteomyelitis and septic arthritis—a single disease. J Bone Joint Surg [Br] 1986; 68:268–274.
18. Emslie K, Nade SML. Acute haematogenous staphylococcal osteomyelitis: evaluation of cloxacillin therapy in an animal model. Pathology 1984; 16:441–446.
19. Emslie KR, Nade SML. Acute haematogenous staphylococcal osteomyelitis: a description of the natural history in an avian model. Am J Pathol 1983;110:333–345.
20. Deysine ME, Isenberg HD, Steiner G. Chronic haematogenous osteomyelitis: studies on an experimental model. Int Orthop 1983;7:69–78.
21. Deysine ME, Rafkin H, Russell R, Teicher I, Aufses AH. The detection of acute experimental osteomyelitis with 67-Ga citrate scanning. Surg Gynecol Obstet 1975;141:40–42.
22. Matsuoka M. Haematogenous osteomyelitis induced by strain SMU-0611 of Staphylococcus warneri in mice. Nippon Seikeigeka Gakkai Zasshi 1991;65:1112–1119.
23. Emslie K, Nade SML. Acute haematogenous staphylococcal osteomyelitis: the effect of surgical drilling and curettage on an avian model. Pathology 1986;18:227–233.
24. Alderson M, Nade S. Natural history of acute septic arthritis in an avian model. J Orthop Res 1987;5:261–274.

25. Speziale P, Hook M, Wadstrom T. Binding of type II collagen to Staphylococcus aureus. Zentralbl Bakteriol Parasitenkd Infektionskr Hyg 1985; 14(suppl):191–196.
26. Tompkins DC, Hatcher VB, Patel D, Orr GA, Higgins LL, Lowy FD. A human endothelial cell membrane protein that binds Staphylococcus aureus in vitro. J Clin Invest 1990;85:1248–1254.
27. Vercelloti GM, Lussenhop D, Peterson PK, et al. Bacterial adherence to fibronectin and endothelial cells: a possible mechanism for bacterial tissue tropism. J Lab Clin Med 1984;103:34–43.
28. Chen JK, Shapiro HS, Wran JL, Reimers S, Heersche JN, Sodek J. Localisation of bone sialoprotein (BSP) expression to sites of mineralized tissue formation in fetal rat tissues by in situ hybridization. Matrix 1991;11:133–143.
29. Wise DR. Staphylococcal osteomyelitis of the avian vertebral column. Res Vet Sci 1971;12:169–171.
30. Bremell T, Lange S, Yacoub A, Ryden C, Tarkowski A. Experimental Staphylococcus aureus arthritis in mice. Infect Immun 1991;59:2615–2623.
31. Bashinskaya VA. Experimental osteomyelitis and some problems of its pathogenesis. Bull Eksp Biol Med 1960;48:38–44.
32. Yamaguchi H, Takeuchi H, Torikata C, Ashizawa M, Shiobara H. Experimental osteomyelitis induced by repeated administration of soluble immune complexes: consideration of the fundamental pathogenesis of osteomyelitis. Int Arch Allergy Appl Immunol 1975;49:763–773.
33. Brondolo W, Frassi GA. La vascularizzione dell'osso nella osteomielite sperimentale. Arch Orthop 1962;75:1427–1443.
34. Pryjma K, Zembala M, Grov A, Heczko PB. Cellular immunity to staphylococcal antigens 1. Delayed hypersensitivity and intracellular killing activity of peritoneal exudate cells in guinea pigs immunized with staphylococcal antigens. In: Jeljaszewicz J, ed. Staphylococci and staphylococcal diseases. Stuttgart: Gustav Fischer Verlag, 1976:861–871.
35. Haldeman KO. Acute osteomyelitis: a clinical and experimental study. Surg Gynecol Obstet 1934;59:25–31.
36. Scheman L, Janota M, Lewin P. The production of experimental osteomyelitis. JAMA 1941;117:1525–1529.
37. Norden CW, Kennedy E. Experimental osteomyelitis. 1. A description of the model. J Infect Dis 1970;122:410–418.
38. Norden CW, Kennedy E. Experimental osteomyelitis. II. Therapeutic trials and measurement of antibiotic levels in bone. J Infect Dis 1971;124:565–571.
39. Crane LR, Kapdi CC, Wolfe JN, Silberberg BK, Lerner AM. Xeroradiographic, bacteriologic, and pathologic studies in experimental staphylococcal osteomyelitis. Proc Soc Exp Biol Med 1977;156:303–314.
40. Johansson A, Svensson O, Blomgren G, Eliasson G, Nord CE. Anaerobic osteomyelitis. A new experimental rabbit model. Clin Orthop 1991;265: 297–301.
41. Lambe DW, Ferguson KP, Mayberry-Carson KJ, Tober-Meyer B, Costerton JW. Foreign-body-associated experimental osteomyelitis induced with Bac-

teroides fragilis and Staphylococcus epidermidis in rabbits. Clin Orthop 1991;266:285–294.
42. Norden CW, Myerowitz RL, Keleti E. Experimental osteomyelitis due to Staphylococcus aureus or Pseudomonas aeruginosa: a radiographic-pathological correlative analysis. Br J Exp Pathol 1980;61:451–460.
43. Graham GD, Lundy MM, Frederick RJ, Berger DE, O'Brien AW, Brown TJ. Predicting the cure of osteomyelitis under treatment: concise communication. J Nucl Med 1983;24:110–113.
44. Hartshorne MF, Graham GD, Lancaster J, Berger DE. Gallium-67/technetium-99m methylene diphosphonate ratio imaging: early rabbit osteomyelitis and fracture. J Nucl Med 1985;26:272–277.
45. Norris SH, Watt I. Radionuclide uptake during the evolution of experimental osteomyelitis. Br J Radiol 1981;54:207–211.
46. Rinsky L, Goris ML, Schurman DJ, Nagel DA. 99-technetium bone scanning in experimental osteomyelitis. Clin Orthop 1977;128:361–366.
47. Dahners LE, Funderburk CH. Gentamicin-loaded plaster of Paris as a treatment of experimental osteomyelitis in rabbits. Clin Orthop 1987;219:278–282.
48. Gomis M, Herranz A, Aparicio P, Alonso MJ, Prieto J, Martinez T. An experimental model of chronic osteomyelitis caused by Escherichia coli treated with cefotaxime. J Antimicrob Chemother 1990;26(suppl A):15–21.
49. Jacob E, Setterstrom JA, Bach DE, Heath JR, McNiesh LM, Cierny G. Evaluation of biodegradable ampicillin anhydrate microcapsules for local treatment of experimental staphylococcal osteomyelitis. Clin Orthop 1991;267:237–244.
50. Mader JT, Wilson KJ. Comparative evaluation of cefamandole and cephalothin in the treatment of experimental Staphylococcus aureus osteomyelitis in rabbits. J Bone Joint Surg [Am] 1983;65:507–513.
51. Norden CW. Experimental osteomyelitis. IV. Therapeutic trials with rifampin alone and in combination with gentamycin, sisomycin, and cephalothin. J Infect Dis 1975;132:493–499.
52. Norden CW. Experimental osteomyelitis. V. Therapeutic trials with oxacillin and sisomycin alone and in combination. J Infect Dis 1978;137:155–160.
53. Norden CW, Budinsky A. Treatment of experimental chronic osteomyelitis due to Staphylococcus aureus with ampicillin/sulbactam. J Infect Dis 1990;161:52–53.
54. Norden CW, Dickens DR. Experimental osteomyelitis. III. Treatment with cephaloridine. J Infect Dis 1973;127:525–528.
55. Norden CW, Keleti E. Treatment of experimental staphylococcal osteomyelitis with rifampin and trimethoprim, alone and in combination. Antimicrob Agents Chemother 1980;17:591–594.
56. Norden CW, Neiderreiter K. Ofloxacin therapy of experimental osteomyelitis caused by Pseudomonas aeruginosa. J Infect Dis 1987;155:823–825.
57. Norden CW, Shinners E. Ciprofloxacin as therapy for experimental osteomyelitis caused by Pseudomonas aeruginosa. J Infect Dis 1985;151:291–294.

58. Van Wingerden GI, Lolans V, Jackson GG. Experimental pseudomonas osteomyelitis. Treatment with sisomycin and carbenicillin. J Bone Joint Surg [Am] 1974;56:1452–1458.
59. Esterhai JL, Clark JM, Morton HE, Smith DW, Steinbach A, Richter SD. Effect of hyperbaric oxygen tension within the medullary canal in the rabbit tibial osteomyelitis model. J Orthop Res 1986;4:330–336.
60. Mader JT, Brown GL, Guckian JC, Wells CH, Reinarz JA. A mechanism for the amelioration by hyperbaric oxygen of experimental staphylococcal osteomyelitis in rabbits. J Infect Dis 1980;142:915–922.
61. Mader JT, Guckian JC, Glass DL, Reinarz JA. Therapy with hyperbaric oxygen for experimental osteomyelitis due to Staphylococcus aureus in rabbits. J Infect Dis 1978;138:312–318.
62. Mayberry-Carson KJ, Tober-Meyer B, Smith JK, Lambe DW, Costerton JW. Bacterial adherence and glycocalyx formation in osteomyelitis experimentally induced with Staphylococcus aureus. Infect Immun 1984;43:825–833.
63. Moskvin VI. On the experimental model of osteomyelitis. Eksp Khir 1960;5:57–62.
64. Thomas VL, Sanford BA, Keogh BS, Triplett RG. Antibody response to Staphylococcus aureus surface proteins in rabbits with persistent osteomyelitis after treatment with demineralized bone implants. Infect Immun 1989;57:404–412.
65. Andriole VT, Nagel DA, Southwick WO. A paradigm for human chronic osteomyelitis. J Bone Joint Surg [Am] 1973;55:1511–1515.
66. Andriole VT, Nagel DA, Southwick WO. Chronic staphylococcal osteomyelitis: an experimental model. Yale J Biol Med 1974;1:33–39.
67. Worlock P, Slack R, Harvey L, Mawhinney R. An experimental model of post traumatic osteomyelitis in rabbits. Br J Exp Pathol 1988;69:235–244.
68. Worlock P, Slack R, Harvey L, Mawhinney R. The prevention of infection in open fractures. An experimental study of the effect of antibiotic therapy. J Bone Joint Surg [Am] 1988;70:1341–1347.
69. Rodeheaver GT, Rukstalis D, Bono M, Bellamy W. A new model of bone infection used to evaluate the efficacy of antibiotic-impregnated polymethylmethacrylate cement. Clin Orthop 1983;178:303–311.
70. Kondell PA, Granstrom M, Heimdahl A, Mollby R, Nord CE. Experimental mandibular Staphylococcus aureus osteomyelitis: antibody response and treatment with dicloxacillin. Int J Oral Maxillofac Surg 1986;15:620–628.
71. Triplett RG, Branham GB. Treatment of experimental mandibular osteomyelitis with hyperbaric oxygen and antibiotics. Int J Oral Surg 1981;10(suppl 1):178–182.
72. Passl R, Muller C, Zielinski CC, Eibl MM. A model of experimental post traumatic osteomyelitis in guinea pigs. J Trauma 1984;24:323–326.
73. Kempf JE, Herrick JA. Effect of penicillin in experimental staphylococcus osteomyelitis in rats. Proc Soc Exp Biol Med 1945;58:100–102.
74. Hamblen DL. Hyperbaric oxygenation: its effect on experimental staphylococcal osteomyelitis in rats. J Bone Joint Surg [Am] 1968;50:1129–1141.

75. Zak O, Zak F, Rich R, Tosch W, Kradolfer F, Scheld WM. Experimental staphylococcal osteomyelitis in rats: therapy with rifampin and cloxacillin alone or in combination. In: Periti P, Grassi GG, eds. Current chemotherapy and immunotherapy. Washington: American Society for Microbiology, 1982:973–974.
76. Power ME, Olson ME, Domingue PA, Costerton JW. A rat model of Staphylococcus aureus chronic osteomyelitis that provides a suitable system for studying the human infection. J Med Microbiol 1990;33:189–198.
77. Nelson DR, Buxton TB, Luu QN, Rissing JP. The promotional effect of bone wax on experimental Staphylococcus aureus osteomyelitis. J Thorac Cardiovasc Surg 1990;99:977–980.
78. Rissing JP, Buxton TB, Fisher J, Harris R, Shockley RK. Arachidonic acid facilitates experimental chronic osteomyelitis in rats. Infect Immun 1985; 49:141–144.
79. Rissing JP, Buxton TB, Horner JA, Shockley RK, Fisher JF, Harris R. Synergism between Bacteroides fragilis and Staphylococcus aureus in experimental tibial osteomyelitis. J Lab Clin Med 1987;110:433–438.
80. Rissing JP, Buxton TB, Weinstein RS, Shockley RK. Models of experimental chronic osteomyelitis in rats. Infect Immun 1985;47:581–586.
81. Markowa J, Marek A, Skrochowska M. Experimental bacterioviral osteitis. Bull Pol Med Sci Hist 1966;9:127–128.
82. Varshney AC, Singh H, Gupta RS, Singh SP. Experimental model of staphylococcal osteomyelitis in dogs. Indian J Exp Biol 1989;27:816–819.
83. Fitzgerald RH. Experimental osteomyelitis: description of a canine model and the role of the depot administration of antibiotics in the prevention and treatment of sepsis. J Bone Joint Surg [Am] 1983;65:371–380.
84. Petty W, Spanier S, Shuster JJ, Silverthorne C. The influence of skeletal implants on the incidence of infection. Experiments in a canine model. J Bone Joint Surg [Am] 1985;67:1236–1244.
85. Petri WH, Schaberg SJ. The effects of antibiotic supplemented bone allografts on contaminated partially avulsive fractures of the canine ulna. J Oral Maxillofac Surg 1984;42:699–704.
86. Feldenzer JA, McKeever PE, Schaberg DR, Campbell JA, Hoff JT. The pathogenesis of spinal epidural abscess: microangiographic studies in an experimental model. J Neurosurg 1988;69:110–114.
87. Takenaka Y, Kahan A, Amor B. Experimental autoimmune spondylodiscitis in rats. J Rheumatol 1986;13:397–400.
88. Fraser RD, Osti OL, Vernon-Roberts B. Iatrogenic discitis: the role of intravenous antibiotics in prevention and treatment. An experimental study. Spine 1989;14:1025–1032.
89. Bardenheier JA, Morgan HC, Stamp WG. Treatment and sequelae of experimentally produced septic arthritis. Surg Gynecol Obstet 1966;122: 249–254.
90. Bhawan J, Roy S. Pathology of experimental pyogenic arthritis. Indian J Med Res 1973;61:1604–1613.

91. Goldenberg DL, Chisholm PL, Rice PA. Experimental models of bacterial arthritis: a microbiologic and histopathologic characterization of the arthritis after the intra-articular injection of Neisseria gonorrhoeae, Staphylococcus aureus, group A streptococci, and Escherichia coli. J Rheum 1983;10:5–11.
92. Johnson AH, Campbell WG, Callahan BC. Infection of rabbit knee joints after intra-articular injection of Staphylococcus aureus. Am J Pathol 1970; 60:165–204.
93. Lewis GW, Cluff LE. Synovitis in rabbits during bacteremia and vaccination. Bull Johns Hopkins Hosp 1965;116:175–190.
94. Riegels-Nielsen P, Frimodt-Moller N, Sorensen M, Jensen JS. Antibiotic treatment insufficient for established septic arthritis. Staphylococcus aureus experiments in rabbits. Acta Orthop Scand 1989;60:113–115.
95. Riegels-Nielsen P, Frimodt-Moller N, Steen Jensen J. Rabbit model of septic arthritis. Acta Orthop Scand 1987;58:14–19.
96. Rigdon RH. Pathogenesis of arthritis following the intravenous injection of staphylococci in the adult rabbit. Am J Surg 1942;55:553–561.
97. Roy S, Bhawan J. Ultrastructure of articular cartilage in pyogenic arthritis. Arch Pathol 1975;99:44–47.
98. Schurman DJ, Hirshman HP, Nagel DA. Antibiotic penetration of synovial fluid in infected and normal knee joints. Clin Orthop 1978;136:304–310.
99. Schurman DJ, Johnson BL, Amstutz HC. Knee joint infections with Staphylococcus aureus and micrococcus species: influence of antibiotics, metal debris, bacteremia, blood, and steroids in a rabbit model. J Bone Joint Surg [Am] 1975;57:40–49.
100. Schurman DJ, Mirra J, Ding A, Nagel DA. Experimental E. coli arthritis in the rabbit. A model of infectious and post infectious synovitis. J Rheumatol 1977;4:118–128.
101. Wang Y, Xu J, Xue D. Experimental study of acute suppurative bone and joint infection. II. Suppurative arthritis. Chin Med J [Engl] 1983; 96:907–912.
102. Tissi L, Marconi P, Mosci P, et al. Experimental model of type IV Streptococcus agalactiae (Group B streptococcus) infection in mice with early development of septic arthritis. Infect Immun 1990;58:3093–3100.
103. Daum RS, Davis WH, Farris KB, Campeau RJ, Mulvihill DM, Shane SM. A model of Staphylococcus aureus bacteremia, septic arthritis, and osteomyelitis in chickens. J Orthop Res 1990;8:804–813.
104. Lindberg L. Experimental staphylococcal arthritis in golden hamsters. Acta Path Microbiol Scand 1969;76:117–125.
105. Barridge BD, Bishr M, Kahn F, Allen JL. Experimental arthritis induced by atypical strains of Streptococcus pyogenes. J Med Microbiol 1988; 27:23–31.
106. Curtiss PH, Klein L. Destruction of articular cartilage in septic arthritis. I. In vitro studies. J Bone Joint Surg [Am] 1963;45:797–806.
107. Smith RL, Merchant TC, Schurman DJ. In vitro cartilage degradation by

Escherichia coli and Staphylococcus aureus. Arthritis Rheum 1982;25: 441–446.
108. Mahowald ML, Peterson L, Raskind J, Raddatz DA, Shafer R, Gerding D. Antigen-induced experimental septic arthritis in rabbits after intra-articular injection of Staphylococcus aureus. J Infect Dis 1986;154:273–282.
109. Daniel D, Akeson W, Amiel D, Ryder M, Boyer J. Lavage of septic joints in rabbits: effects on chondrolysis. J Bone Joint Surg [Am] 1976;58:393–395.
110. Beltran J, McGhee RB, Shaffer PB, et al. Experimental infections of the musculoskeletal system: evaluation with MR imaging and Tc-99mMDP and Ga-67 scintigraphy. Radiology 1988;167:167–172.
111. Chandnani VP, Beltran J, Morris CS, et al. Acute experimental osteomyelitis and abscesses: detection with MR imaging versus CT. Radiology 1990;174:233–236.
112. Hoskinson JJ, Daniel GB, Patton CS. Indium-111 chloride and three-phase bone scintigraphy: a comparison for imaging experimental osteomyelitis. J Nucl Med 1991;32:67–75.
113. Abiri MM, DeAngelis GA, Kirpekar M, Abou AN, Ablow RC. Ultrasonic detection of osteomyelitis. Pathologic correlation in an animal model. Invest Radiol 1992;27:111–113.
114. Rouse MS, Tallan BM, Henry NK, Steckelberg JM, Wilson WR. Animal models as predictors of outcome of therapy with broad spectrum cephalosporins. J Antimicrob Chemother 1992;29(suppl A):39–45.
115. Khardori N, Wong E, Nguyen H, et al. Effect of subinhibitory concentrations of clindamycin and trospectomycin on the adherence of Staphylococcus epidermidis in an in vitro model of vascular catheter colonization. J Infect Dis 1991;164:108–113.
116. Mayberry-Carson KJ, Tober-Meyer B, Lambe DW, Costerton JW. An electron microscopic study of the effect of clindamycin therapy on bacterial adherence and glycocalyx formation in experimental Staphylococcus aureus osteomyelitis. Microbios 1986;48:189–206.
117. Dworkin R, Modin G, Kunz S, Rich R, Zak O, Sande M. Comparative efficacies of ciprofloxacin, perfloxacin, and vancomycin in combination with rifampin in a rat model of methicillin-resistant Staphylococcus aureus chronic osteomyelitis. Antimicrob Agents Chemother 1990;34:1014–1016.
118. Henry NK, Rouse MS, Whitesell AL, McConnell ME, Wilson WR. Treatment of methicillin-resistant Staphylococcus aureus experimental osteomyelitis with ciprofloxacin or vancomycin alone, or in combination with rifampin. Am J Med 1987;82(suppl 4A):73–75.
119. Mader JT, Adams K. Comparative evaluation of daptomycin (LY146032) and vancomycin in the treatment of experimental methicillin-resistant Staphylococcus aureus osteomyelitis in rabbits. Antimicrob Agents Chemother 1989;33:689–692.
120. Southwood RT, Rice JL, McDonald PJ, Hakendorf PH, Rozenbilds MA. Infection in experimental hip arthroplasties. J Bone Joint Surg [Br] 1985; 67:229–231.

121. Burke JF. The effective period of preventive antibiotic action in experimental incisions and dermal lesions. Surgery 1961;50:161–168.
122. Patel H, Nade SML. Acute staphylococcal septic arthritis: the effect of cloxacillin therapy in an avian model. J Orthop Res 1988;6:63–72.
123. Niinikoski J, Hunt TK. Oxygen tensions in healing bone. Surg Gynecol Obstet 1972;134:746–750.

PART TWO

Diagnosis and Management

CHAPTER 4

Clinical Evaluation

Awareness of Musculoskeletal Infection

The diagnosis of infection must be based on suspicion that such a process is taking place. After open wounds, open fractures, or any surgical procedure, the risk of infection is the single most important complication clinicians must seek, usually during the postinjury or the postoperative period. Indicators of infection are: (a) failure of the patient to follow the normal progress to recovery; (b) local signs of inflammation about the site where the skin was breached; (c) systemic signs of infection, such as abnormal elevation of body temperature and increased pulse rate; and (d) pain.

In patients whose resistance to infection is decreased, any deviation from normal level of well-being must be considered as possibly due to infection. An elderly patient who becomes confused without obvious cause must be suspected of having an infection. Loss of sensation in a paraplegic often heralds the presence of a urinary tract infection by increased muscle tone and "spasm" in the legs. In such a case, in which normal homeostasis has been disturbed, despite the fact that pain (the usual signal) has been suppressed, good clinicians will be guided to infection as a diagnosis.

Pain is the usual signal that something is wrong. In most of the conditions discussed in this book, patients consult physicians because of pain. Evaluation of patients, therefore, requires analysis of the pain. If there is no obvious portal of entry of micro-organisms to bone, joints, or soft tissues, it should be assumed that hematogenous dissemination has occurred from a site not obvious.

In addition to the cardinal feature of pain, there is often a history of fever and loss of function of the affected part. Other useful local signs are swelling, tenderness, joint effusion, and erythema. There may be evidence of weight loss, dehydration, rash, skin infection, respiratory sepsis, meningitis, throat, skin, ear, or dental sepsis. Host compromise may accompany malnutrition, diabetes mellitus, neoplasia, sickle-cell anemia, renal and liver disease, steroid therapy, drug abuse, immune disorders, and vascular disease. The presence of cannulae, shunts, or prostheses may predispose to infection.

Pain and Musculoskeletal Infections

The hallmark of pain due to infection is its constancy. In the musculoskeletal system, constant pain means infection or neoplasia. *Constant pain,* once started, has not left the patient. The level of pain due to infection might fluctuate, depending on posture or movement of the affected part, and in relation to analgesic drugs or time of day, but it does not ever disappear. "Is the pain there all the time?" must be asked immediately after the questions: "Where is the pain?" "When did it start?" If the pain is constant, further questioning must be directed at determining whether infection or neoplasm is the cause.

Even in acute osteomyelitis, septic arthritis, or pyomyositis, onset of pain is not sudden, as in a fracture or muscle rupture. Onset is gradual (over a few hours, days, or even weeks), depending on the nature of the infective process. The severity of the pain is usually an index of the time between its onset and the report of the symptom to a clinician.

In addition to these questions about pain, patients must be asked what makes it better or worse and what has been done about the pain since its onset. Questions about the level of function—"Can you walk? Can you move the joint? When could you last do so?"—also give an idea about the rapidity of change in the tissues caused by the infective process.

A child who complains of pain in a limb and cannot say exactly where the pain is should be asked to point to the site of pain. For example, a child who points to the metaphyseal region of a bone is very likely to have osteomyelitis. Obviously, other possible causes of pain must be excluded—is there evidence of injury, repetitive strain (e.g., jogging causing stress fracture), or other disease?

Adults with back pain due to infection must also be quizzed in the same way. Lumbago is a common symptom. If infection is suspected from the constancy of pain, the simple question—"Is this pain like, or unlike, the pain that you have had for a long time?"—often is sufficient to confirm that infection may be superadded to a degenerative disorder of the spine. Such must be suspected if there is an exacerbation of pain after recent (within 3 mo) dental extraction, cystoscopy, or other surgical manipulation.

Inflammation

Infection in bone evokes an inflammatory response in and around the bone. The deep site of bones in the body may mask the cardinal signs of inflammation from the examining clinician and delay confirmation of suspected diagnosis. Musculoskeletal inflammation can be considered under two headings—revealed and concealed.

Revealed Inflammation

Where there has been a recent open wound, infection and inflammation are usually revealed, even if the primary site (if that can ever be determined) is in bone or joint. The organisms enter from without, and have a path to follow through disrupted tissues. Therefore, within a few days, the cardinal signs of acute inflammation are usually seen in the skin. There are other useful clinical signs—unexpected pyrexia; increasing pain after surgery; and importantly, unexplained swelling of the digits at a distance from the septic focus. The response to a deep infection is often reflected in decreased venous and lymphatic return. A serous or hemoserous discharge through an otherwise normally healing wound is another sign of tissue edema and may precede a purulent discharge by some days.

In hematogenous osteomyelitis, the classic signs of acute inflammation may not be present at the time an intramedullary abscess in bone commences. Local metaphyseal tenderness, found in an identical place on repeated gentle palpation, is the clinical sign to raise suspicion. The classic signs of acute inflammation—redness, warmth, and swelling—usually do not appear until there is pus in the tissues outside the bone.

In acute septic arthritis, warmth about the infected joint, tenderness limited to the joint, and very restricted movement of the joint usually appear early in the infective process in the more superficially accessible joints. Although raised body temperature is usual in childhood bone and joint infections, it may not be manifest in adults or neonates.

Concealed Inflammation

When the spine, pelvis, or hip are the focus of infection, which is not uncommon, the signs of acute inflammation may be concealed. In chronic inflammation, a discharging sinus may present at a distance from the infectious focus. A "cold" abscess in the groin associated with spinal tuberculosis or a "hot"abscess in the groin associated with psoas or iliacus pyomyositis are good examples.

Even in concealed sites, inflammation can be suspected. Most acutely inflamed sites and some chronic sites are made more painful by movement, particularly if a joint is involved. The natural response of the body is to splint the part against such movement by muscle contraction—both agonists and antagonists having increased tone at the same time. This response is not part of the normal physiology of muscle action but is protective.

In spinal infection, clinical clues to inflammation are the "rigidity" of the spine, the intense contraction of the spinal muscles, and the difficulty in carrying out such relatively simple yet essential movements as turning in bed or getting out of a bed or a chair. Such "rigidity" should alert clinicians to infection in concealed sites.

Differential Diagnosis

To experienced clinicians, the history given by the patient is the most important part of the diagnostic exercise. After taking a complete history, the list of possible causes of the symptoms is usually quite small. Diagnosis requires that the tissue involved is identified and the pathological process clarified. If an etiological agent is obvious, then diagnosis is all the easier.

Less experienced clinicians perhaps place more reliance on physical examination, imaging, and laboratory aids, until they are familiar with the natural evolutionary history of a disease. Perhaps the differential diagnostic list of such a clinician is a little longer. The physical examination is most useful in confirming that one of the diagnoses postulated from history-taking does exist and the others do not. Special investigations do not usually cause surprises in bringing to light a suspected diagnosis; they confirm site, size, and activity and are a guide to treatment.

With respect to musculoskeletal infections, the most important differential diagnosis is neoplasia, which, like infection, causes constant pain. Limb pain may be due to metastases or primary neoplasms. The age of the patient is also a guide to neoplasia: Childhood osteomyelitis can have similar symptoms to osteosarcoma, Ewing's tumor, neuroblastoma, secondary Wilm's tumor, and leukemia.

Not all patients tell the whole truth, and in the case of suspected gonococcal infection or opportunistic infection in drug abusers, clinicians must specifically ask if these possibilities exist.

A further aspect apparent on clinical evaluation is the effect of the local process on normal homeostasis. A child with osteomyelitis may have a fever and vomit, causing caloric malnutrition and dehydration with metabolic dysfunction. To proceed with urgent operative surgery in such a child risks death. The degree of variation from normal homeostasis must be assessed, and the treatment schedule must be arranged to reverse that situation.

Clinical evaluation also requires that the history is carefully documented and the physical signs are recorded accurately. The decision to operate on a child with osteomyelitis is often made on the basis of failure to improve with nonoperative treatment. Such comparisons must be made on an objective basis.

Many aspects of clinical evaluation defy written recording—the well-being of a patient is something an observer can gauge but not define. Therefore, it is important that the evaluation of a child with osteomyelitis be repeatedly carried out by the same experienced clinician—this task cannot be delegated.

The Usual Clinical Course

Most infections, whether treated or untreated, follow predictable courses that clinicians must clearly understand. It is important to know what the usual clinical course is, because failure of progress along that course is a signal for concern regarding initial diagnosis and patient compliance with therapy, or an indication that some intervention is necessary.

Pain, fever, body weight, and patterns of movement must all be taken into account, as well as laboratory tests. Often there is a phase difference in radiological signs (e.g., bone loss apparently progressing while systemic improvement of the patient is taking place as a result of treatment). Experienced clinicians place much more reliance on clinical evaluation than imaging or laboratory tests. Evaluation must also be continued for a considerable period; and patients must be told what to look for and report without delay.

"Typical" Acute Osteomyelitis or Septic Arthritis

The typical presentation of acute osteomyelitis or septic arthritis is a child aged under 15 years with fever, prostration, pain, and loss of function around a major joint. Inquiry may elicit a history of trauma in up to 40%: this feature was noted by Nathan Smith (1) in 1827 and has been generally accepted since, but its true relevance has never been determined. Tenderness, warmth, swelling, and joint effusion are usually present. Specific local bony tenderness is characteristic of osteomyelitis. A painful joint effusion usually indicates septic arthritis, but sympathetic effusion of a nearby osteomyelitis may cause confusion. Septic arthritis may be an intrinsic joint infection or may spread from osteomyelitis (2), particularly in younger children. A "proven" diagnosis requires demonstration of an infecting organism from the local lesion. Although it is good practice to institute provisional antibiotic management on a "best-guess" principle in probable osteoarticular infection if no organism can be identified, aspiration of the suspected area should be carried out promptly before treatment is begun and without waiting for the results of other laboratory investigations, which at best can only raise the diagnosis to the "probable" level.

Subacute Osteomyelitis

The subacute presentation of osteomyelitis is characterized by a long history (usually > 14 days) of symptoms dominated by pain. Such pain is rarely severe. Fever is slight or absent, and constitutional symptoms rare. Loss of function is usually minimal but may be dramatic in spinal disease in childhood.

Chronic Osteomyelitis

Chronic osteomyelitis is distinguished from acute osteomyelitis by the characteristic histopathological signs of chronic inflammation, which are potentially detectable by morbid anatomists, but not clinicians.

The clinical features of chronic osteomyelitis are primarily a history (with or without external evidence of acute osteomyelitis in the past); either hematogenous or from a contiguous source; and a relapse of pain, erythema, swelling, fluctuation, and serous or purulent discharge from a sinus, either singly or in any combination. The duration between primary infection and first or subsequent relapse may be short, long, or very long (i.e., many years). There may be no symptoms or signs, mild discomfort, or persistence of sinus discharge between relapses. Chronic osteomyelitis is often borne stoically for long periods by affected individuals, dependent mainly on level of pain or inconvenience caused by the volume or odor of discharge.

Because cure of chronic osteomyelitis cannot be guaranteed, the major purpose of the clinical evaluation is to decide whether a simple or radical treatment should be instituted. Infrequent episodes of acute inflammation with attendant symptoms may require infrequent antibiotic therapy of short duration. Patients with a chronic malodorous discharging sinus, in whom the possibility of malignant change needs consideration, must be carefully assessed regarding institution of radical surgery with, frequently, long periods of rehabilitation.

The Atypical Clinical Course

The atypical course of osteomyelitis requires a knowledge of the typical course. If, however, the course is atypical, the diagnosis must be reassessed—sometimes infection supervenes on another condition in bone. Ewing's tumor and osteomyelitis in the same bone are not unknown. The patient may have abandoned prescribed drugs or taken them at times that reduce absorption. Infection may have been the presenting feature of immune incompetence due to a systemic disease, but that disease may not itself have been apparent at the time of initial diagnosis of infection. Unusual organisms may also provoke clinical syndromes that are atypical.

Fever and pain after treatment of open wounds should alert clinicians to the fact that necrotic tissue may still be present in the wound and anaerobic infection is imminent. Rapid intervention may prevent death from gas gangrene.

In the management of infections of the musculoskeletal system, clinical evaluation has an important role. Experienced clinicians must re-examine their patients frequently. If responsibility for care is to be delegated to others, they must be informed of the likely progress and what to do if such progression is not observed.

Special Situations Relating to Age or Immune Status

Neonates and Infants

Observation is a particularly important first step in neonates and young children. Very young children with fever and a serious illness may not manifest classic local signs (3). Careful attention to six observations—(a) quality of cry, (b) reaction to parental stimulation, (c) variation of sleeping and waking, (d) color, (e) hydration, and (f) response to social overtures—is highly predictive for severe sepsis, including septic arthritis.

In young infants, the history should include a search for possible sources of infection in pregnancy or during delivery (e.g., maternal syphilis, gonorrhea, streptococcal infection, or candidiasis) and an obstetric and nursing history. Particular sources of infection include omphalitis (4); pustular dermatitis and paronychia (5); purulent rhinitis (6); infected operative sites, including circumcision (7); intramuscular injection (8); scalp vein needle; umbilical catheterization; and heel puncture (9).

Physical examination should confirm the general observations and concentrate on local examination of the affected limb, exclusion of other potential sites of infection, and the general status of the child. Pseudoparalysis (i.e., limitation of spontaneous movement of the affected limb) may be obvious and is the most common sign of bone and joint infection in neonates (10). Some limitation of passive motion with pain is usual but may be surprisingly slight compared with older children. In a small child, the amount of soft-tissue swelling may be dramatic, which may cause confusion in diagnosis.

The likelihood of skeletal sepsis in a young child with a highly febrile illness is quite small. One study (11) found that 79% of highly febrile children had respiratory infection: Only 1% had bone and joint infection. In a subacute presentation with joint pain, history and physical examination may demonstrate the cause (12). The rash of Henoch-Schönlein purpura is characteristic; endocardial involvement suggests rheumatic fever, lupus erythematosus, or subacute bacterial endocarditis. Rash and fever associated with joint pain are most suggestive of an autoimmune disorder. If a joint effusion is present and associated with fever, aspiration should be performed.

Musculoskeletal Infections in the Elderly

In the elderly joint involvement may not be obvious; the only manifestation may be general illness with rigor (13,14). Any swollen joint should be aspirated without hesitation, and, in patients with rheumatoid arthritis, it is important to remember that multiple joints may be septic (15). In osteomyelitis in older patients, in contrast, local symptoms dominate (16), and diabetes is often present.

Fever of Unknown Origin

Fever of unknown origin is an illness characterized by a temperature of 38.3°C or greater on multiple occasions that lasts three weeks or longer and remains undiagnosed after one week of evaluation in hospital (17). In adults, infection accounts for up to one third of all fevers of unknown origin. Tuberculosis, mainly in extrarespiratory sites, accounts for 4 to 11% (18). Musculoskeletal infection is a rare explanation of prolonged fever.

Immunosuppressed Patients

Bone and joint involvement was relatively uncommon in immunosuppressed patients with infection (19). Symptoms and physical signs may be muted to some extent. In patients with human immunodeficiency virus infection, particularly those manifesting the acquired immunodeficiency syndrome, mycobacterial infection (i.e., tuberculosis or other strain) does involve bones and joints (20). This subject is discussed in detail in Chapter 12.

Hemodialysis

Episodic pyrexial reactions may occur during dialysis, and these reactions are frequently bacteremic. Osteomyelitis, particularly of ribs and thoracic spine, occasionally occurs; localizing signs appear to be unusual and the diagnosis is sometimes made incidentally.

Infectious arthritis tends to be localized to the sternoclavicular, sacroiliac, and acromioclavicular joints, rather than the large peripheral joints (21). Diagnostic confusion may occur with gout (22), renal osteodystrophy, and Charcot's arthropathy (23). For more detail, refer to Chapter 18.

Sickle-Cell Disease

The clinical features of osteomyelitis in children with sickle-cell disease differ from typical osteomyelitis in a number of ways. Multiple infected sites are common, and involvement of the hands and feet is frequent. Some authors (24), however, suggest that infarction (i.e., sequestration crisis) in long bones is at least 50 times more common than bacterial osteomyelitis but may resemble it closely, with bone pain, swelling, tenderness, warmth, and erythema. Fever is likely to be higher in osteomyelitis, but the great majority of fevers in children with sickle-cell disease are caused by bacterial pneumonia or viral syndromes (25,26). This issue is addressed in Chapter 12.

Special Situations Relating to Anatomical Site

Pelvis

In the pelvis, the sacroiliac joint and adjacent bone is the most frequent location of sepsis. The fact that the morbidity of pelvic osteomyelitis prior to antibiotic therapy was as high as 40% (27) points to the difficulty in clinical diagnosis. Although clinicians were consulted within 1 to 2 weeks of onset of symptoms, delay in diagnosis was common (up to 12 weeks). Children are usually over the age of seven. The majority of presentations are acute, with fever, systemic signs, and pain. There are three characteristic syndromes (28,29).

Abdominal Syndrome

These patients have signs more typical of appendicitis (i.e., right iliac fossa tenderness, guarding, and occasionally a mass). The focus is usually close to the sacroiliac joint, and the subperiosteal abscess is deep to the iliacus.

Gluteal Syndrome

Pain is felt in the buttock and a palpable mass may be present. In these children, the subperiosteal abscess is deep to the glutei.

Lumbar Disk Syndrome

Lumbar disk syndrome is the most common presentation (29), emphasizing back, hip, and thigh pain, and inability to walk. Straight leg raising is limited and painful. There is a subgroup in which hip pain dominates (30). It is presumed that in this group, pus has spread into the pelvis and irritates the femoral nerve or the sciatic plexus.

In all these presentations, compression of the pelvis is a useful physical sign, producing pain on the affected side. Gaenslen's test—abducting the flexed and externally rotated hip—often helps identify the sacroiliac joint as the site of pathology.

Leukocytosis is not common, but a markedly raised erythrocyte sedimentation rate (ESR) is the rule. *Staphylococcus aureus* is the most frequent cause. Initial radiographs are often normal, but new bone formation causing radiodensity or erosion of bone appears subsequently. Prognosis is good for recovery after antibiotic treatment and surgical drainage.

Pelvic osteomyelitis in the same site also occurs in adults. There are few reported series of patients (31), although most orthopedic surgeons have seen a case. The features are similar to that in childhood. Indiscriminate use of antibiotics may have modified the clinical course.

Radioisotope scanning is useful in diagnosis and should be carried out at any hint of this diagnosis to prevent unnecessary abdominal surgery, pointless neurological evaluation, or unnecessary delay in treatment. Magnetic resonance imaging is also useful and may show the direction of anatomical tracking of pus, which can relate to the syndromes described.

Clavicle

Osteomyelitis of the clavicle is often associated with multiple sites of infection, similar to other flat bones. Although most frequently hematogenous in origin, it has also been reported after subclavian venipuncture. Differential diagnosis includes fracture or neoplasm. In reported cases, there has been difficulty in identifying organisms following repeated attempts at culture after biopsy. Nonspecific chronic inflammation may be seen, and considerable enlargement of the clavicle is common—usually there is fever, local tenderness, and swelling. In the acute phase, treatment should follow conventional lines; however, chronic multifocal osteomyelitis frequently involves one or both clavicles. This topic is addressed in Chapter 16.

Calcaneum

Osteomyelitis of the calcaneum usually follows a puncture wound, which is often unnoticed. Pain is the principal symptom, associated with a limp. Infection is not usually suspected. Leukocytosis is uncommon, but the ESR is usually raised. Radiographs show predominantly lytic changes. The usual causative organisms are *S. aureus* or *Pseudomonas aeruginosa*. Heel pain in active children is not uncommon and is usually diagnosed as apophysitis (Sever's) or tendonitis. Lack of systemic symptoms delays the correct diagnosis.

The Cervical Spine

Severe unremitting neck pain and stiffness with torticollis are characteristic in cervical spine infection. Pain may radiate to the shoulder girdle.

Mastoid

This complication of otitis media is now relatively rare (32). The features are pain in the ear, deafness, pyrexia, edema, tenderness, and perhaps some reddening behind the ear. The postauricular sulcus may be obliterated.

Maxilla

The clinical features of osteomyelitis of the maxilla in newborns include fever, edematous eyelids, and swelling and redness of the cheek (33). Pus is almost always present in the nostril, and the nose may be deviated to the opposite side.

Mandible

Osteomyelitis in the mandible is usually of dental origin (34). There is severe dental pain, and eating may be difficult. Fever and regional adenopathy are present. Paresthesia or anesthesia may affect the lip. Swelling and reddening of skin and mucosa may occur as a late feature.

The Sternoclavicular Joint

Typically, a painful, tender swelling of the sternoclavicular joint is associated with a feverish illness and pain on movement of the shoulder girdle, but swelling may be slow to appear, and the presentation may be as chest pain (35).

Ribs

In the ribs, osteomyelitis generally has a subacute presentation (36): swelling of the rib is usual. Before chemotherapy, tuberculosis was considered the most common cause of osteitis in a rib. If costal cartilages are involved, typhoid should be considered. Many pathogens, however, may occasionally give rise to rib osteomyelitis. Actinomycosis with chronic draining sinuses is now uncommon because antibiotics tend to confine the disease to the lungs (37). Osteomyelitis of the first rib can present as torticollis (38).

Infections of the Hand

Antibiotics have resulted in a change of emphasis in hand infections. Late, extensive, tissue space infections have given way to a range of superficial soft-tissue infections, infectious tenosynovitis, human bites, and occasional osteoarticular sepsis from other sources. With the exception of boils and carbuncles, most patients recall a preceding trivial injury, the position, type, and timing of which may be highly predictive (39). In the hand, the loose connective tissue and skin of the dorsum allow gross edema to occur. This edema is not predictive of site—it is seen in dorsal cellulitis, web space infections, and deep palmar space infections.

In a classic monograph on this subject, Kanavel (40) listed the signs of tendon sheath infection.

1. The finger is held in slight flexion: any attempt at extension is exquisitely painful, and active flexion is minimal.
2. The finger is uniformly swollen and red.
3. Tenderness is present along the line of the sheath.

When the ulnar bursa is involved, either by direct infection or, more rarely, by extension from the little finger, swelling and tenderness extend above the wrist and the whole hand is held in flexion (41).

Septic arthritis is usually a consequence of minor penetrating joint injury, often from a tooth. The clinical features (39) are swelling disproportional to the skin lesion; restricted joint movement, which is often slow to develop; and, in the established case, instability. Human punch injuries, in which there is a break in the skin in the region of a metacarpophalangeal joint, almost always enter that joint. Septic arthritis with mixed organisms often follows and such "small" injuries should not be dismissed without adequate surgical toilet.

Infections of the Foot

Two distinct syndromes are characteristic in the foot. Penetrating injuries, particularly common in children, may give rise to chronic soft-tissue infection with secondary osteomyelitis. The history identifies the initial injury. There is typically a period of 2 to 3 days when the initial pain settles, only to worsen thereafter. Local pain, swelling, and erythema are prominent, but systemic signs are unusual (42). Although tetanus is now rare in vaccinated communities, its occasional appearance as a complication of penetrating injuries should not be forgotten.

The second group of patients have osteomyelitis or septic arthritis associated with vascular insufficiency. Most are over 50 years of age. Local symptoms dominate the presentation. There may be ulcers on the sole or over bony prominences, and cellulitis and subcutaneous abscesses are frequently found. Diabetes mellitus is common in such patients (see Chapter 11).

Suspicion of osteomyelitis in unusual sites should evoke a careful search for proof. In the absence of pus, antibiotic treatment can be commenced and used as sole treatment. If the response is not rapid, then exploration for biopsy and drainage if pus is found is indicated. Neoplasia in children can present in a similar manner to osteomyelitis.

The Urgency of Intervention

Two forms of intervention should be considered: diagnostic and therapeutic. If the clinical history and findings on examination are clearly those of infection, no further diagnostic tests are necessary. Therapy should not be delayed. Confirmation of diagnosis should of course be sought, identification of the causative organism should not be ignored, and localization and extent of infection should be delineated precisely.

For example, in classic acute hematogenous osteomyelitis, the child should be admitted to hospital, rested in bed with the painful limb splinted, and blood cultures taken. Rehydration by the intravenous route should be started and antibiotic therapy commenced. Blood tests are usually done, but the blood can be drawn when the intravenous line is set up. Radiography can also follow such treatment (although it is not usually a cause for delay). Radioisotope imaging is not a necessary investigation before treatment starts, and the findings will not be appreciably altered by treatment.

Whether surgery to release pus is indicated will be dictated by the presence of pus on clinical evaluation. Rehydration, caloric replacement, and antibiotic drugs are more important than urgent surgery to release pus. Surgery can be delayed for several hours. The same rules apply to acute septic arthritis, but arthrocentesis should be done early because it is a guide to appropriate antibiotic therapy.

In contrast, in subacute, chronic, or unusual presentation of musculoskeletal sepsis, diagnosis must precede treatment. Little is to be lost if antibiotics are withheld for a few days, but much is lost if they are administered in inappropriate doses without a clear diagnosis. In the absence of features of septicemia or high fever, pain should be managed by rest, splintage, and analgesic drugs until the diagnosis is clear.

References

1. Smith N. Observations on the pathology and treatment of necrosis. Phil Month J Med 1827;1:11–19;66–75.
2. Brodie BC. Pathological and surgical observations on disease of the joints. London: Longman, 1818.
3. McCarthy PL, Wasserman D, Spiesel SZ, et al. Evaluation scales to identify serious illness in febrile children. Pediatrics 1982;70:802–809.
4. Dennison WM, McPherson DA. Haematogenous osteitis of infancy. Arch Dis Child 1952;27:375–381.
5. Thomson J, Lewis IC. Osteomyelitis in the newborn. Arch Dis Child 1950;25:273–279.
6. Linblad B, Ekengren K, Aurelius G. The prognosis of acute haematogenous osteomyelitis and its complications during early infancy after the advent of antibiotics. Acta Paediatr Scand 1965;54:24–32.
7. Green M, Nyhan WL, Fousek MD. Acute haematogenous osteomyelitis. Pediatrics 1956;17:368–381.
8. Aractingi TR. Etude de 32 cas d'osteomyelite de Nouveaune. Rev Chir Orthop 1961;47:50–63.
9. Edwards MS, Baker CJ, Wagner KH, et al. An etiologic shift in infantile osteomyelitis: the emergence of the group B streptococcus. J Pediatr 1978; 93:578–583.
10. Weissberg ED, Smith AL, Smith DH. Clinical features of neonatal osteomyelitis. Pediatrics 1974;53:505–510.
11. Wright PF, Thompson J, McKee KT, et al. Patterns of illness in the highly febrile young child: epidemiologic, clinical and laboratory correlates. Pediatrics 1981;67:694–700.
12. McCarthy PL, Wasserman D, Spiesel SZ, et al. Evaluation of arthritis and arthralgia in the pediatric patient. Clin Pediatr 1980;19:183–190.

13. Brewerton DA. Rheumatic disorders. In: Rossman I, ed. Clinical geriatrics. Philadelphia: Lippincott, 1979:451–459.
14. Vincent GM, Amirault JD. Septic arthritis in the elderly. Clin Orthop 1990;251:241–245.
15. Kellgren JH, Ball J, Faibrother RW, et al. Suppurative arthritis complicating rheumatoid arthritis. Br Med J 1958;1:1193–1200.
16. Norden CW. Osteomyelitis. In: Mandell GL, Douglas RG, Bennet JE, eds. Principles and practice of infectious disease. New York: Wiley, 1978: 946–956.
17. Petersdorf RG, Belson PB. Fever of unexplained origin. Medicine 1961; 40:1–30.
18. Esposito AL, Gleckman RA. A diagnostic approach to the adult with fever of unknown origin. Arch Intern Med 1979;139:575–579.
19. Cohen J. Infection and immunosuppression. Q J Med 1982;51:1–15.
20. Hughes RA, Rowe IF, Shanson D, Keat ACS. Septic bone joint and muscle lesions associated with human immunodeficiency virus infection. Br J Rheumatol 1992;31:381–388.
21. Mathews M, Shen FH, Lindner A, et al. Septic arthritis in hemodialized patients. Nephron 1980;25:87–91.
22. Caner JEZ, Decker JL. Recurrent acute (gouty) arthritis in chronic renal failure treated with periodic hemodialysis. Am J Med 1964;36:571–582.
23. Leonard A, Comty CM, Shapiro FL, et al. Osteomyelitis in haemodialysis patients. Ann Intern Med 1973;78:651–658.
24. Keely K, Buchanan GR. Acute infarction of long bones in children with sickle-cell anemia. J Pediatr 1982;101:170–175.
25. Kravis E, Fleischer G, Ludwig S. Fever in children with sickle-cell hemoglobinopathies. Am J Dis Child 1982;136:1075–1078.
26. Al-Salem AH, Ahmed HA, Qaisaruddin S, Al-Jam'a A, Elbashier AM, Al-Dabbous I. Osteomyelitis and septic arthritis in sickle-cell disease in the eastern province of Saudi Arabia. Int Orthop 1992;16:398–402.
27. Young F. Acute osteomyelitis of the ilium. Surg Gynecol Obstet 1934; 58:986–994.
28. Edwards MS, Baker CJ, Granberry WM, et al. Pelvic osteomyelitis in children. Pediatrics 1978;61:62–67.
29. Beaupre A, Carroll N. The three syndromes of iliac osteomyelitis in children. J Bone Joint Surg [Am] 1979;61:1087–1092.
30. Morgan A, Yates AK. The diagnosis of acute osteomyelitis of the pelvis. Postgrad Med J 1966;42:74–78.
31. Delbarre F, Rondier J, Delrieu F, et al. Pyogenic infection of the sacro-iliac joint; a report of thirteen cases. J Bone Joint Surg [Am] 1975;57:819–825.
32. Ransome J. Acute suppurative otitis media and acute mastoiditis. In: Kerr AG, ed. Scott-Brown's Otolaryngology (otology). London: Butterworth's, 1987:203–214.
33. Cavanagh F. Osteomyelitis of the superior maxilla in infants. Br Med J 1960;1:468–472.

34. Donohue WM, Abelardo LM. Osteomyelitis of the jaw. Can Med Assoc J 1970;103:748–750.
35. Seviour PW, Dieppe PA. Sternoclavicular joint infection as a cause of chest pain. Br Med J 1984;288:133–134.
36. Levinsohn EM, Sternick A, Echeverria TS, et al. Acute haematogenous osteomyelitis of the rib. Skeletal Radiol 1982;8:291–293.
37. McQuarrie DG, Hall WH. Actinomycosis of the lung and chest wall. Surgery 1968;64:905–911.
38. Steinberg GG. Osteomyelitis of the rib presenting as a painful torticollis. J Bone Joint Surg [Am] 1979;61:614–615.
39. Lister GD. The hand. Diagnosis and indications. Edinburgh: Churchill Livingstone, 1977.
40. Kanavel AB. Infections of the hand. Philadelphia: Lea and Febiger, 1933.
41. Pollen AG. Acute infections of the tendon sheaths. Hand 1974;6:21–25.
42. Green NE, Bruno J. Pseudomonas infections of the foot after puncture wounds. South Med J 1980;73:146–149.

CHAPTER 5

Laboratory Investigation

Laboratory investigation is an integral part of the evaluation of patients with suspected infection. Although there is no infallible clinical criterion of infection, it is possible to recognize accurately many specific infectious processes with the aid of laboratory examinations such as blood counts, serology, and microbiological examinations. In this chapter these techniques are reviewed as they apply to patients with presumed infection.

Hematological Investigation

Infection of bone and joints is frequently associated with anemia; however, the finding of anemia is totally nonspecific and its absence does not exclude the presence of infection. The principal response to infection seen in the white blood cells is an increase in their circulating number. The most common cause of a neutrophil leukocytosis is infection. Bacterial infection causes a prompt and fairly marked leukocytosis in the range of 15 to 30 $\times 10^9$/L, although higher values (50–80 $\times 10^9$/L) occur occasionally. Eosinophils and basophils are often reduced in acute infections and may be absent from blood films. In nonpyogenic infections, the leukocytosis is not usually as pronounced; cell counts may be normal or slightly elevated. In an overwhelming infection, the marrow may fail to respond and leukopenia may occur. Similarly, acute pyogenic infection in a debilitated patient with poor resistance may not be followed by leukocytosis. During childhood, infection usually causes a sharp increase in the leukocyte count. In young children, there is sometimes an increase in lymphocytes in response to an infection that in adults causes a neutrophil leukocytosis (1).

Infection causes an increase not only in the total number of cells but also in the proportion of younger cells, which results in a "shift to the left" in the differential count (i.e., the proportion of neutrophils with one or two lobes is increased). In severe infections, a moderate number of metamyelocytes and a few myelocytes and promyelocytes may be found in a blood film. In mild infections, a shift to the left may be found without an increase in the total count.

Severe infections are sometimes accompanied by toxic and degenerative changes in the neutrophils, affecting granules, cytoplasm, and nucleus, either singly or together. Changes in the granules are the most common toxic effect; they consist of disappearance of the normal neutrophil granules and appearance of toxic basophilic granules.

Although some infections may cause a leukopenia below the normal level of 4×10^9/L, this condition is rarely found in those infections that involve the musculoskeletal system, unless it is part of an overwhelming severe infection in elderly or debilitated subjects.

The Erythrocyte Sedimentation Rate

Probably the most used test in monitoring progress is the erythrocyte sedimentation rate (ESR). If the level is raised at the time of commencing treatment, a regular gradual decrease that parallels clinical improvement is expected. However, there is no direct relation between the ESR and the severity of infection. Despite clinical improvement, there may be a transient increase in ESR. Although in the long term the ESR generally returns to normal levels, this change may occur quite slowly. The ESR should not be used as a guide to duration of treatment or as an indication for intervention. The ESR is elevated in 90% of patients who have serious musculoskeletal infections, such as diskitis, osteomyelitis, and septic arthritis (2). In general, if the ESR does not decrease after antimicrobial treatment of osteomyelitis, factors such as undrained pus should be sought as an explanation.

C-Reactive Protein

As a marker of acute phase response to inflammation, C-reactive protein (CRP) has been known for many years (3) and is normally present in blood in very small amounts (4). It appears, however, in response to a number of injurious stimuli that have an inflammatory component. It lacks specificity: It can be demonstrated in a number of infectious diseases, rheumatic fever, rheumatoid arthritis, and myocardial infarction. Levels also increase after surgery. In such circumstances, the plasma concentration of most acute phase proteins may double, whereas the CRP concentration may be increased by as much as 100-fold or more.

The rate of CRP synthesis and secretion increases within hours of an acute injury or the onset of inflammation, probably under the influence of humoral mediators such as leukocyte endogenous pyrogen and prostaglandin E_1. A level of less than 10 mg/L, with a median value in healthy adults of 800 μg/L, is normal. Peak levels after stimulation starts may reach as much as 300 mg/L within 24 to 48 hours (3). Bacterial infections are a prominent (but not the only) cause of levels greater than 100 mg/L (5). CRP becomes detectable within 6 to 24 hours. Once initiated, the induction process involves progressive recruitment of liver cells to CRP synthesis and, consequently, an increase in serum levels. An elevated serum concentration of CRP is unequivocal evidence of an active tissue-damaging process. After a variable period following the stimulus, CRP levels usually decrease sharply (6). The CRP level invariably increases after major surgery, but with an uncomplicated normal recovery, decreases toward normal over 7 to 10 days. Absence of this decrease or a secondary increase in CRP provides early warning of intercurrent infection or thromboembolic complications. Recently introduced methods of precise quantitative assessment of CRP have made the detection of CRP a more useful test (7).

Confirmation of infection after joint replacement is often difficult in the assessment of pain from the region of surgery. The changes in levels of CRP following total hip arthroplasty are an increase to a peak 2 days after operation and a decrease to normal levels by 21 days, although at 7 days, the level is slightly raised (8). Alteration in this normal pattern may be useful in predicting infection, but its worth has not been tested. In a study of 117 patients who had undergone hip or knee arthroplasty (9), it was found that on the first postoperative day, CRP increased significantly above preoperative levels, reaching a peak on day 2. By the time of discharge from hospital, the levels were almost normal, but still raised. Six or eight weeks after operation, CRP levels were not significantly different from those before operation. The levels were not related to age, sex, previous history of major surgery, smoking, which joint was replaced, indication for surgery, or the use of cement. A raised level 2 months or more after operation may be a good guide to deep infection. One study to determine the value of CRP in infected hip arthroplasty (10) found that it exceeded 20 mg/L in all, whereas in cases of nonseptic loosening, the level was less than 20 mg/L. Together with a raised ESR, it could be a useful guide to infection after hip replacement. However, not all infected patients had both values raised simultaneously.

It would appear that the most useful role of CRP estimations is to determine whether a person with an underlying disease (e.g., leukemia or malignancy) has a superimposed infection. If constant pain in concealed site suggests inflammation or malignancy, then increased CRP levels may be a guide to infection.

Relation of ESR and CRP

The disadvantages of serum CRP and ESR tests are that they are nonspecific and may increase in response to several diseases with acute inflammatory reactions. The correlation between CRP and ESR is often poor. The ESR tends to increase more slowly than CRP; thus measurement at a single time point after an acute stimulus would not be expected to correlate well. Overall, CRP is a more useful but nonspecific indicator of inflammation, infection, and necrosis because it increases faster than the ESR and is not affected by other red cell or plasma parameters. A critical review (7) concluded that CRP has little value as a differential diagnostic test in the acute clinical situation. It has a useful role in monitoring certain clinical problems, such as early identification of secondary infections and response to treatment in some bacterial infections and chronic inflammatory conditions. In these situations, it is more useful than the ESR.

Microbiological Investigations in Bone and Joint Infection

The key to appropriate therapy in bone and joint infections is identification of causative organisms. Certain factors govern the likelihood with which this identification is achieved. These factors include the manner in which specimens are obtained; the speed with which they are taken to the laboratory; and the accuracy and relevance of the clinical information given to the microbiologist regarding suspected diagnosis, source of the specimen, prior antimicrobial therapy, among others.

Specimen Collection and Processing

1. The specimens selected should be likely to yield the organisms causing the disease. For example, in osteomyelitis, sinus tract cultures are less likely to yield pathogens than are cultures of pus or direct aspiration of bone (11).

2. An adequate quantity of material for culture should be submitted to the microbiology laboratory. Not infrequently, 10 mL of pus are found and a swab is sent to the microbiology laboratory; sending more rather than less should be axiomatic.

3. The techniques of collecting specimens must avoid contamination by organisms normally found on the skin and mucous membranes.

4. Material for culture should be delivered rapidly to the microbiology laboratory so that fastidious organisms do not die or are not overgrown by other organisms.

5. Wherever possible, specimens for culture should be obtained before antimicrobial therapy is begun.

The details of specimen collection procedures and processing are generally available from each hospital microbiology laboratory. It is beyond the scope of this text to review these factors in detail, but such manuals should be consulted and discussed by microbiologists and clinicians if questions arise when diagnostic procedures are being undertaken.

Types of Specimens for Collection in Musculoskeletal Infections

In any febrile patient, blood should be cultured for the diagnosis of bacteremia. Specific procedures for the amount of blood to be collected and the medium to be inoculated are usually provided by the microbiology laboratory. If unusual pathogens such as mycobacteria or *Brucella* are suspected, the microbiology laboratory should be consulted for the best way to obtain specimens and to process them in the laboratory.

Musculoskeletal infections are usually due to bacteria and sometimes to fungi. Unopened or undrained abscesses are excellent sources of organisms; adequate amounts of material should be sent to the microbiology laboratory for both culture and microscopy. Swabs of sinus tracts are generally unsatisfactory (11). Swabs of ulcers may also be misleading; it has been suggested that curettings or biopsy specimens taken from the undermined edge or base are more appropriate (12,13). Cultures taken from wounds, particularly if pus is obtained, provide important information as to the cause of underlying infection.

If routine cultures fail to grow organisms and the specimen has been carefully taken following the principles enunciated, consideration should be given to other pathogens. Histological examination may be extremely useful; the presence of granulomas should suggest other pathogens and consultation with the microbiology laboratory should prompt a search for mycobacteria, *Brucella,* and fungi.

If a joint is inflamed or swollen, synovial fluid should be aspirated and an adequate quantity sent to the microbiology laboratory (14). Gross examination should record color, turbidity, and clot. White and red blood cell counts should be performed. Gram's stain should be done on an air-dried smear, and the remainder of the fluid should be used to seed culture plates. If the Gram stain reveals no organisms or the white blood cell count differential is predominantly lymphocytes, pathogens other than the usual bacterial species should be considered, and appropriate tests should be performed for mycobacteria, fungi, or other organisms endemic to a given area.

Identification of Organisms

It is beyond the scope of this chapter to review details of the techniques for identifying micro-organisms; however, there are certain basic principles by which laboratories provide both preliminary and definitive identification of etiological agents.

1. Specimens, either unstained or stained, can be examined microscopically. The value of rapid diagnosis, on the basis of a carefully performed and examined Gram's stain of specimens, is to allow a more rational choice of empiric antimicrobial therapy.

2. Organisms are identified by their growth patterns and biochemical responses after they have been isolated by appropriate culture techniques.

3. Immunological techniques for detection of antigens or antibodies directly in body fluids, tissues, or from organisms isolated from cultures may be used for identification.

4. Organisms may be identified by DNA probes that can detect the intact organism or its genetically encoded characteristics.

Serological Tests

In certain instances, cultures may be unavailable or unrewarding because of the lack of developed tests, safety concerns about attempting to isolate certain organisms, or the need for special skills and facilities, which many laboratories do not possess. Cultures may also be negative in the face of prior antimicrobial therapy. In such circumstances, detection of antibodies may be of diagnostic use; however, antibody responses to infections are often quite variable. In addition, a single elevated antibody titer is usually insufficient to distinguish between active or old infection; the absence of an elevated antibody titer may simply be a reflection of the lack of antigenicity of the organism or that insufficient time has elapsed for an antibody response to have developed. In general, serological testing should be performed simultaneously, with both an acute phase and a convalescent specimen taken at least one week apart. The generally accepted criterion for infection is a four-fold or greater increase in antibody titer. Bacterial diseases for which serological tests may be useful include *Brucella,* tularemia, *Legionella,* leptospirosis, rickettsial disease, *Salmonella,* group A streptococcal infection, syphilis, *Psittacosis,* and mycoplasma infections.

Antibiotic Susceptibility Testing

Susceptibility tests are usually performed for organisms with unpredictable susceptibility to antimicrobial agents or frequently with any isolated organism that is believed to be clinically significant. Susceptibility tests are usually performed according to standardized criteria, but techniques may vary from laboratory to laboratory. Standards for testing rapidly growing aerobic and facultatively anaerobic bacteria are established; standards for testing anaerobic bacteria, mycobacteria, and fungi are being developed, although many microbiology laboratories have established procedures for performing these tests. Many laboratories report the susceptibility of bacterial isolates as either susceptible (i.e., the bacterial strain is amenable to treatment with that agent in ordinary dosage) or resistant (i.e., the strain is unaffected by high concentrations of antibiotic and therefore unlikely to respond to conventional doses). Some laboratories that perform dilution tests report minimal inhibitory concentrations and also indicate what concentration is likely to be susceptible or resistant. Measurement of the minimal bactericidal concentration generally remains a tool for evaluation of new antimicrobial agents and is not used in routine microbiological evaluation in hospital laboratories. Serum bactericidal tests are infrequently performed in musculoskeletal infections, although some clinicians use them to assess the adequacy of antibiotic therapy in the management of osteomyelitis (15,16).

References

1. DeGruchy CC. Clinical haematology in medical practice. Oxford: Blackwell Scientific, 1960.
2. Schulak DJ, Rayhack JM, Lippert FG, Convery FR. The erythrocyte sedimentation rate in orthopaedic patients. Clin Orthop 1982;167:197–202.
3. Pepys MB. C-reactive protein fifty years on. Lancet 1981;1:653–656.
4. Sipe JD. The acute phase response to inflammation: the erythrocyte sedimentation rate (ESR) and C-reactive protein (CRP) and other plasma protein responses to tissue injury. In: Cohen AS, ed. Laboratory diagnostic procedures in the rheumatic diseases, ed 3. Orlando: Grune & Stratton, 1985:77–94.
5. Morley JJ, Jushner I. Serum c-reactive proteins in disease. Ann NY Acad Sci 1982;389:406–418.
6. McIntyre SS, Schultz D, Kushner I. Biosynthesis of c-reactive protein. Ann NY Acad Sci 1982;389:76–87.
7. Young B, Gleeson M, Cripps AW. C-reactive protein: a critical review. Pathology 1991;23:118–124.
8. Aalto K, Osterman K, Peltola H, Rasanen J. Changes in erythrocyte sedimentation rate and c-reactive protein after total hip arthroplasty. Clin Orthop 1984;184:118–120.
9. Choudhry RR, Rice RPO, Triffitt PD, Harper WM, Gregg PJ. Plasma viscosity and c-reactive protein after total hip and knee arthroplasty. J Bone Joint Surg [Br] 1992;74:523–524.
10. Sanzen L, Carlsson AS. The diagnostic value of c-reactive protein in infected hip arthroplasties. J Bone Joint Surg [Br] 1989;71:638–641.
11. Mackowiak P, Jones S, Smith J. Diagnostic value of sinus tract culture in chronic osteomyelitis. JAMA 1978;239:2772–2775.
12. Lipsky B, Pecoraro RR, Wheat J. The diabetic foot, soft tissue and bone infection. Infect Dis Clin North Am 1990;4:409–432.

13. Sapico F, Canawati H, Witte J, et al. Quantitative aerobic and anaerobic bacteriology of infected diabetic foot. J Clin Microbiol 1980;12:413–420.
14. Cohen AS, Goldenberg D. Synovial fluid. In: Cohen AS, ed. Laboratory diagnostic procedures in the rheumatic diseases, ed 3. Orlando: Grune & Stratton, 1985:1–54.
15. Prober C, Yeager A. Use of the serum bactericidal titer to assess the adequacy of oral antibiotic therapy in the treatment of acute hematogenous osteomyelitis. J Pediatr 1979;95:131–135.
16. Weinstein M, Stratton C, Hawley H, et al. Multicenter collaborative evaluation of a standardized serum bactericidal test as a predictor of therapeutic efficacy in acute and chronic osteomyelitis. Am J Med 1987;83:218–222.

CHAPTER 6

Diagnostic Imaging

The site of pain and the identification of tenderness are the usual clues to the site of infection. *Location of the site of infection* can be helped greatly by imaging techniques that display abnormalities in the anatomy and physiology of tissues. Confirmation that the changes seen on the images obtained are due to infection is done by location and identification of organisms.

This chapter reviews the methods of imaging available to clinicians to support diagnosis and to aid treatment. *Location and identification of organisms,* the proof of infection, is addressed in Chapter 5.

Locating the Site of Infection

Radiology

To interpret radiographs, it is important to understand the way tissues react to infection and the pathological changes that take place.

Conventional Radiography

Both bones and soft tissues must be examined. In acute hematogenous osteomyelitis, the earliest stages of the infection have no radiological signs (the small intramedullary abscess cannot be detected). Once there is spread of pus or edema outside the bone, the swelling in the soft tissue may be seen if the plane of the radiographic beam is sufficiently tangential so that the bone does not obscure the swelling. Initially, there is separation of lucent tissue planes from underlying metaphyseal bone, followed within a few days by muscle swelling and obliteration of soft-tissue shadows. Deep muscles and soft tissues are affected first, followed by involvement of more superficial muscle and subcutaneous tissues. Such changes are visible during the first week after initiation of infection.

The changes that occur in bone are those of destruction, or failure of formation, of metaphyseal bone, and repair—which may be seen easily as a result of periosteal osteogenic activity or, less easily, initially at least, within the medulla. The response of periosteum and bone marrow to any type of insult or injury is to form bone. Therefore, the presence of such bone is not diagnostic of adjacent bone infection. Furthermore, the bony changes detected are smaller than those visible on pathological observation (1).

In children, bone destruction is seen as an ill-defined lucency in the metaphysis, adjacent to the physis. Lateral spread may show bone loss

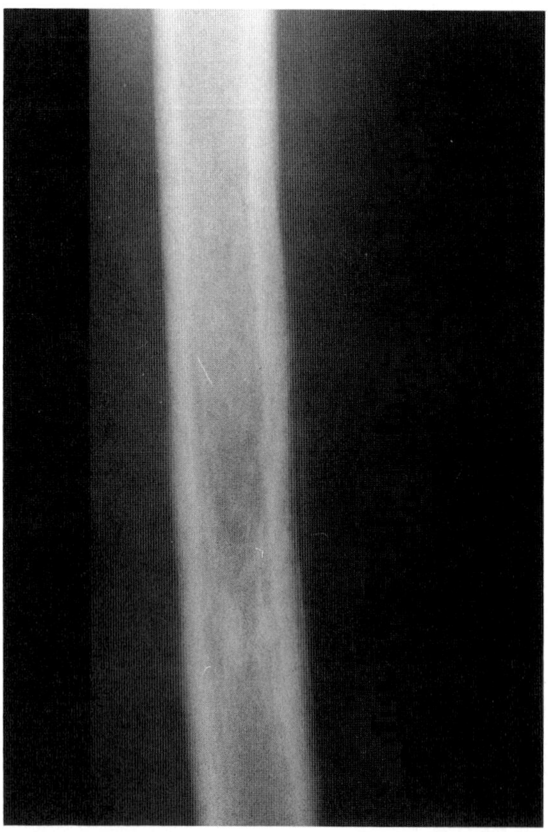

Figure 6-1. *Osteomyelitis of humeral diaphysis approximately one week after onset of symptoms. Note the osteopenia of the diaphysis and two thin lines of bone formed from periosteum parallel to the diaphysis but separated from it by a radiolucent zone. This type of bone formation is a response to "irritation" of the normal bone and is not specific to sepsis.* (Radiograph provided by Dr. G.K. Chapman.)

in the adjacent cortex. The response of periosteum to nearby sepsis is the laying down of bone, parallel to the cortex in the metaphysis, separated by a thin lucent line (Figure 6-1). The shape of newly formed bone on plain radiographs is often curved—furthest away from the cortex near the center of the infective focus and merging with the cortex at a distance from it—not unlike a cone or a trumpet, enveloping the septic site. In relation to the disuse, there may be regional osteopenia of the bone, involving up to one third of the whole bone in a diffuse, nonfocal manner. An effusion may be present in an adjacent joint.

In infants with absent or partial ossification of epiphyses, recognition of bone destruction is much more difficult, and the periosteal response is most obviously seen (Figure 6-2). Soft-tissue changes are important in this age group (Figure 6-3).

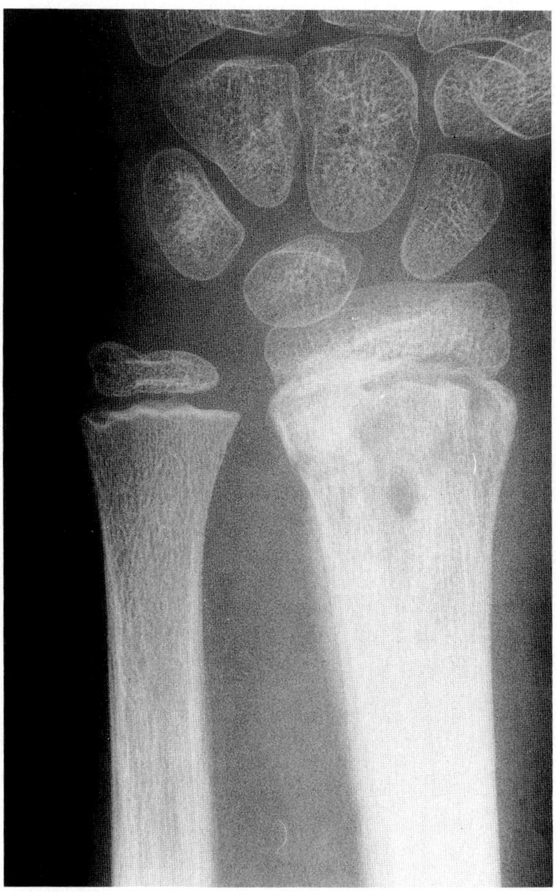

Figure 6-2. *Osteomyelitis of distal radius. Note the periosteal lines seen on the upper edges of the radius and the ulna; the lines on the radius are thicker in terms of newly formed bone in relation to the infective process. There is a destructive lytic area in the radial metaphysis. In addition, there is relative osteopenia of the carpal bones, epiphyses, and the distal part of the ulna.*

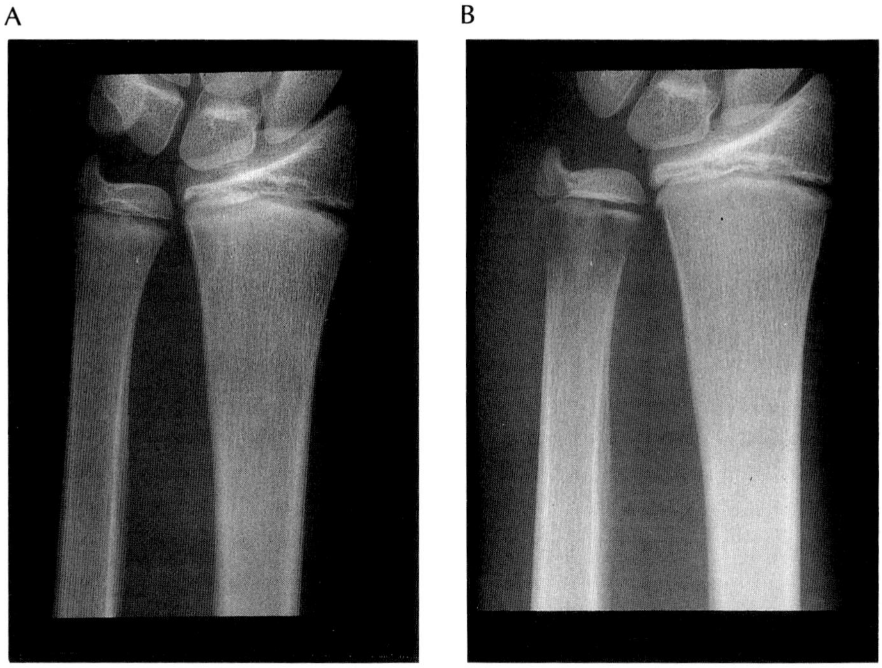

Figure 6-3. *(A) This 13-year-old boy gave a 2-day history of pain and swelling on the ulnar side of his wrist. There are no osseous changes, but the skin contour shows the swelling clearly. (B) Six days later, there are obvious changes in the ulna underlying the swelling of metaphyseal loss of bone due to the osteomyelitic process.* (Radiographs provided by Dr. G.K. Chapman.)

In contrast, soft-tissue changes are more difficult to detect in adults. Bone destruction produces lucent areas of varying sizes, often not clearly defined but merging into surrounding trabeculae. Cortical resorption is often seen as endosteal scalloping, intracortical lucency, or tunneling (Figure 6-4). There is usually a periosteal bone-forming response, less marked than in children or infants. Encapsulation of abscess by medullary new bone produces a dense shell of bone about the septic site. Deposition of bone on necrotic trabeculae causes an increased density—the sequestrum. Such increased density can also appear on radiographs if ischemia and granulation tissue prevent the normal mechanisms of removal of dead bone from taking place, and if surrounding areas become osteopenic, leading to relative increased density of the sequestrum (Figure 6-5). The presence of an area of

A B

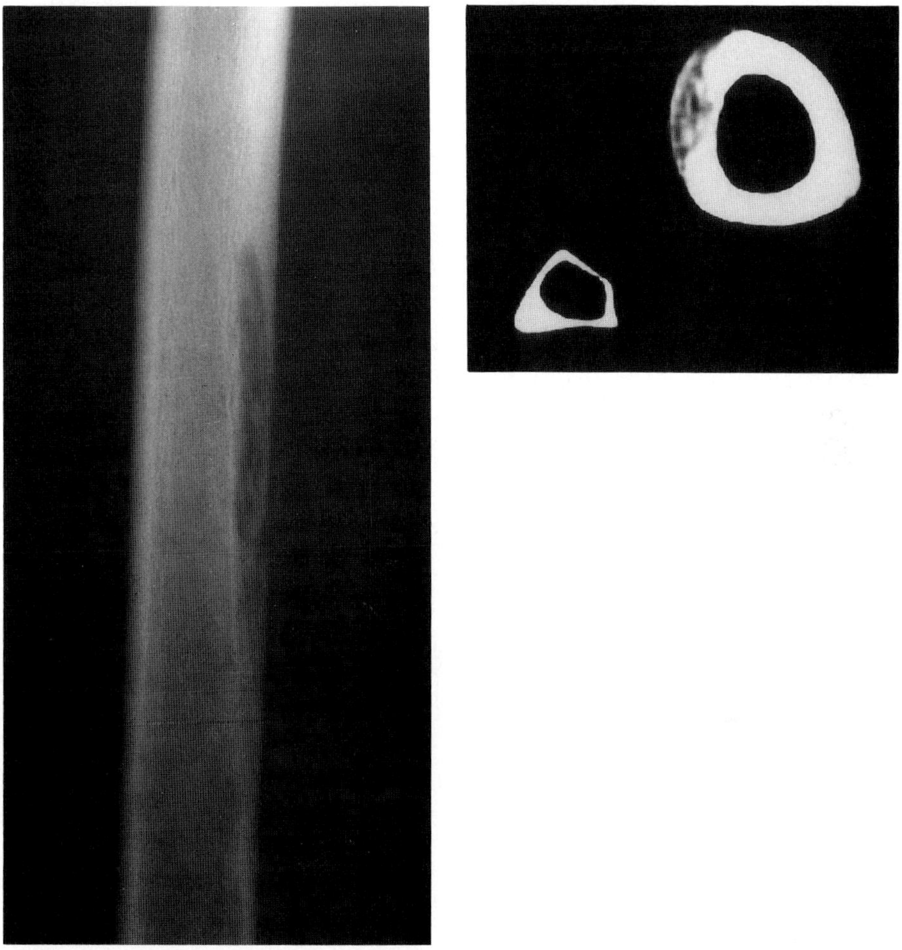

Figure 6-4. *(A) Cortical resorption and tunneling of microabscesses in adult osteomyelitis are not often associated with a significant periosteal reaction producing bone in plain radiographs. Computerized tomography (B) shows the extent of the bone destruction in the cortex of a tibia.*

increased density within an infected bone, although called a sequestrum, may indicate dead bone, living reactive new bone, or both. Another feature of bone sepsis may be loss of cortical continuity on its external surface without clear cut margins (Figure 6-6).

The combination of periosteal bone formation and cortical and cancellous bone destruction is usual in both inflammation and neoplasia

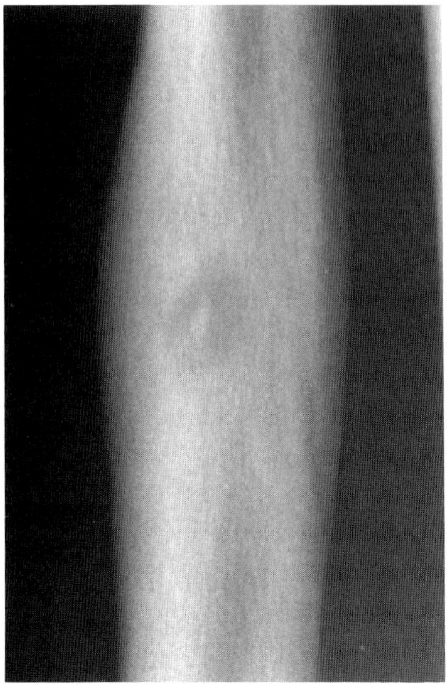

Figure 6-5. *Note the lucent zone representing an abscess, in the center of which is an area of increased radiodensity representing a focus of dead bone—the sequestrum. The diaphysis of the bone shows a uniform fusiform thickening due to reactive bone formation by periosteal activity.*

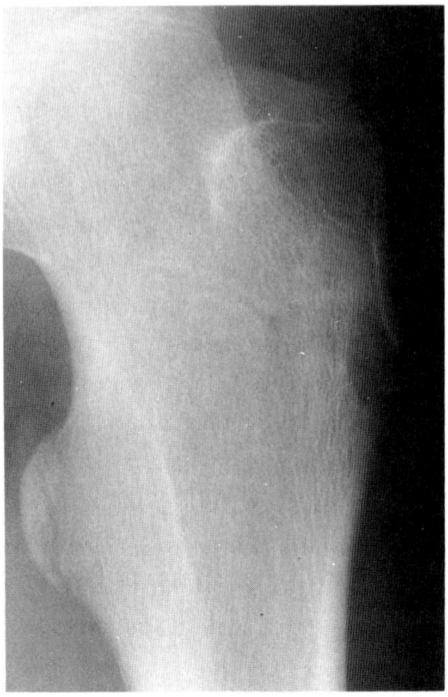

Figure 6-6. *Just below the greater trochanter of this adolescent femur, there is a break in the continuity of the cortex and underlying loss of bone. There is no discernible reactive bone formation by periosteum. The most likely cause of bone loss is osteomyelitis.*

involving bones. The balance of the two changes often leads to the diagnosis. In pyogenic bone infection, the periosteal response is about equal in amount to the erosion, whereas in malignant neoplasia, there is a greater imbalance between the two—either a slight periosteal reaction with marked erosion or a gross reaction with slight erosion.

These generalizations do not hold in atypical manifestations of either neoplasm or infection; they are also not applicable in flat bones, tarsal bones, carpal bones, and vertebrae. Nevertheless, the principle is a useful starting base for interpretation of radiographs, considered together with clinical features.

Acute Hematogenous Osteomyelitis: In typical long bone osteomyelitis, the earliest radiographic change is a faint hazy shadow around the shaft of bone due to pus and edema, which is often unnoticed. The first reliable radiographic evidence is a small area of erosion and periosteal reaction (Figure 6-7) between 10 and 14 days after onset of symptoms. The erosion may precede the reaction, the reverse may occur, or both may appear simultaneously. The erosion may consist of single or multiple poorly demarcated translucent zones (Figure 6-8), circular or elongated, which may be separated by zones of bone that appear radiographically normal. The periosteal new bone is a thin linear shadow parallel to the cortex but separated from it by a translucent zone 2 to 10 mm wide. The linear shadow may lie over an erosion or be separated from it by normal cortex, arising at a different level

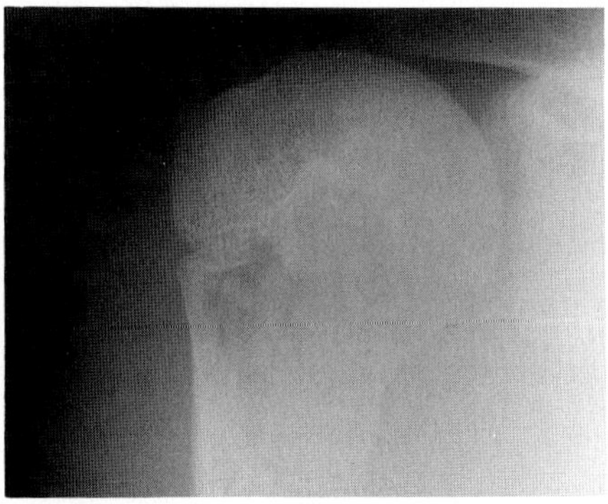

Figure 6-7. *In the metaphysis of this humerus, adjacent to the growth plate is an area of poorly defined lucency. There is no discernible periosteal reaction, although radionuclide bone scanning may provide evidence of bone formation at this stage, which is likely to be seen within one week of onset of symptoms.*

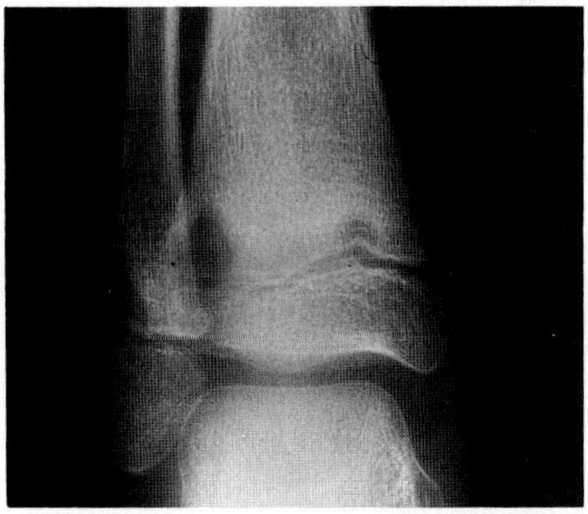

Figure 6-8. *Adjacent to the growth plate in the tibial metaphysis are two lucent zones separated by apparently normal bone. The lucency indicates that bone has been removed by the infective process or its consequences, but the infection may involve the whole metaphyseal region. It is not possible to predict the effect of the infection on the growth plate. There has been no obvious bone formation by periosteal activity. Plain radiography is not a sensitive test of small amounts of bone formation.*

from the erosion (see Figure 6-2). Such changes are usually metaphyseal. If treatment is effective at an early stage, the new bone continues to spread, whereas the erosion becomes stationary and eventually reossifies. The periosteal response is more prominent until normal shape of bone returns as remodeling occurs.

If the infection is not controlled, erosion and the periosteal response occur together and worsen. Sometimes the periosteal response has an onion-skin appearance (i.e., bone deposits separated by narrow translucent zones) (Figure 6-9); sometimes the response is striate, at right angles to the shaft, and the striations are joined at the periphery in the so called close-feathering pattern.

As healing takes place, the living bone regains its normal density. Cavities filled with fibrous tissue are seen as areas of lucency within

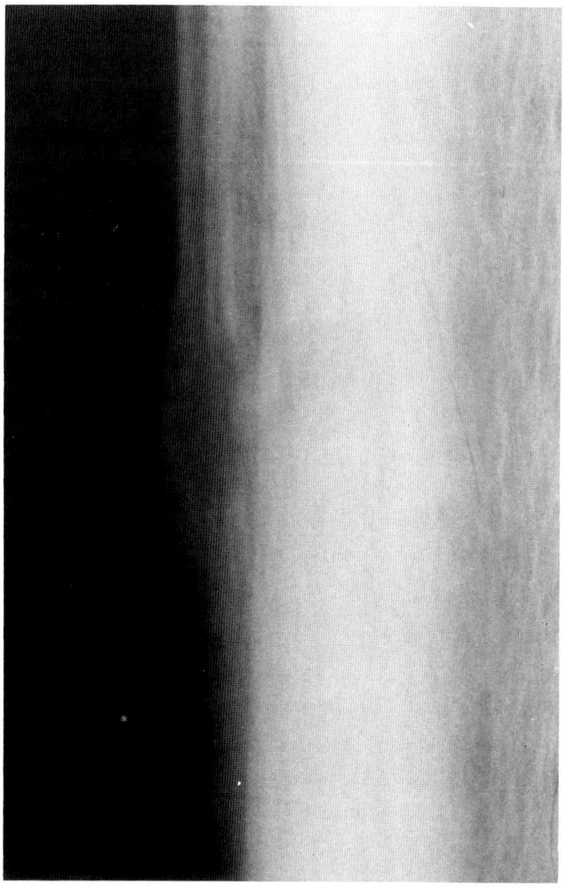

Figure 6-9. *Peripheral to the cortex is a zone of bone in which there is striation not unlike an onion skin, with alternate layers of bone and fibrous tissue. In the central portion, there is a radiolucency suggesting that there may be purulent material in this region. The newly formed bone from a response of periosteum to the infection tapers to blend imperceptibly with the original diaphyseal cortex inferiorly.*

thickened and dense bone of irregular contour (Figure 6-10). Such radiodensity may persist for a long time even though the infection has been controlled (Figure 6-11). In infants and children, normal growth and remodeling of bone may allow reconstitution of normal anatomy. In adolescents or adults, radiological changes often persist despite clinical resolution. Sequestra may appear by about the third week after onset.

Clinical evidence of control of infection must be taken as the response to therapy. The evolution of radiological changes may show an increase in bone reaction, which is part of the healing process, not evidence of persisting infection. It may take months until normal bone appearance is restored.

Osteomyelitis due to direct spread from adjacent infection has different radiological patterns: The direction of spread is opposite to that of hematogenous (medullary) osteomyelitis. The bones most of-

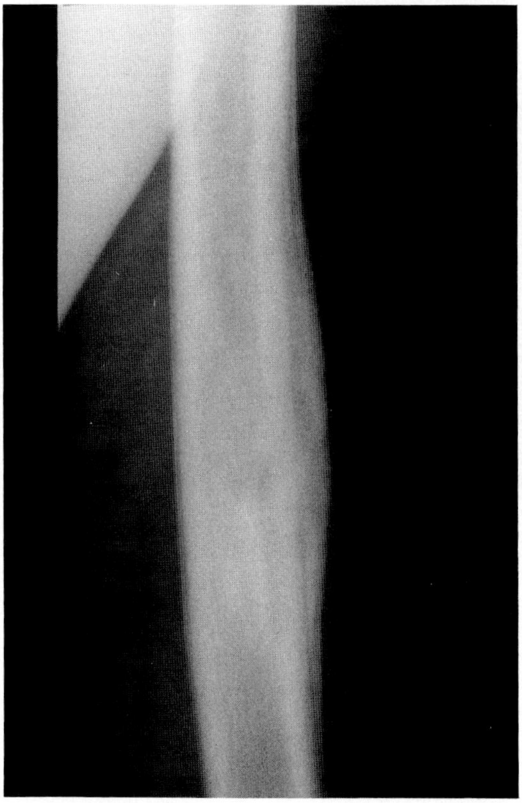

Figure 6-10. *Same patient as in Figure 6-1, six weeks later when clinically normal after treatment with antibiotics. Considerably more bone has formed as a result of periosteal activity on opposite sides of the diaphysis. There is still a zone of separation of the newly formed bone from the diaphysis depicted as a lucency and comprised of granulation or fibrous tissue.* (Radiograph provided by Dr. G.K. Chapman.)

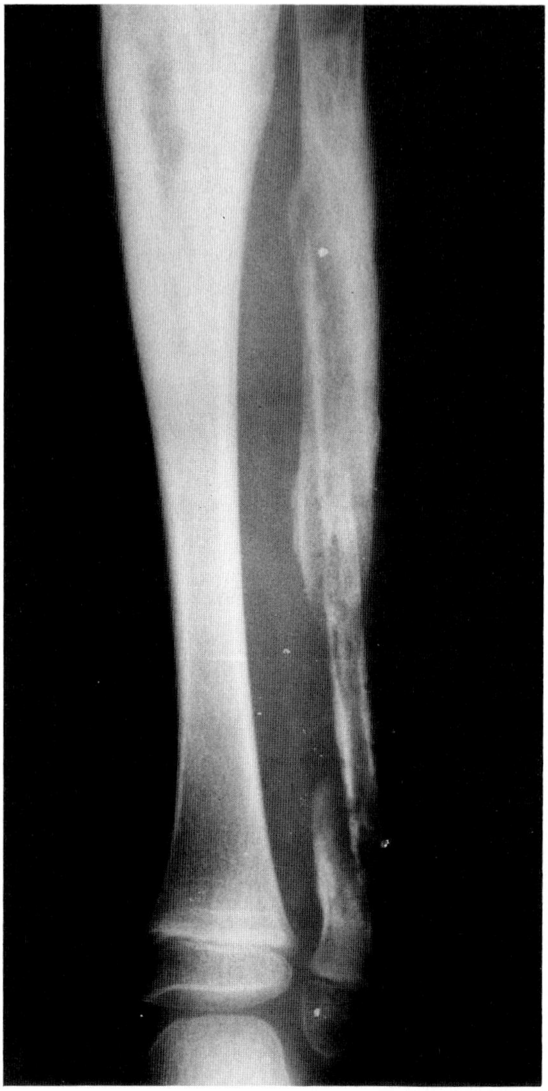

Figure 6-11. *The central part of the fibula is a necrotic sequestrum, which in its upper half is surrounded by newly formed living bone called the involucrum. Absence of soft-tissue swelling indicates that the infection is controlled. The involucrum of new bone is part of the healing response and may proceed for months after abortion of the acute infection. This process is accompanied by intense uptake of bone-seeking radiopharmaceutical, which would not be indicative of acute osteomyelitis. Note that the pathological fracture of the lower end of the fibula remains unhealed.*

ten involved are the terminal finger phalanges, the skull, the mandible, and the ribs.

In the terminal phalanges and the skull, the principal change is erosion, with very little periosteal reaction (Figure 6-12). In the fingers (Figure 6-13), the erosion may completely obliterate the bone outline; however, during repair, the trabecular pattern reappears quite quickly, in contrast to the skull, in which it is slow.

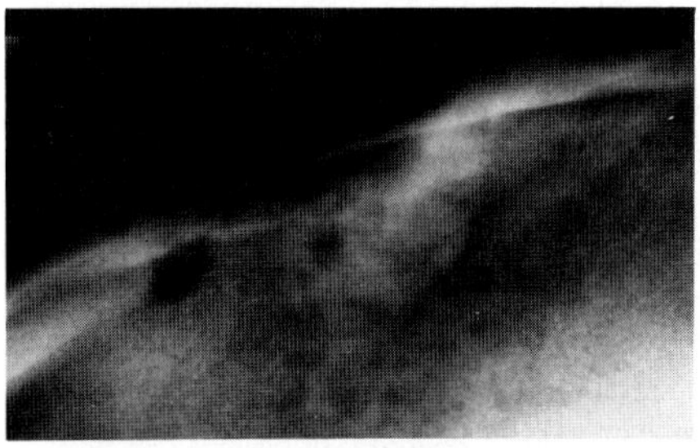

Figure 6-12. *Osteomyelitis of the skull, which occurred after removal of a skin tumor and infection of the wound. Note the loss of calvarial bone and surrounding zone of bone formation. Unless the radiographic beam is tangential to the skull surface, this appearance may not be obtained.* (Radiograph provided by Dr. K.J. Sherbon.)

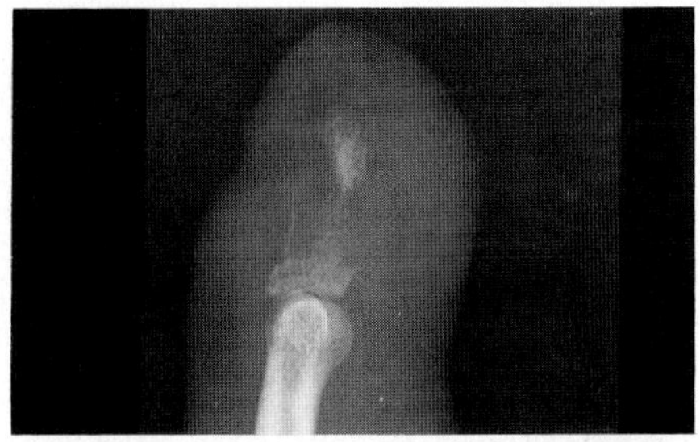

Figure 6-13. *Osteomyelitis of the terminal phalanx of a finger. The finger tip is swollen and there is an irregularity in the skin on the palmar aspect indicating a discharging sinus. Note the marked loss of bone substance in the terminal phalanx, which still retains its shape. The middle phalanx is not involved in the infective process, which most likely was a sequel to a puncture wound of the finger. The combination of soft-tissue swelling, a sinus, and bone loss are clues to the diagnosis.* (Radiograph provided by Dr. K.J. Sherbon.)

The soft-tissue abscesses are usually visible. The periosteal bone-forming response is usually greater than the destructive response. The lytic areas in bone cortex often precede the appearance of lytic areas in the medulla. Cortical erosions are usually ill defined.

Bone infection following direct implantation of organisms (e.g., after puncture wounds or bites) produces similar radiographic appearances to that after contiguous spread (Figure 6-14).

In the mandible, erosion plus increased bone density around an infected tooth are more common than the periosteal reaction. If there is no obvious dental cause, actinomycosis must be considered. In contrast, when ribs are involved, the periosteal response is far more prominent than bone destruction.

When there is infection in relation to open fractures or following bone surgery, erosion and the periosteal reaction are slight, but there is absence or delay in appearance of the normally expected mineral-

A B C

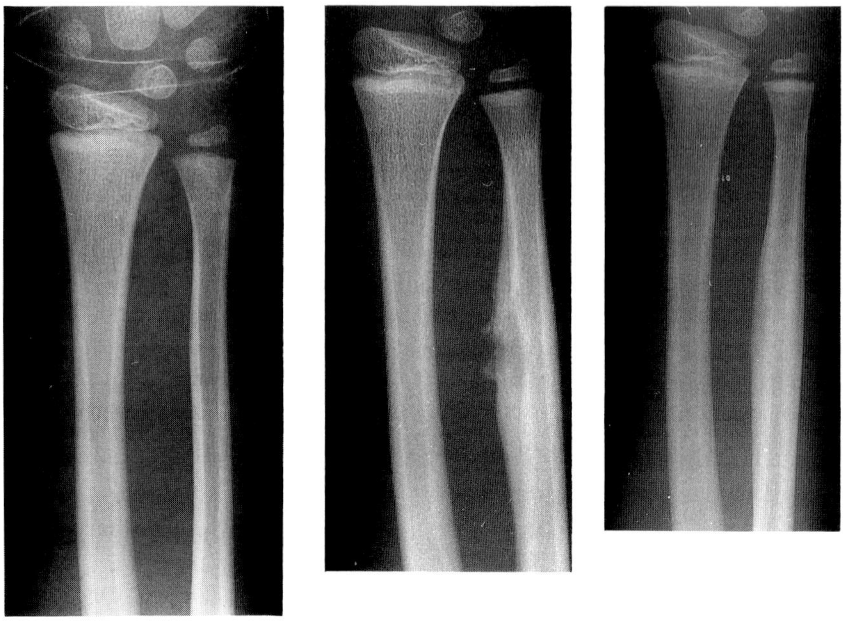

Figure 6-14. *(A) Bandaging obscures the gas in the soft tissues of the forearm of this child who was bitten by a dog. (B) Radiographs two months later show a localized area of periosteal bone formation with patchy osteolysis. There is evidence of both bone destruction and bone formation. Culture grew* Pasteurella *species. Following resection of the infected area (C), bone healing occurred, leaving as evidence a small fusiform swelling of cortical bone.*

ization in callus. Paradoxically, the appearance of fluffy callus after rigid internal fixation ("irritation callus") indicates loss of rigidity, usually from infection. If there is erosive change, either in cancellous or cortical bone, it is highly suspicious of infection. A similar interpretation should be investigated with regard to erosion seen about metallic implants.

Subacute Osteomyelitis: In subacute osteomyelitis, there has been more time for both the destructive and the repair processes to advance. A Brodie's abscess (2) has a characteristic appearance on radiographs (Figure 6-15). A metaphyseal lucency is surrounded by a clearly defined bony wall. It is usually spherical in shape. If a track

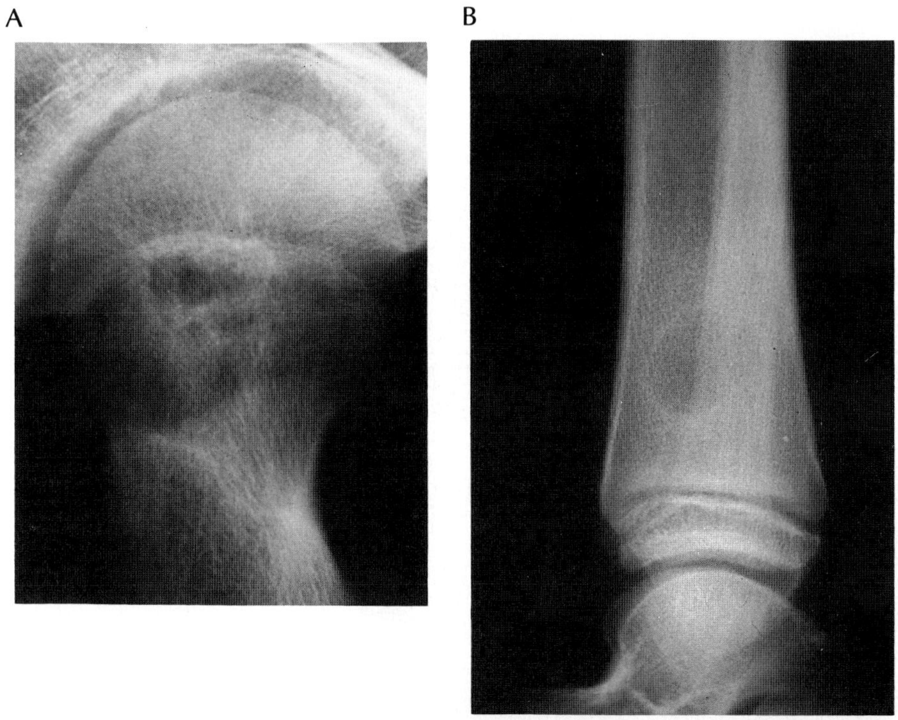

Figure 6-15. *Typical appearances of a Brodie's abscess. (A) A metaphyseal lucency adjacent to the growth plate with a circular circumferential zone of increased radiodensity due to medullary bone formation around the infective focus. (B) The cavity within the tibial medulla has appeared to migrate proximally due to bone growth adjacent to the physis, which has occurred since the time of formation of the abscess. Such a finding need not be associated with clinical symptoms or signs.*

connecting it to the physeal region can be detected, then osteomyelitis is the most likely cause. Diaphyseal abscesses do occur, located in the central or subcortical trabecular bone, or in the cortex (Figure 6-16). Sometimes a central sequestrum is present. The appearance of a lucent lesion with surrounding new bone and a periosteal reaction is similar to an osteoid osteoma or a stress fracture.

Sequestra may appear in medullary or cortical sites. They are usually sharply defined and have various shapes. Sequestra move toward the surface along sinuses and may be evident as extrusions through gaps in the bone cortex.

Sometimes the periosteal and intramedullary new bone-forming

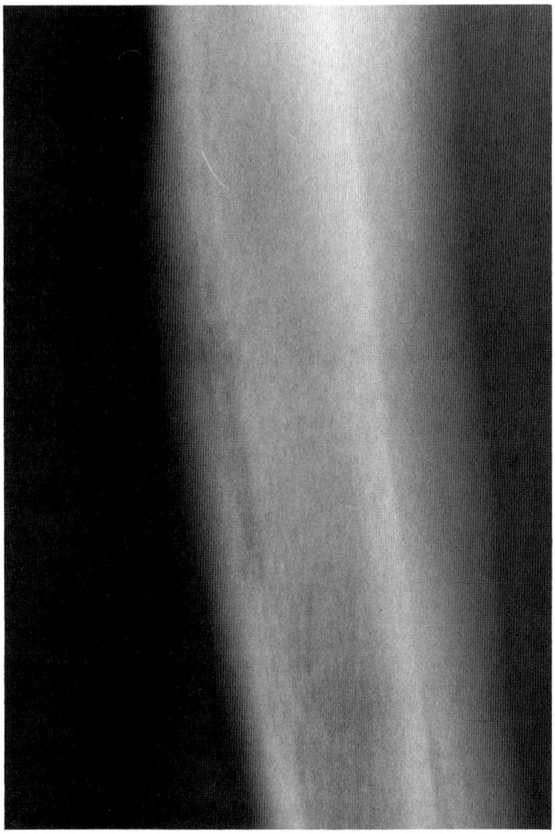

Figure 6-16. *Note the streaky linear erosion within the cortex, presumably due to microabscesses. Other cortical lesions may show relatively uniform destruction of the cortex, described as type III subacute osteomyelitis in the classification of Gledhill and Roberts.*

response is great, with the production of large involucra (Figure 6-17), especially in neonates, or dense thickening in the bone cortex (Figure 6-18).

Often a clear diagnosis of infection cannot be made on a single radiological examination. Repeated investigations after a reasonable period, determined by the nature of the symptoms and disease process, often are very useful as they indicate the dynamic nature of the underlying pathology.

Although clinical and radiological features usually lead to a confident diagnosis of osteomyelitis, aggressive bone destruction not balanced by repair may simulate malignant neoplasms, such as Ewing's tumor (Figure 6-19), osteosarcoma in children, reticulum cell sarcoma, or skeletal metastases. Neoplasms tend to permeate into surrounding bone, whereas infection has some delineation of its margins.

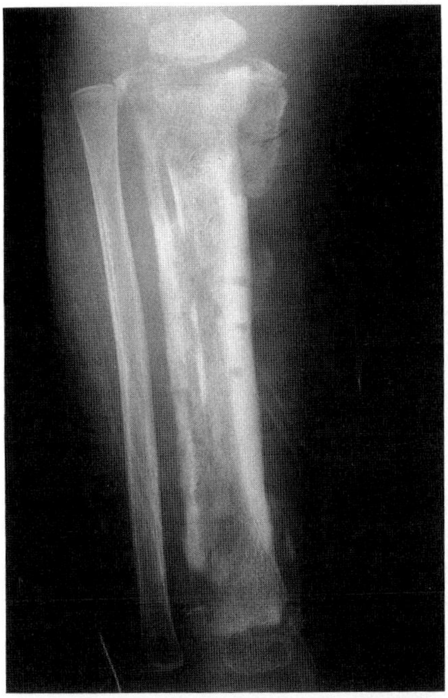

Figure 6-17. *Note the extent of involucrum surrounding almost the entire length of the tibia. Much of the original tibia appears to be a sequestrum in which three drill holes seem to have been made. The involucrum in this patient is a consequence of bone formation by the periosteum. At the lower end of the tibial involucrum, there is a break in the continuity of the bone, called a* cloaca.

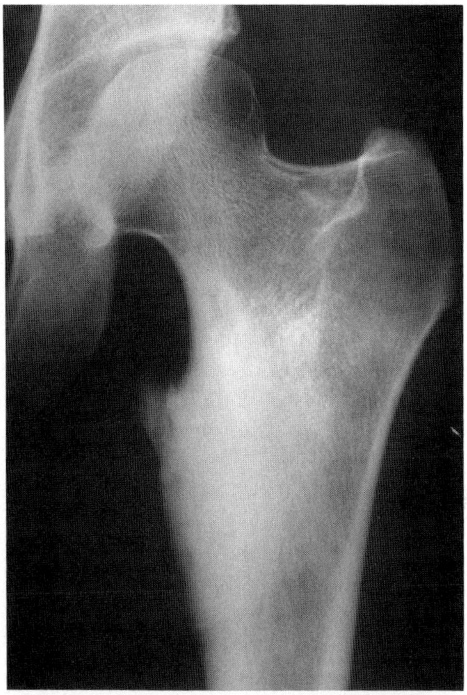

Figure 6-18. *Biopsy of this dense lesion of the proximal femur revealed reactive changes of newly formed bone, which showed a chronic inflammatory infiltrate compatible with chronic osteomyelitis.*

Periosteal proliferation and bone formation are not specific for infection. Lytic foci in the metaphysis of a child's bone usually signify infection. In an adult, other considerations are giant cell tumor, intraosseous ganglion, or subchondral cyst. Increased bone density over a widespread area may also have a variety of causes (e.g., malignant tumors, fibrous dysplasia, Paget's disease) or be related to ischemic necrosis of bone.

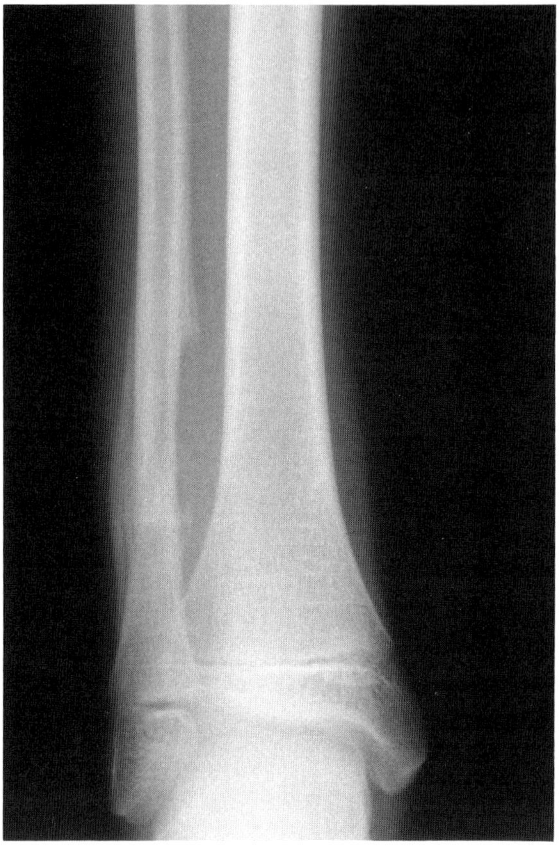

Figure 6-19. *This lesion of the distal fibular diaphysis was identified in a child with a low-grade fever, pain, and a raised erythrocyte sedimentation rate. A subacute infection was considered in the differential diagnosis, but biopsy showed Ewing's tumor. Radiological appearances in the two conditions can be identical.*

Chronic Osteomyelitis: Chronic osteomyelitis frequently produces a combination of periosteal new bone together with increased density of underlying bone, suggesting bone deposition on the endosteal (medullary) surface. The periosteal build-up of bone causes a change in the bone shape (i.e., spindle-like if the diaphysis is involved) (Figure 6-20). The periosteal bone is often dense and merged imperceptibly with the adjacent cortex; it is, however, an involucrum.

Sometimes there are destructive changes or erosions, but the combination of bone formation and destruction may obscure each other in conventional radiographs. Computerized tomography may be helpful in interpretation of such lesions (Figure 6-21).

Sequestra are the hallmark of chronic osteomyelitis—denser than the surrounding decalcified bone and surrounded by a translucent

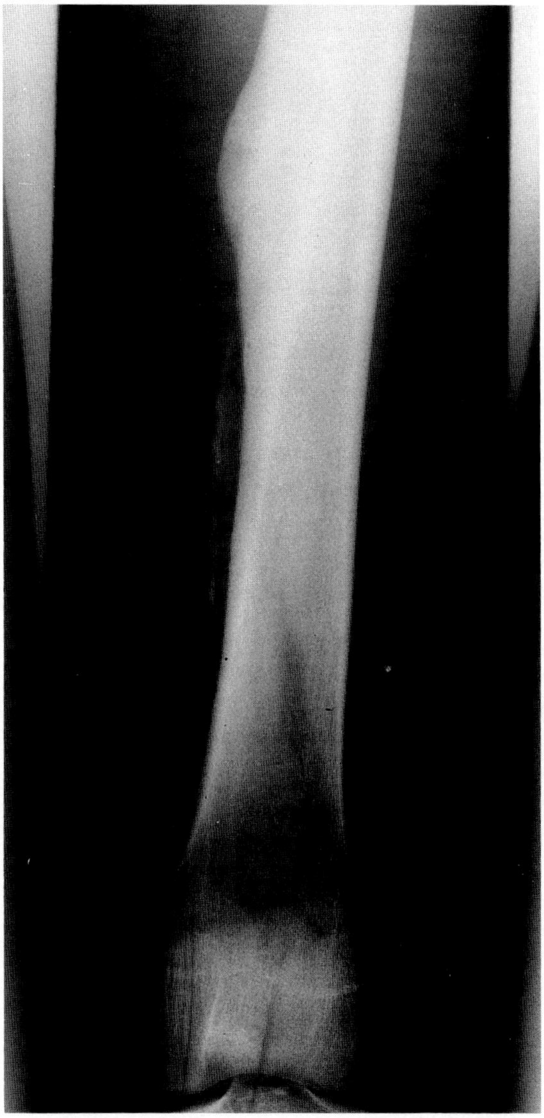

Figure 6-20. *In this case of chronic osteomyelitis of the femur, the bone has a spindle shape in its diaphysis due to production of involucral bone as a consequence of the infection. Below the spindle is a thin zone of involucrum produced by the periosteum, perhaps lifted from the diaphyseal cortex by pus or granulation tissue. Should more such bone form in the future, the length of the spindle-shaped swelling would increase as the involucrum was incorporated into the femoral diaphysis.*

zone, which in turn is demarcated by a radiodense zone. Because of the combination of shadows and the often central portion of sequestra, they may not always be apparent on routine radiographs—which show chronic osteomyelitis—but will be demonstrated by computerized tomography (Figure 6-22).

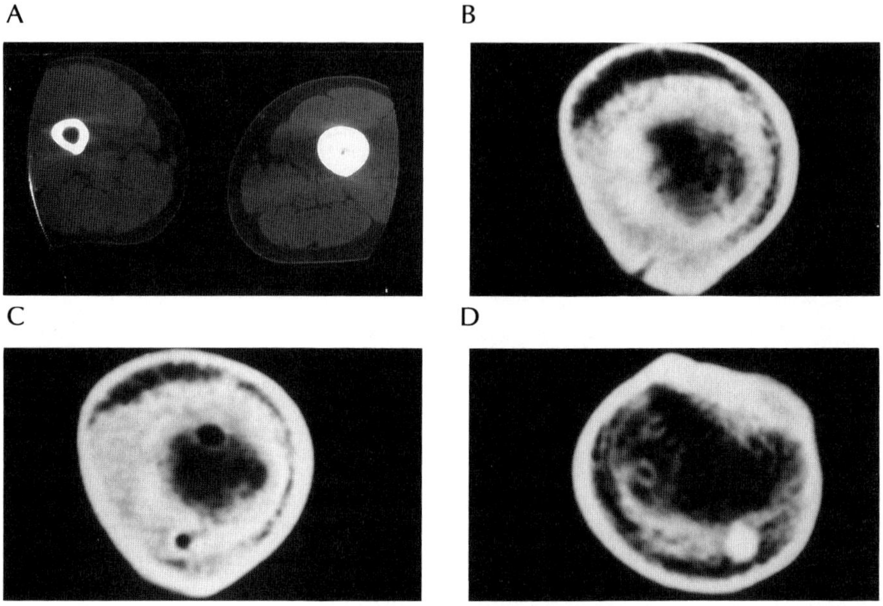

Figure 6-21. *Computerized tomography of both femurs shows the changes that occur in chronic osteomyelitis of the femur. (A) Note the amount of involucral bone that has formed both within the medullary cavity and from periosteal activity, thereby increasing the diameter and circumference of the bone. (B) The original femur can be seen inside the involucral femur; they are separated by granulation or fibrous tissue. It is possible that there are remaining but dormant septic foci in the bone (C), one adjacent to the medullary cavity and the other tunnelling within the cortex of the original femur. The infection obviously first occurred many years ago, as evidenced by the smooth remodeling of the circumference of involucral bone. (D) An island of dense bone, which would give the appearance of a sequestrum on plain radiography.*

A localized chronic bone abscess may not evoke a marked periosteal response; however, there is usually a rather inconspicuous linear shadow at the same level as the loss of the medullary trabecular pattern.

Septic Arthritis: The radiological features of septic arthritis also parallel the pathological changes that occur. Edema and hypertrophy of synovium with intra-articular fluid production can be seen as a swollen joint limited by capsular attachments and containing a homoge-

A B C

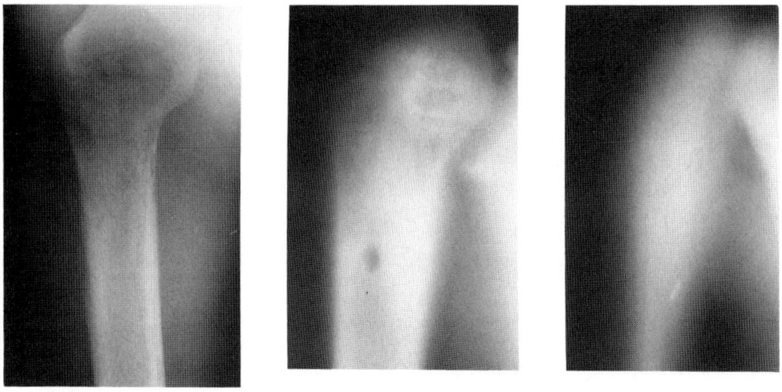

Figure 6-22. *(A) Active chronic staphylococcal osteomyelitis of the proximal humerus of a 14-year-old boy showing generalized osteopenia and a small periosteal bone-forming reaction. (B) Plain tomography reveals an unexpected cloaca. (C) Another tomographic plane reveals a small sequestrum of dense bone.*

neous soft-tissue shadow. Disuse osteopenia of bone adjacent to the infected joint appears quite quickly. Bone destruction, initially in the form of erosions next to the cartilaginous articular margin, can be detected long before similar changes in the cartilage are evident radiographically. It is only when so much articular cartilage is lost that the subchondral bone ends can approximate each other, that evidence of cartilage loss is confirmed. Once "loss of joint space" has occurred, bone erosion of subchondral distribution may be seen.

In all varieties of septic arthritis, involvement of adjacent osseous structures produces the changes characteristic of osteomyelitis. At a late stage, dystrophic calcification in a periarticular distribution may appear.

Although gas-forming organisms may cause septic arthritis and cause radiographic lucencies due to gas within the joint, a more usual cause of such a finding is a prior arthrocentesis that allowed air to enter the joint, or an open wound that has ruptured the joint capsule. Such findings after trauma demand surgical joint toilet if septic arthritis is to be prevented.

Accumulation of fluid within a joint, capsular distension, and loss of articular cartilage may allow subluxation or dislocation of an infected joint. In infants, in whom congenital hip dysplasia, neurological disorders, or trauma may also cause hip subluxation or dislocation, the radiological signs alone are not usually sufficient to diagnose presence or absence of infection.

Infants pose a problem in the radiological location of joint infection because their epiphyses are either nonossified or partially ossified. The limits of the cartilaginous articulation are not clear on radiographs. Furthermore, in childhood, epiphyseal ossification may show irregular patterns while developing normally. The later effects of joint sepsis, particularly if unrecognized initially, include destruction of epiphyses. Comparison with the opposite side, which should develop simultaneously, is often a useful ploy in radiographic assessment of abnormalities of joints in infants and children (Figure 6-23).

In adults, a significant number of septic joints occur in joints with

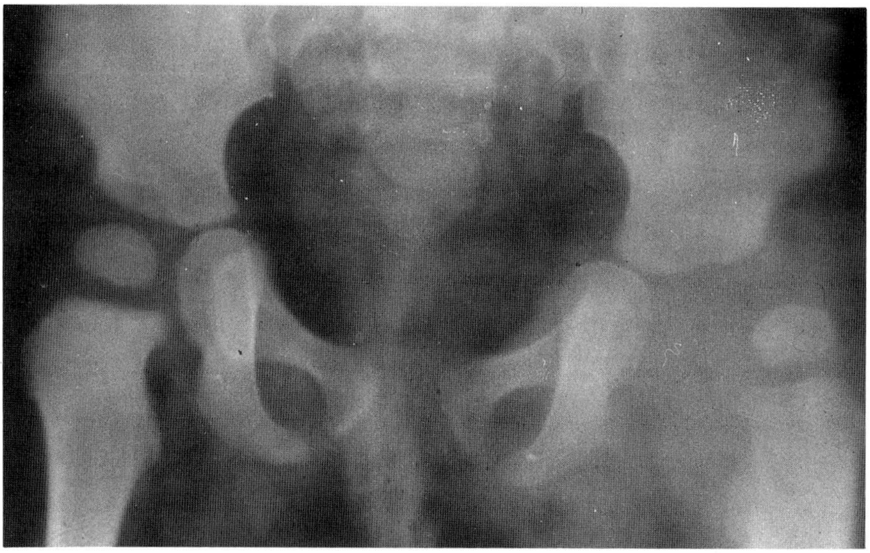

Figure 6-23. *Plain radiography of the pelvis of a neonate shows that the left femur is laterally displaced from the acetabulum when compared with the normal right side. There is also increased density of soft tissues. This finding is highly suggestive of infective arthritis of the hip. It is likely that the clinical signs would have been pseudoparalysis of the limb and swelling. However, the systemic signs of sepsis seen in older children may not be found in neonatal bone and joint sepsis.*

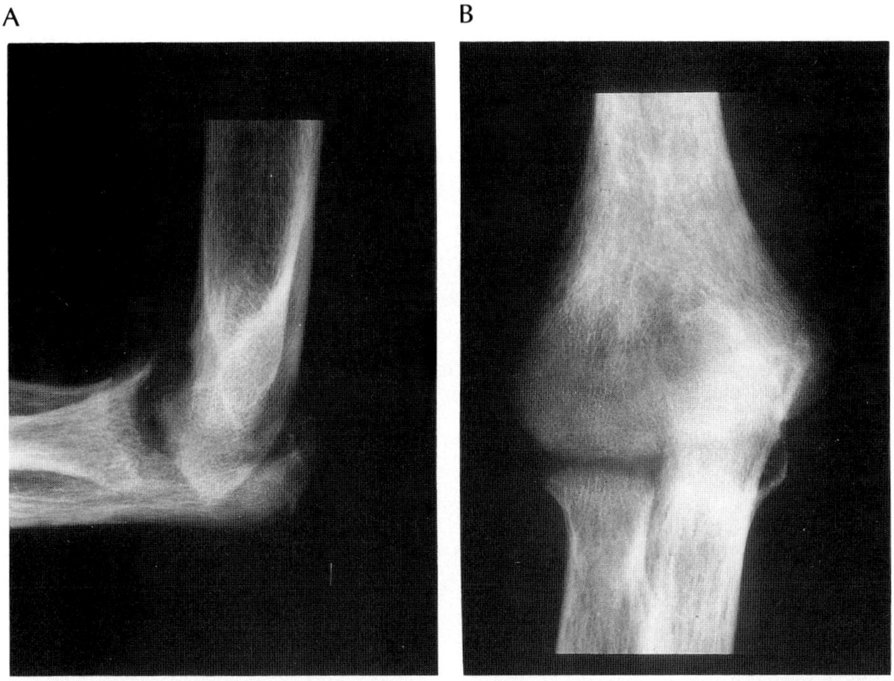

Figure 6-24. *(A) Lateral and (B) anteroposterior views of an elbow in which the articular surface and subchondral bone are missing. There is more bone loss than would be expected in acute septic arthritis in an adult, and the density of adjacent bone is not suggestive of rapid loss of bone substance. This man had rheumatoid arthritis that caused much of the loss of articular cartilage and subchondral bone, as well as a super-added subacute infection of the joint. Rheumatoid joints are prone to infection, whether arthrocentesis has been performed, and in any acute flare-up of such a joint, infection may occur.* (Radiograph provided by Dr. K.J. Sherbon.)

pre-existing pathology (Figure 6-24). Rheumatoid arthritis is a prime example of a disease with joints at risk—either by the hematogenous route or by direct implantation—because these patients frequently undergo arthrocenteses and intra-articular injection of drugs. Because of the popularity of diagnostic arthroscopy and surgical manipulations associated with it, joint sepsis, particularly of knee and shoulder, might be expected to increase. The radiological signs of the pathology for which the arthroscopy was done might be present, as well as evidence of sepsis, making radiological diagnosis of the latter more difficult.

The earliest change is often a slight opacity of the joint, compared with the opposite side, and swelling of the soft-tissue shadows about the joint. The "joint space" may be increased in width due to effusion.

If treatment is not instituted, patchy decalcification appears deep in the bone, consisting of translucent areas 3 to 5 mm in diameter and scattered at larger intervals. This decalcification may extend for several centimeters along the length of the bone. Eventually, small linear shadows of periosteal new bone may appear adjacent to the shaft of one of the long bones forming the joint, usually close to the joint but outside the capsular attachment. As recovery occurs, the osteopenia is reversed and the periosteal bone fuses with the cortex and becomes absorbed.

In tuberculous arthritis, the most characteristic changes (Figure 6-25), in addition to diminished "joint space," are periarticular low-density shadowing (due to thickened synovium and capsule) and effusion, articular cortical erosion, and a generalized but severe osteopenia of nearby bones. These generally observed changes are

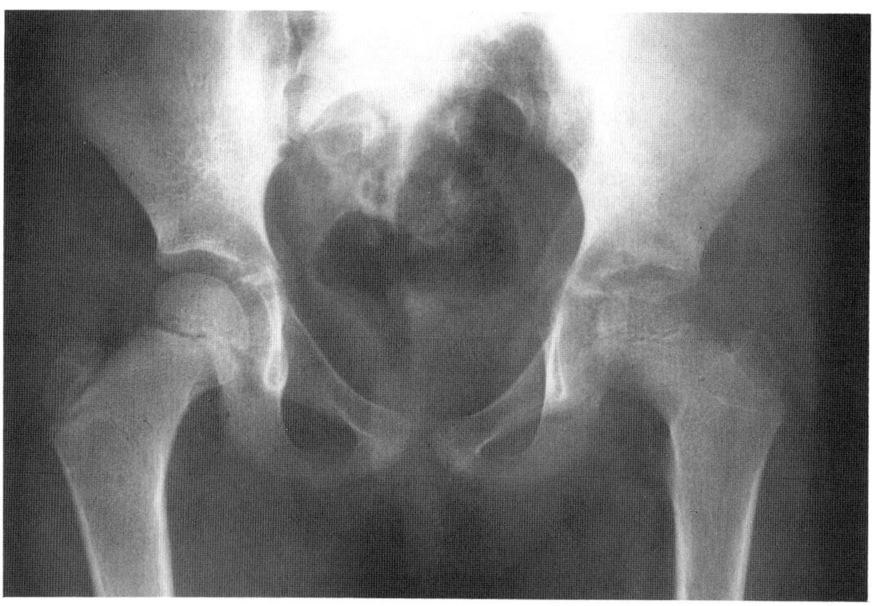

Figure 6-25. *Typical early stage tuberculosis of the left hip. The articular cartilage is narrower than normal and there is osteopenia of both proximal femur and acetabular region of the pelvis.*

modified by the age of the patient, the virulence of the infection, and the joint involved.

With soft-tissue infections, the principal role of radiography is to exclude underlying bone infection. Swelling of soft tissues is usually easily detected, and the plane of swelling—skin in cellulitis, bursae (e.g., in olecranon bursitis), or muscle (e.g., if in a limb or psoas)—can often be determined. The presence of gas in the soft tissues means that a gas-forming organism is present, there has been communication with air outside, or a fistula with the gastrointestinal tract has formed.

Magnification Radiography

Use of a magnifying glass to examine conventional radiographs or use of magnification techniques to produce an enlarged image of the site under examination on the film are sometimes useful. The earliest signs of bone destruction or formation may be more apparent with magnification than naked eye examination. Small osteolytic foci in osteomyelitis, minor disruption of subchondral bone in septic arthritis (particularly in small joints of hands, wrists, or feet), and slight periosteal reaction may be detected.

Tomography

Plain radiographs are a two-dimensional image of all tissues that impede the passage of x-ray beams from generator tube to film. Therefore, detail in the center of a medullary cavity may be obscured by overlying structures, causing difficulty in diagnosis. Although radiographs in two or more planes help to avoid such confusion and help observers build up a three-dimensional picture of what is happening, tomography is often useful in bone and joint disease.

By producing sequential tomographic cuts, a clearer location of lucency or opacity can be determined. The major role of this form of tomography in infections is detection of sequestra in chronic osteomyelitis. Their density, as well as surrounding lucent granulation tissue, allow accurate localization. The state of subchondral bone can also be detected by tomography. It is useful for assessing the extent of bone destruction in spinal osteomyelitis and hence, confirming suspicion of infection prompted by minor changes on plain radiographs.

Computerized axial tomography is a major advance in radiological detection of musculoskeletal disorders. It now enables precise location of bone destruction and production, as well as accurate portrayal of the extent of soft-tissue swelling or loss. Soft tissues can be seen as well as bone. Several parallel "cuts" allow a three-dimensional image to be built up. The extent of a pathological process is much better defined; thus, therapy can be planned with precision. Those inexperienced in its use may be surprised to learn the extent of a pathological process, formerly not visible on conventional radiographs.

Sinography

When chronic discharging sinuses are present (e.g., in chronic osteomyelitis) their path, extent, and volume may be detected by injection of radiopaque contrast agents through a small catheter into the cutaneous opening (Figure 6-26). This technique may provide a useful guide to surgical treatment. The risks of introducing infection at the time of sinography appear to be remote.

Magnetic Resonance Imaging

Magnetic resonance imaging (MRI) has several advantages over other imaging modalities. It is faster to perform, has a much better spatial

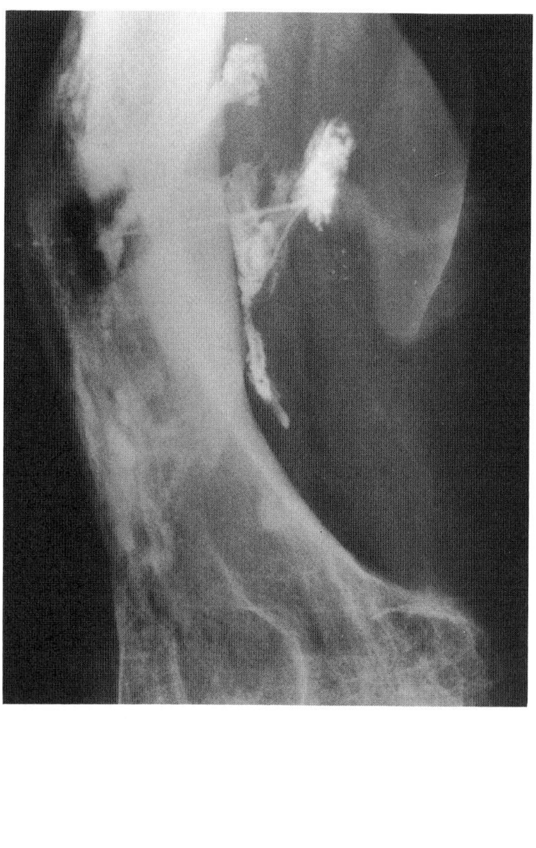

Figure 6-26. *By insertion of a catheter into a sinus and injection of radiopaque contrast medium, the extent of a cavity containing fluid in a bone with chronic osteomyelitis can be shown. This technique may be a useful guide to the planning of surgery. It frequently shows a serpiginous track with many diverticula extending a considerable distance from the opening of the sinus.*

resolution than radioisotope bone scanning, and uses no ionizing radiation, thus it is possible to use in pregnancy. However, the nature of the image produced depends on the skills of the operator. Unlike conventional radiography, there is not a sole image produced from the part of the body under study; the choice of image type may display, or disguise, the true pathology.

To determine the effectiveness of MRI in evaluating infection, the following questions must be answered: (a) Can MRI detect infection as early or earlier than isotope studies? (b) Which pulse sequences and MRI techniques are most specific? (c) Can treatment and healing be effectively monitored? (3)

MRI examination requires at least T1- (spin echo [SE] 500/20 or inversion recovery) and T2- (SE with long TE > 60 and TR > 2,000) weighted sequences to provide the necessary contrast between normal and abnormal tissues and to detect characteristic subtle abnormalities. The characteristic appearance of acute osteomyelitis (symptoms less than 2 weeks) shows abnormal focal dark signal intensity within the marrow on T1-weighted SE images (Figure 6-27) and abnormal brighter-than-fat signal intensity on T2-weighted (Figure 6-28) and short T1 inversion recovery (STIR) images. On the STIR images, signal from normal, unaffected marrow fat is suppressed, whereas pathologically involved marrow appears exceedingly bright (4). Cortical bone appears normal. Muscle and fascial planes around the affected bone demonstrate diffuse increased signal intensity on T2-weighted and STIR images, representing edema.

In chronic osteomyelitis, MRI demonstrates a well-defined rim of low signal intensity surrounding the area of focal active disease. This "rim sign," which appears if the symptoms have been present more than four weeks, is dark with use of all sequences (T1-weighted, STIR, and T2-weighted). In addition to the characteristic "rim sign," chronic osteomyelitis of long bones is further characterized by remodeling of cortical bone. Invariably, marrow changes are less extensive than cortical abnormalities, and often normal fat marrow intensity refills large segments of the remodeled medullary cavity. The area of active infection is clearly distinguished from normal regenerative marrow by signal characteristics described for acute osteomyelitis. Sinus tracks can be identified as an area of high signal intensity, with disruption of the cortex and a contiguous path to the skin. The soft-tissue changes in chronic osteomyelitis are limited to the area around the

A B

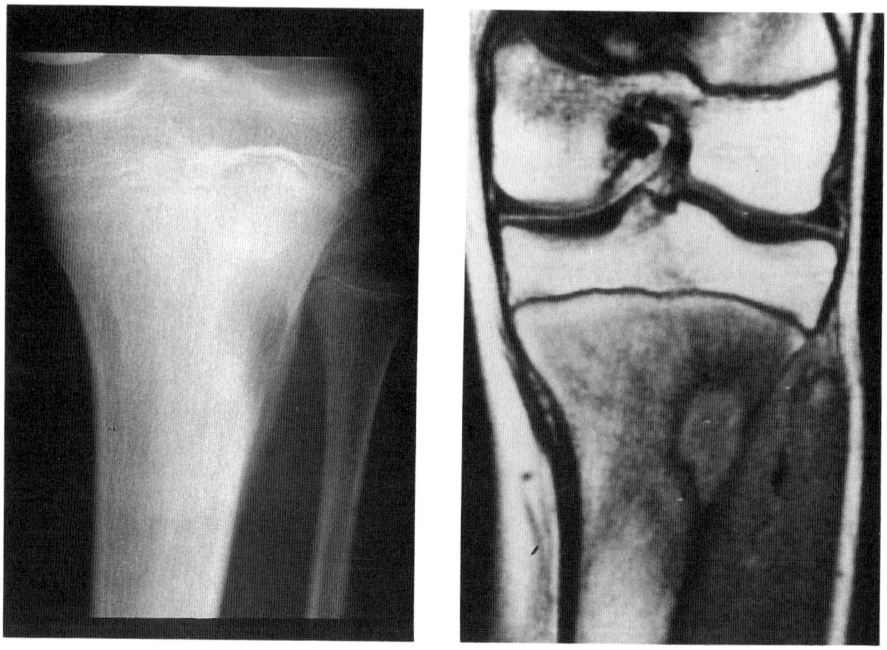

Figure 6-27. *(A) This 16-year-old boy had pain below his knee for two weeks. In the lateral side of the proximal tibial metaphysis is a radiolucent zone with surrounding periosteal reaction on plain radiography. This area was subjected to magnetic resonance imaging. (B) In the T1-weighted image, the same region shows darker than normal appearance of bone marrow surrounding a clearly circumscribed zone, which is causing some bulging of the bone cortex.* (Provided by Dr. G.K. Chapman.)

sinus track and are not as extensive or diffuse as the juxtacortical edema seen in acute hematogenous osteomyelitis (4).

The specificity of MRI in diagnosing osteomyelitis needs to be more clearly defined. The only reliable image feature noted to date has been increased signal in medullary bone with a well-defined lucent margin (Figure 6-29). Infection must be present for several weeks to allow this reactive margin to develop (3).

In diabetic feet with infected marrow, signal intensities are low on T1-weighted images and high on T2-weighted and STIR images (Figure 6-30). Subcutaneous and cutaneous edema are characteristic and more extensive than in nondiabetic infections. The "rim sign" is not a feature.

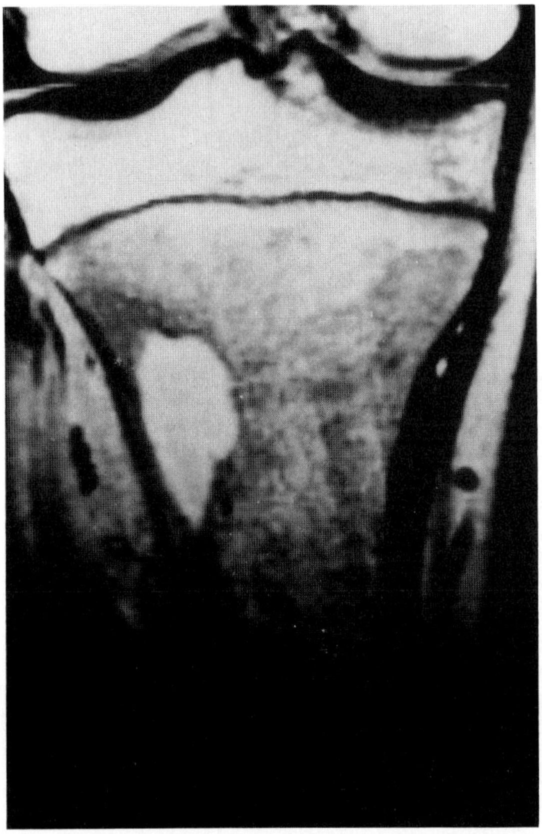

Figure 6-28. *On T2-weighted images, the same region shows brighter-than-fat signal intensity in the marrow and changes in adjacent muscle and fascia due to edema.* (Provided by Dr. G.K. Chapman.)

In septic joints, the synovial fluid shows very low (lower than muscle) signal intensity on T1-weighted images and high signal intensity on T2-weighted and STIR images. Superimposed osteomyelitis shows the changes described. Patients with septic arthritis but without osteomyelitis demonstrate abnormal signal intensity in the marrow on both sides of the joint (on both T1-weighted and STIR images), which can be misinterpreted as signs of osteomyelitis (4).

When clinical signs support osteomyelitis, there will still be some patients who do not have an infective process (e.g., fracture, gout, sickle-cell disease, lymphoma, malignant histiocytoma, metastatic disease). MRI invariably demonstrates abnormal marrow with decreased signal intensity on T1-weighted images and increased marrow intensity on STIR images. The morphological appearances (i.e., rim sign, soft-tissue edema, or cortical abnormalities) may be more reliable

A B

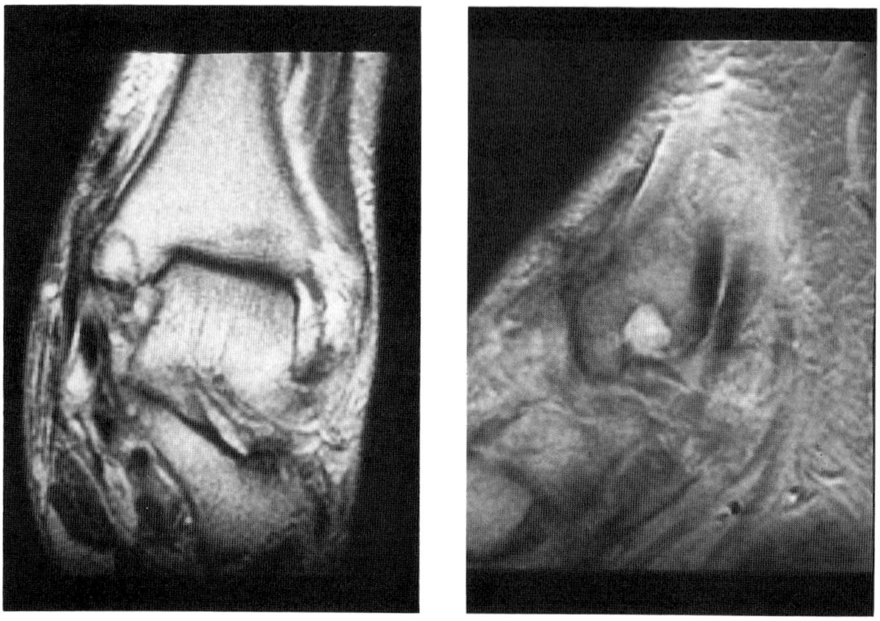

Figure 6-29. *Magnetic resonance images of osteomyelitis of the medial malleolus. T2-weighted images ([A] [spin-echo, 2,000/20 coronal] and [B] spin echo, 2,000/60 sagittal]) show a focal area of osteomyelitis with a well-defined margin. This appearance does not occur in the early stage of the infection.* (Provided by Dr. T.H. Berquist.)

than marrow signal intensity changes in differentiating these patients from those with infection. A fracture or a bone infarct may be indistinguishable from infection.

The morphological appearance of osteomyelitis on MRI varies depending on location, mechanism, and duration of infection. There is an overlap between the appearance of acute and chronic osteomyelitis. Healing osteomyelitis appears normal on MRI unless there is a complication, such as ischemic necrosis. A study of all three conditions with specific reference to soft tissues, cortex, and marrow (5) found that the best predictors of acute osteomyelitis were poorly defined soft-tissue planes, absence of cortical thickening, and poor interface between normal and infected marrow. In contrast, chronic osteomyelitis was suggested by the presence of well-defined soft-tissue abnormality, thickened cortex, and a relatively good interface be-

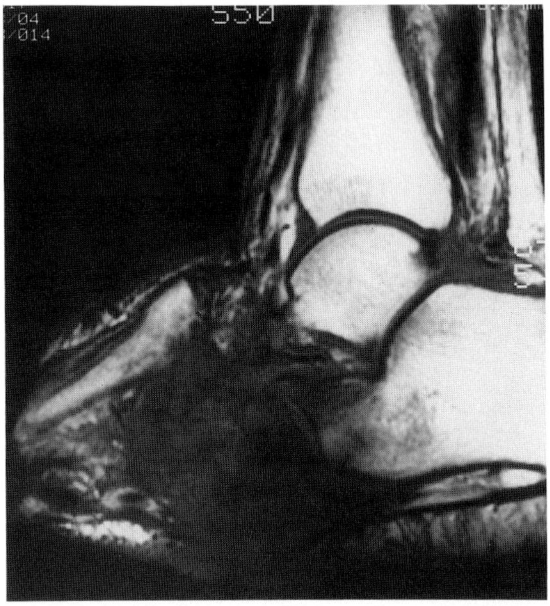

Figure 6-30. *T1-weighted image reveals forefoot amputation, normal signal in distal tibia, talus, and posterior calcaneus. The interior portion of calcaneus has edema. The remainder of the tarsal bones are destroyed and replaced by a dark, heterogeneous inflammatory mass.*

tween normal and diseased marrow. The appearance of osteomyelitis did not depend on the anatomical site of infection.

The MRI appearance of vertebral osteomyelitis is characteristic (Figure 6-31), and the technique is as least as accurate and sensitive as radionuclide scanning. The T1-weighted images show a confluent decreased signal intensity at the involved vertebral bodies and the intervening disk, whereas the T2-weighted images demonstrate increased signal intensity (Figure 6-32). In addition, the normal biconcave configuration of the disk changes and the normal internuclear cleft is lost. Abscesses cause an abnormal area of low signal intensity on a T1-weighted image and a relatively increased signal intensity on T2-weighted images because of increased fluid content. MRI can delineate paraspinal abscesses as distinct entities separate from adjacent spinal cord, psoas muscle, and other surrounding paravertebral tissues (Figure 6-33). Although soft-tissue topography is shown better by MRI than by computed tomography (CT) because of its higher contrast resolution, some disadvantages of MRI can be recognized (6). Tuberculous abscesses are often characterized by macroscopic calcifications. These "rice bodies," often seen on CT, may not be appreciated on MRI, in which they appear as small areas of

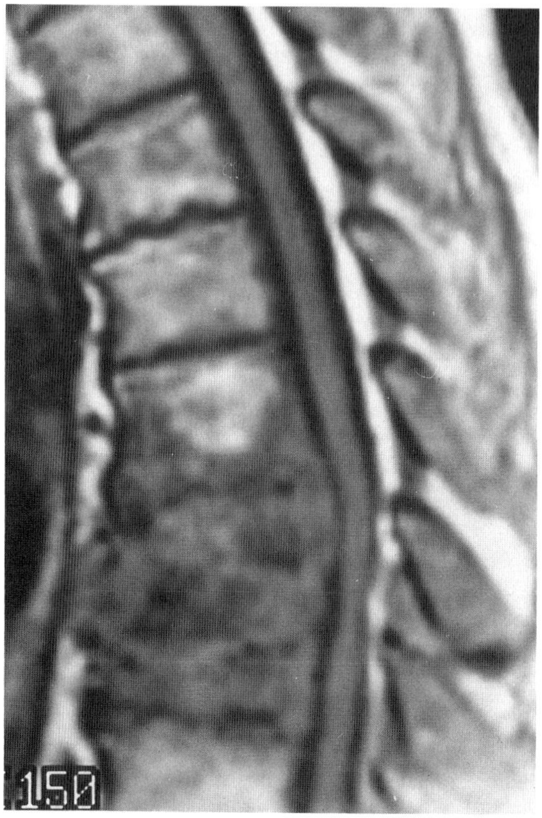

Figure 6-31. *Sagittal T1-weighted magnetic resonance image of thoracic spine. There is destruction of the adjacent end plates and loss of height of the T8 and T9 vertebral bodies. The extension of the paravertebral soft tissues anteriorly (grey) and posteriorly into extradural fat are well shown. The extradural component extends from T7 to the T9–T10 level, causing considerable compression of the thecal sac.* (Provided by Dr. K.J. Sherbon.)

signal void. Metastatic disease is distinguished from vertebral osteomyelitis by the lack of involvement of the intervertebral disk, much as on plain radiographs (7).

Septic sacroiliitis is difficult to diagnose, and traditional imaging techniques have been CT and nuclear imaging. One study of six patients to compare the diagnostic effectiveness of MRI against other methods (8) showed that abnormalities could be detected in all six on MRI, making it more useful than CT or nuclear scanning when this condition was suspected. Accurate prediction of eradication of infection cannot yet be made from MRI data (8).

Radioisotope Imaging

There are many reports of the use of radioisotope imaging techniques in musculoskeletal infections. For review of the subject, readers are

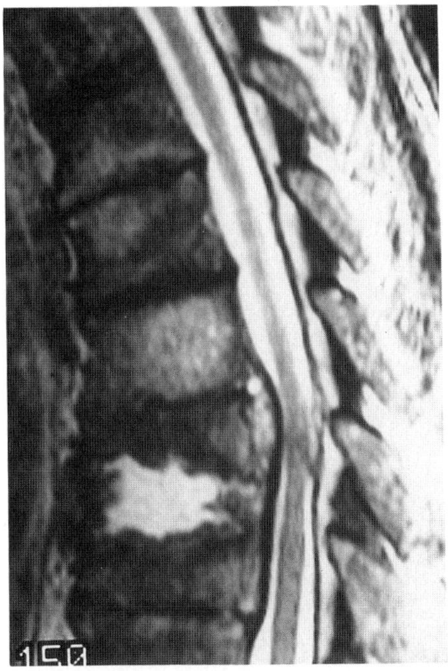

Figure 6-32. *Sagittal T2-weighted magnetic resonance image of thoracic spine of same person in Figure 6-31. There is an abnormal area of fluid signal (white) in the T8–T9 intervertebral disk and the T9 vertebral body. Also, the T7 vertebral body has a speckled grey appearance, indicating a greater than normal fluid content. The anterior paravertebral extension is not seen as well as on the T1-weighted image, but the intraspinal extradural edematous bulge is well seen compressing the spinal cord.* (Provided by Dr. K.J. Sherbon.)

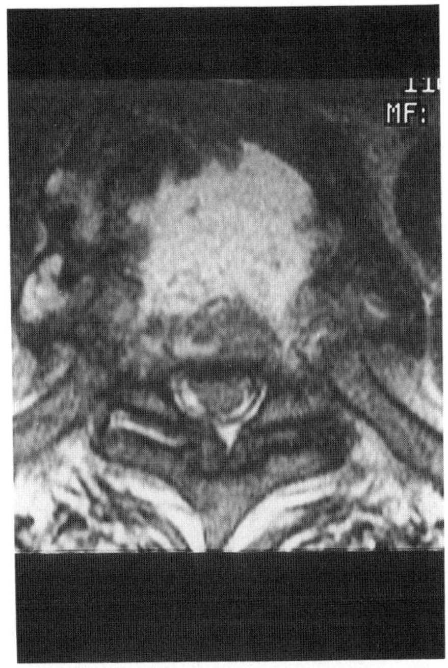

Figure 6-33. *Axial T1-weighted magnetic resonance image through T9 of the patient depicted in Figures 6-31 and 6-32. There is increased fluid (pale) within the vertebral body, which has an irregular contour. The thecal sac is distorted, losing its normal circular shape. This 87-year-old man had a history of back pain of fairly sudden onset three months earlier. The images clearly show destruction of bone and intervertebral disks, with paravertebral edema and spinal cord compression characteristic of vertebral osteomyelitis.* (Provided by Dr. K.J. Sherbon.)

referred to articles by Kirshner and Simon (9) and Merkel and colleagues (10).

Radioisotopes can either be injected as part of a simple molecule or be attached to nonradioactive molecules and act as markers of where the molecules are distributed in the body. They provide knowledge not only of the anatomical sites at which the isotopes aggregate, but also of the physiological processes occurring at such sites. Although the precise mechanisms of distribution are not always known, clinical experience with the use of such radiopharmaceuticals has proved very valuable in the management of patients with musculoskeletal infection.

The radiation sources most useful in this regard are technetium-99m (^{99m}Tc), gallium-67 (^{67}Ga), and indium-111 (^{111}In).

Mechanisms of Isotope Distribution

^{99m}Tc-Phosphate Compounds: ^{99m}Tc is a radionuclide that has no specificity for bone. To acquire organ specificity, it must be linked to a carrier molecule whose biodistribution localizes it in a given organ. For the skeleton, ^{99m}Tc is usually linked to a phosphorous compound.

The commonly used radiopharmaceutical is ^{99m}Tc-methylene disphosphonate (MDP). Most of the ^{99m}Tc-MDP is cleared from the vascular compartment within 15 minutes. ^{99m}Tc-MDP scans are usually made in three phases. Scanning (i.e., detection of emission sites of gamma rays) done during this "early" period can show sites where the blood flow pattern is increased. Immediately after injection of the radiopharmaceutical, the isotope gives an anatomical picture of vessels that is not as clear as an opaque contrast angiogram. Within a few minutes, a second scan reflects the relative vascularity of the area, the radiopharmaceutical having diffused out of capillaries. This is a nonspecific representation of accumulation of the technetium phosphate in the extravascular compartment during equilibration in areas where "vascularity" is increased.

After an initial equilibration phase, the ^{99m}Tc-MDP is taken up by bone-forming activity in the skeleton. Approximately 4 hours after intravenous injection, approximately 30% to 40% of the radiopharmaceutical has been excreted in the urine and 55% to 60% is retained in the skeleton. Scanning at this time reflects increased osteoblast activity more than alterations in blood flow.

The combination of scanning in both the early and delayed periods after injection allows anatomical and physiological interpretations that are often useful in determining underlying pathology.

A common diagnostic problem referred to Departments of Nuclear Medicine is the child with an "irritable hip." Many of these conditions, such as Legg-Calvé-Perthes' disease, osteomyelitis, slipped capital femoral epiphysis, and hemarthrosis, have a specific and recognizable pattern on bone scan. A significant number of patients have a photopenic or "cold" area involving the femoral head and proximal growth plate, as well as part of the neck of the femur in the blood pool phase, with mildly decreased uptake in these structures in the delayed scans. In a review (11) of 55 patients with a "cold hip" (Figure 6-34) on bone scan over a seven-year period, 12 of 15 patients treated surgically (22% of the total) had pus in the hip joint. The conclusion was that a ^{99m}Tc-MDP "cold hip" is an indication for surgical arthrolavage.

Despite its usefulness, radionuclide imaging has four important limitations (12). First, in some patients, multiple "hot spots" are detected at an "early" stage of *S. aureus* septicemia but do not progress to osteomyelitis; they are probably areas of aborted infection. Nevertheless, scans limited to clinically suspect areas should never be done, because whole-body imaging may detect sites that are clinically nonsuspicious. Second, there are numerous studies, experimental and clinical, in which osteomyelitis has been confirmed bacteriologically and histologically, even though scans were initially negative or normal (false-negative results) (13). Third, radionuclide imaging sometimes does not allow differentiation of cellulitis from osteomyelitis, especially if the early "blood pool" imaging is not done at the same time as the "uptake" image. Finally, bone scanning does not differentiate the bone repair of infection from the bone repair of fracture or neoplasm, and ^{99m}Tc-MDP scans are not useful indicators of healing or "progress."

Gallium Compounds: Although ^{67}Ga has been used for a number of years to localize inflammatory lesions, its mechanism of accumulation at such sites is unclear. It is available as a sodium citrate complex. There is some support for three mechanisms—(a) direct uptake by leukocytes, (b) uptake by bacteria, and (c) protein bonding to tissues. Interpretation of discrete sites of ^{67}Ga distribution is that an inflam-

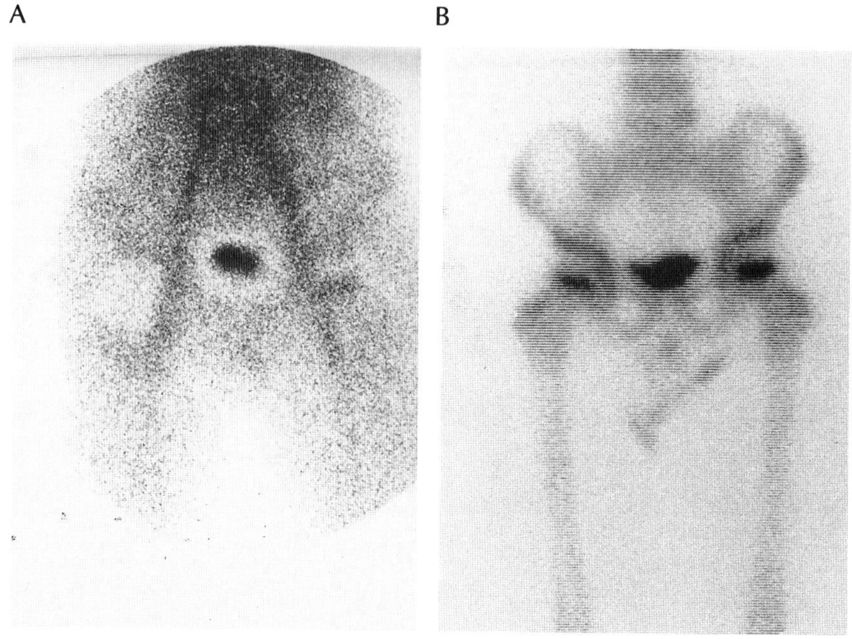

Figure 6-34. *Radioisotope scans using ^{99m}Tc-MDP in a child with discomfort about the right hip. The blood pool phase (A) was obtained after the dynamic phase done at the time of injection of the radiopharmaceutical, with the patient supine and the legs held together. All of the structures within the right hip joint show decreased uptake, most notably the proximal growth plate of the femur. The 2-hour delayed anterior image (B) also demonstrates a right "cold hip" sign. There was some uptake of radiopharmaceutical since it was injected because the patient was lying in a comfortable position with the hip flexed, perhaps decreasing intra-articular pressure and allowing some blood flow into the hip. However, it is clear that less isotope has been taken up by the right femoral head. The "cold hip" sign should be regarded as an indicator of infective arthritis.* (Provided by Dr. R. Uren.)

matory process is occurring; however, it is not specific for bone infection. Gallium is also taken up at sites of new bone formation, tumors, and noninfectious processes, and hence leads to false-positive results. Its level of specificity is not high. False-negative results also occur. ^{67}Ga citrate imaging for the diagnosis of acute septic arthritis is not generally considered useful.

Indium Compounds: Techniques have been developed for labeling leukocytes with ^{111}In. Isolation of patients' leukocytes, labelling, and re-injection allows for scanning to be repeated, because of the 67 hour half-life of ^{111}In. Leukocytes accumulate at sites of abscesses by chemotaxis, and their detection by repeated scanning for ^{111}In distribution may well prove to be a useful technique. Nearly 100 mL of venous blood is required, and it takes about 3 hours to isolate and label the leukocytes. Scanning is usually done 18 to 24 hours after the cells are reinjected. Sites with focal accumulation higher than surrounding bone are interpreted as infected sites. However, for unexplained reasons, this technique is less sensitive in detection of spinal infection than other sites (14).

Immunoglobulins: Recent preparations of IgG immunoglobulin have been labelled with ^{99m}Tc and ^{111}In, and their use has been advocated for the detection of foci where a specific humoral response is occurring to an infective inflammation (15–18). The role of such radionuclides has not yet been fully evaluated for the diagnosis of musculoskeletal infection.

Clinical Applications

The usefulness of radioisotope imaging in bone and joint diseases is determined by the physician's knowledge of how the radiopharmaceutical is localized to skeletal tissues and how the technique will answer questions of physiology and pathology.

For example, in classic acute osteomyelitis, ^{99m}Tc-phosphate compounds have been found to be highly sensitive for early detection before radiographic changes in bone are apparent, but the diagnosis can be made without a bone scan. In vague bone pain, particularly in the axial skeleton, in an aged person with some degenerative changes, scanning techniques may be very useful in deciding whether the pain is due to infection, arthritis, or neoplasia (Figure 6-35).

In most patients with osteomyelitis, bone scintigrams become positive within 48 to 72 hours of the onset of clinical symptoms, thereby preceding radiological changes (9).

Cellulitis is often a differential diagnostic problem. Three-phase scintigraphy is effective in separating these two conditions, because cellulitis does not cause an increased uptake in bone but does show

A B

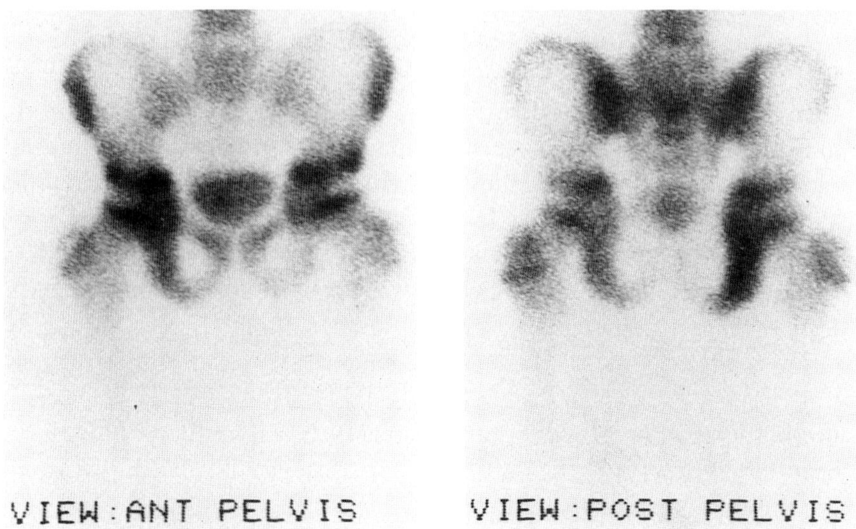

Figure 6-35. *(A) Radioisotope scanning with ^{99m}Tc-MDP showed that there was asymmetrical uptake of the radiopharmaceutical, with relative increase in the right ischium. (B) A posterior scan (with the detector gamma camera nearer the ischium) shows more clearly the anatomical site of new bone formation, making the diagnosis of osteomyelitis likely but not proving it. A site such as the ischium is not easily accessible to clinical examination, and infection there may be concealed. In such a clinical situation, the radionuclide scan can be very useful in revealing the site of pathology.*

increased uptake in the first phase (19). Bone infarction can also be distinguished.

In neonates, the three-phase bone scan is not nearly so useful. It is possible to perform sequential ^{99m}Tc and ^{67}Ga scans to try and increase specificity for musculoskeletal infection. The technetium scan is done four hours after isotope injection, and the gallium scan is done 48 to 72 hours after isotope injection. Interpretation of such scans requires experience and is based on the spatial location and relative intensity of isotope (20, 21). They are also of little use in detection or confirmation of post-traumatic and postsurgical osteomyelitis because they accumulate wherever bone is being produced regardless of stimulus. Although ^{67}Ga- or ^{111}In-labeled leukocytes might be potentially useful in accurately determining infection, their sensitivity is not 100%. Experience is accumulating and other radiopharmaceuticals will doubtless be developed to aid in these difficult clinical problems.

The problems of pain following prosthetic joint replacement and differentiation of loosening without infection from sepsis are increasingly difficult. Use of ^{111}In-labeled leukocytes appears to have increased the sensitivity of detection of sepsis in this situation to that formerly achieved with technetium and gallium scanning. In one study (22), the findings at operation done because of a painful total hip prosthesis were compared with the scintigraphic appearances using all three of the isotopes (^{99m}Tc, ^{67}Ga, ^{111}In) in normal radiopharmaceutical tests. ^{111}In-labeled white cells had a predictive value of more than 90% for infection as a cause of such hip pain.

Although abnormal radionuclide scans with each of the agents mentioned may be found in septic arthritis, there is really no place for such investigations if that diagnosis is suspected.

Ultrasound

The use of high frequency sound waves and the recording of their reflection from interfaces of two dissimilar tissues in the body has become a useful diagnostic tool in medicine. Unfortunately, the characteristic bone conduction of ultrasound prevents its use for detection of cavities within bone. In assessment of soft-tissue swellings, however, fluid-filled cysts or abscesses may be detected and their size measured accurately by this method, which is free from the hazards of ionizing radiation.

Use of ultrasound imaging has been advocated (23) for the diagnosis of lesions of bone and as an adjunct to conventional radiology. It can be used to diagnose fractures in infancy, separation of epiphyses, osteomyelitis, to measure distraction in leg lengthening, and to assess fracture healing. In infants, hip ultrasound has been used to visualize the cartilaginous structures that cannot be demonstrated directly by a radiograph. It is less well recognized that ultrasound can now provide a range of information in a broad age range and is not limited by the presence of fully ossified bone. This technique requires a different approach to that used in the infant hip but is simple and rapid to perform. High resolution linear array ultrasound equipment is required, using frequencies of 5 MHz or greater. Small effusions in joints can be detected. Ultrasound examination can be usefully employed to differentiate between transient synovitis, hemarthrosis, pyarthrosis, osteomyelitis, and the synovitis associated with other forms of acute or chronic arthritis. Much of the information provided is in addition to that obtained from standard radiographs or bone scans. It has a particularly useful role in the assessment of children with painful hips (24). A concise but useful review of the place of ultrasound in clinical orthopedics (25) states that it is the practice of the authors to ask referring clinicians to give them "carte blanche" to solve a clinical problem with the most appropriate imaging methods at their disposal. They used ultrasound as the first adjunct to the clinical examination and found that it was often not necessary to proceed to more expensive techniques.

Ultrasound is now becoming a very useful tool in the detection of osteomyelitis, or in its exclusion by absence of well-defined anechoic or partially echogenic fluid collections adjacent to bone. Although there is not yet a lot written about the value of ultrasound in osteomyelitis, it is a technique that is likely to add a great deal to both diagnostic and therapeutic accuracy in osteomyelitis. In a study of 48 patients referred for diagnosis of possible osteomyelitis (26) (with a disease prevalence of 25%), sensitivity was 83%, specificity was 100%, positive predictive value was 100%, and negative predictive value was 95%.

Sonographic criteria for the diagnosis of osteomyelitis are: (a) an abnormal collection of fluid producing an anechoic (echoless) zone adjacent to bone without intervening soft tissues and elevation of the periosteum by 2 mm (27,28); (b) thickening of the periosteum with hypoechoic zones, both superficial and deep, giving the appearance of a "sandwich"; and, (c) swelling of overlying muscle or subcutaneous tissue maximum nearest the bone. These changes occur early and can generally be seen within 24 hours of onset of symptoms. The changes are specific enough to allow osteomyelitis to be differentiated from clinically similar conditions. The ultrasound examination is not complete until the whole circumference of the bone has been examined. The site of "point tenderness" often corresponds to the site of periosteal elevation.

With respect to the hip, a joint effusion is demonstrated by progressive widening of the space between the anterior surface of the femoral neck and the joint capsule (29) (Figure 6-36). Thickening of the synovium can also be assessed. Increasing size of the effusion is recognized by progressive distension and increasing convexity of the joint

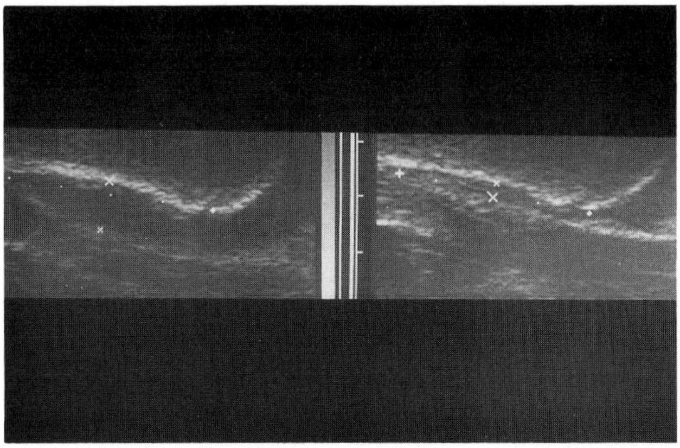

Figure 6-36. *Ultrasound imaging of both hip regions in longitudinal section. The image on the left shows a normal appearance. The femoral head and physis (+) can be seen as well as the neck of the femur (between + and +). The two* x *and* X *marks indicate the distance between the femoral neck and the hip joint capsule (≤2 mm). The image on the right shows the other hip in the same child. Note the markedly increased distance between* x *and* X*, which represents an effusion in the hip joint. Change in size of the effusion can be measured if necessary by serial ultrasound examination.* (Provided by Dr. V. Antico.)

capsule. Ultrasound has been shown to have a sensitivity for detection of hip joint effusions of between 95% and 100%, compared with a radiographic sensitivity of less than 50% (30). The important differentiation of fluid in the hip joint due to infection or a nonseptic condition cannot be made reliably by ultrasound (31), nor can septic arthritis and osteomyelitis always be distinguished by ultrasonography alone (32). Ultrasound is very useful in diagnosis of soft-tissue infection (25). Once identified, abscesses can be drained under local anesthesia and acute septic arthritis can be differentiated from acute synovitis. Soft-tissue abscesses and pyomyositis can usually be diagnosed by ultrasonography and confirmed by needle aspiration guided by ultrasound scanning during the procedure (28).

Although the radioisotope bone scan remains the most sensitive indicator of acute osteomyelitis (with the possible exception of the neonatal period), careful ultrasound examination may demonstrate an unsuspected focus of infection. Deep soft-tissue abscesses may be found adjacent to bone (Figure 6-37), together with periosteal thicken-

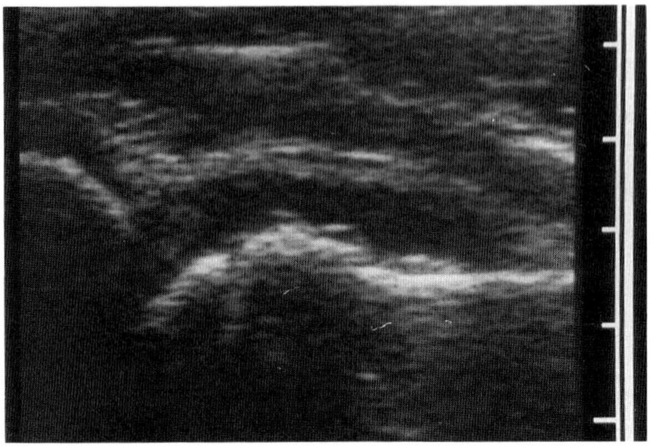

Figure 6-37. *Ultrasound image of a hip region (compare with Figure 6-36). The anterior capsule of the joint shows a double image. That adjacent to the bone is probably fluid, whereas the more anterior band is probably thickened synovium. Because ultrasound imaging delineates interface differences in propagation of sound waves, some care must be taken in interpretation of the images produced on the screen.* (Provided by Dr. V. Antico.)

ing and elevation from the bone (27). In established infections, irregularity and erosion of cortical bone can be demonstrated. With more extensive bone destruction, the cortex will be attenuated or breached, and transmission of sound into the medullary space will lead to reflections from the marrow fat. Ultrasound is particularly useful for detecting and demonstrating subperiosteal collections of pus (Figure 6-38). Such precise localization and information on the extent of the abscess can be of significant help in surgical drainage. A study from Tunisia (33), where osteomyelitis is common, demonstrated that subperiosteal abscesses could be detected by ultrasound in 45 of 50 patients with acute osteomyelitis; pus was confirmed surgically in each. By active drainage of all such abscesses, they found that the rate of progression to chronic osteomyelitis diminished markedly compared with the time when clinical detection of an abscess was the criterion for surgery.

Ultrasound may assist in the diagnosis of children presenting with pain in the hip region referred from another site. Pelvic osteomyelitis may be indicated by deep soft-tissue swelling or abscess formation close to the pelvic wall. Extension of the ultrasound examination to include these areas should be a routine part of the study when no evidence of pathology is found in the hip joint.

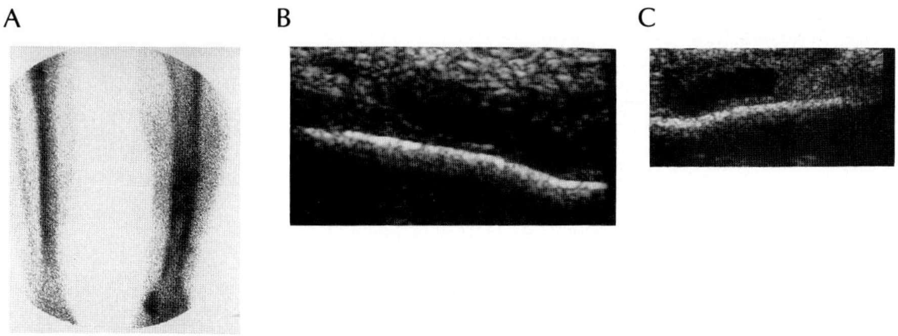

Figure 6-38. *(A) Radionuclide scan with ^{99m}Tc-MDP showing increased uptake of radiopharmaceutical in the diaphysis of the left femur. (B) Ultrasound imaging of this area shows an anechoic area adjacent to the bone without any interposed tissue. Such a collection of fluid is characteristic of pus in osteomyelitis. (C) Another image in the same patient shows that the anechoic region communicates with a serpiginous track through overlying tissue (muscle) and represents a sinus.* (Provided by Dr. V. Antico.)

We believe that ultrasound is an extremely useful aid to enhance clinical evaluation in: (a) all patients who are clinically suspected of having osteomyelitis; (b) predicting osteomyelitis if fluid is demonstrated in contact with bone; (c) differentiating osteomyelitis from soft-tissue abscesses; (d) localization of lesions before aspiration or surgical management; and (e) detecting recurrence of osteomyelitis in patients with chronic osteomyelitis by reaccumulation of fluid and development of sinuses.

For example, there was a delay in diagnosis of osteomyelitis of the ischium in a 15-year-old boy (Figure 6-39). He had pain in the buttock for several weeks, and initial radiographs were normal. Had ultrasound been performed, it is likely that the purulent collection that was subsequently drained would have been detected before the bone changes were evident.

Aspiration and Biopsy

Modern techniques of radiology with biplanar screening and image intensification to reduce radiation exposure have allowed access to the whole body by an exploring needle. Frequently, however, in musculoskeletal sepsis, no such sophisticated equipment is required. Most

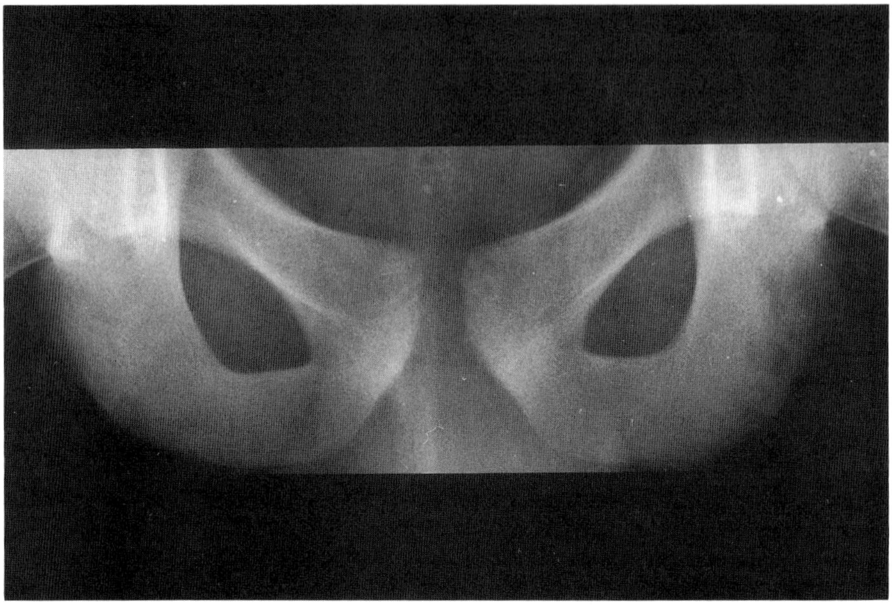

Figure 6-39. *Radiograph of the pelvis of a 15-year-old boy who had buttock pain for several weeks. Radiographs taken two weeks before this one were normal. Note the bone loss in the left ischium. A radioisotope bone scan also showed increased uptake in this area. Ultrasound examination was not performed but should have been because it would have shown the purulent abscess, which was subsequently drained.* (Provided by Dr. G.K. Chapman.)

joints can be entered using standard anatomical landmarks, and tender areas in bone present no problem. Accurate needle positioning in deeper tissues is aided by radiological techniques. The entry of a needle into a suspected site of sepsis allows aspiration of fluid, lavage and aspiration, or biopsy of tissue, depending on the type of needle or trephine used. When radiological control of needle or trephine placement is required, hard copy film should be made to confirm the site of sampling.

Direct aspiration with a syringe is done initially. If fluid is obtained, it should be observed, some smeared on sterile slides for Gram staining and cytology, and some placed in sterile containers and into special culture medium if indicated. If no fluid is obtained, or only small amount, then lavage with a small volume of isotonic sodium chloride (containing no preservatives) may allow a useful sample to be collected on reaspiration.

Biopsy specimens of bone, obtained with a trephine, should be divided, with some sent for histopathological examination, and some for direct culture for bacteria or other organisms.

Monitoring Progress

Radiology

Radiology has much less of a role in monitoring the progress of infection than in confirming the clinical diagnosis and accurately locating its site. The reason for this role is that the extent of the infective process is often much greater than apparent on initial radiographs; second, clinical improvement may be apparent and the disease process may be under control and evolving toward healing, whereas the amount of bone destruction on radiographs and the periosteal response are increasing.

When there has been significant bone loss as a result of infection or its treatment, radiographs are useful to indicate the rate and amount of bone replacement occurring. Especially in the tibia and the femur, the amount of bone seen on radiographs may guide clinicians to the time when they can dispense with external protection for the bone.

Radioisotope Imaging

Because a portion of the administered radioactivity persists for some time within the body, a radionuclide study cannot be repeated at will, or be followed immediately by another imaging study. A second study should be delayed until most of the isotope from a previous study has been excreted or decayed. For ^{99m}Tc complexes, this means approximately two days; for ^{67}Ga, approximately 10 days.

^{67}Ga images can be produced in the presence of ^{99m}Tc activity (because of the higher energy of gallium emissions); if both studies are done at the same time, the ^{99m}Tc imaging should be done before the ^{67}Ga is injected. The screening for ^{67}Ga is done 2 or 3 days later.

Although potentially a useful tool in following the progress of bone infection, there has been little written about the sequential changes of radionuclide scanning that occur during healing of treated musculoskeletal infections. An experimental examination (34) of the problem produced inconclusive results. In the doubtful case of radionuclide scanning suggestive of osteomyelitis, MRI might aid in diagnosis because it shows changes within the bone marrow indicating osteomyelitis. If the bone marrow is normal and there is coexisting soft-tissue abnormality, then osteomyelitis can be excluded (35).

References

1. Resnick D, Niwayama G. Diagnosis of bone and joint disorders. Philadelphia: WB Saunders, 1981.
2. Brodie BC. An account of some cases of chronic abscess of the tibia. Trans Med Chir Soc 1832;17:238–249.
3. Berquist TH. Musculo-skeletal infection. In: Berquist TH, ed. MRI of the musculoskeletal system, ed. 2. New York: Raven, 1990:475–490.
4. Erdman WA, Tamburro F, Jayson HT, Weatherall PT, Ferry KB, Peshock RM. Osteomyelitis: characteristics and pitfalls of diagnosing with MR imaging. Radiology 1991;180:533–539.
5. Cohen MD, Cory DA, Kleiman M, Smith JA, Broderick NJ. Magnetic resonance differentiation of acute and chronic osteomyelitis in children. Clin Radiol 1990;41:53–56.
6. Bell GR, Stearns KL, Bonutti PM, Boumphrey FR. MRI diagnosis of tuberculous vertebral osteomyelitis. Spine 1990;15:462–465.
7. Modic MT, Feiglin DH, Piraino DW, et al. Vertebral osteomyelitis: assessment using MR. Radiology 1985;157:157–166.
8. Klein MA, Winalski CS, Wax MR, Piwnica-Worms DR. MR imaging of septic sacro-iliitis. J Comput Assist Tomogr 1991;15:126–132.
9. Kirschner PT, Simon MA. Radioisotope evaluation of skeletal disease. J Bone Joint Surg [Am] 1981;63:673–681.
10. Merkel KD, Fitzgerald RH, Brown ML. Scintographic evaluation in musculo-skeletal sepsis. Orthop Clin North Am 1984;15:410–416.
11. Uren RF, Howman-Giles R. The "cold hip" sign on bone scan: a retrospective review. Clin Nucl Med 1991;16:53–56.
12. McCoy JR, Morrissey RT, Seibert J. Clinical experience with the Technetium-99 scan in children. Clin Orthop 1981;154:175–180.
13. Berkowitz ID, Wenzel W. "Normal" technetium bone scans in patients with acute osteomyelitis. Am J Dis Child 1980;134:828–830.
14. Schauwecker DS, Park HM, Mock BH, et al. Evaluation of complicating osteomyelitis with Tc-99m-MDP, In-111 granulocytes and Ga-67 citrate. J Nucl Med 1984;25:849–853.
15. Fischman AJ, Rubin RH, Khaw B-A, et al. Detection of acute inflammation

with ^{111}In-labeled nonspecific polyclonal IgG. Sem Nucl Med 1988;18:335–344.
16. Rubin RH, Fischman AJ, Nedelman M, et al. Radiolabeled nonspecific polyclonal human immunoglobulin in the detection of focal inflammation by scintigraphy: comparison with ^{67}Gallium citrate and ^{99m}Technetium labeled albumin. J Nucl Med 1989;30:385–389.
17. Rubin RH, Fischman AJ, Callahan RJ, et al. ^{111}In labeled non-specific immunoglobulin scanning in the detection of focal inflammation. N Engl J Med 1989;321:935–940.
18. Oyen WJC, Claessens RAMJ, van Horn JR, van der Meer JWM, Corstens FHM. Scintigraphic detection of bone and joint infections with ^{111}Indium labeled nonspecific human immunoglobulin. J Nucl Med 1990;31:403–412.
19. Sullivan DC, Rosenfield NS, Ogden J, Gottschalk A. Problems in the scintigraphic detection of osteomyelitis in children. Radiology 1980;135:731–736.
20. Lisbona R, Rosenthall L. Observations on the sequential use of ^{99m}Tc-phosphate complex and ^{67}Ga imaging in osteomyelitis, cellulitis and septic arthritis. Radiology 1977;123:123–129.
21. Tumeh SS, Aliabadi P, Weissman BN, McNeil BJ. Chronic osteomyelitis: bone and gallium scan patterns associated with active disease. Radiology 1986;158:685–688.
22. Gomez-Luzuriaga MA, Galan V, Villar JM. Scintigraphy with Tc, Ga and In in painful total hip prostheses. Inter Orth 1988;12:163–167.
23. Steiner GM, Sprigg A. The value of ultrasound in the assessment of bone. Br J Radiol 1992;65:589–593.
24. Dorr U, Zieger M, Hauke H. Ultrasonography of the painful hip. Prospective studies in 204 patients. Pediatr Radiol 1988;19:36–40.
25. O'Keeffe D, Mamtora H. Ultrasound in clinical orthopaedics. J Bone Joint Surg 1992;74:488–494.
26. Abiri MM, Kirpekar M, Ablow RC. Osteomyelitis: detection with US. Radiology 1989;172:509–511.
27. Howard CB, Einhorn M, Dagan R, Nyska M. Ultrasound in diagnosis and management of acute haematogenous osteomyelitis in children. J Bone Joint Surg [Br] 1993;75:79–82.
28. Nath AK, Sethu AU. Use of ultrasound in osteomyelitis. Br J Radiol 1992;65:649–652.
29. Zieger M, Dorr U, Schultz R. Ultrasonography of hip joint effusions. Skeletal Radiol 1987;16:607–611.
30. Marchal G, Van Holsbeeck M, Raes M, et al. Transient synovitis of the hip in children: role of ultrasound. Radiology 1987;162:825–828.
31. Wingstrand H, Egund N, Lidgren L, Sahlstrand T. Sonography in septic arthritis of the hip in the child: report of four cases. J Pediatr Orthop 1987;7:206–209.
32. Taneja K, Mittal S, Marya S, Mehrotra G, Shiv V, Bhargava S. Acute osteomyelitis: early diagnosis by ultrasonography. Aust Radiol 1992;36: 77–79.

33. Dargouth M, Essadam H, Ben Hamida H, et al. The value of ultrasound in acute osteomyelitis. Fr J Orthop Surg 1989;3:174–180.
34. Graham GD, Lundy MM, Frederick RJ, Berger DE, O'Brien AW, Brown TJ. Predicting the cure of osteomyelitis under treatment. J Nucl Med 1983;24:110–113.
35. Unger E, Moldofsky P, Gatenby R, Hartz W, Broder G. Diagnosing of osteomyelitis by MR imaging. Am J Roentgenol 1988;150:605–610.

CHAPTER 7

Principles of Management

As in any disease of known etiology, the first principle of management is prevention. With regard to musculoskeletal infections, prevention is only possible for potential infection, which follows open injury, or for unwelcome infection, which follows elective surgery, such as internal fixation of fractures or joint replacement. For infections that are primarily hematogenous, attempts at prevention can only be made if there is a known portal of entry for micro-organisms, such as vascular access sites. The duration of continuous vascular access should be kept to a minimum, and cannulae should not be left in place "just to keep the vein open."

Prevention of unwelcome infection following elective clean surgery depends on meticulous attention to Listerian principles of asepsis in the operating suite, minimizing the duration of surgery and the area of the open wound, gentle handling of tissues, and the use of antibiotics in prophylactic dosage (in operations where controlled trials have shown them to be effective). The choice of drug used will depend on the most likely pathogen causing an infection and its sensitivity to the antibiotic. It is essential to continue to monitor the microbiology of surgical infection because the causative organisms change with time, as do their antibiotic sensitivities. Treatment with prophylactic antimicrobials must change accordingly. The most likely cause of surgical infection is still *Staphylococcus aureus,* but surgical operations in some operative sites (e.g., the perineum) increase the incidence of infection with other organisms. The appropriate antibiotic is best administered intravenously immediately before surgical incision, preferably at the time of induction of anesthesia. There is not yet sufficient evidence to be able to say whether a single dose is as effective in infection prevention as several doses, but there is agreement that a narrow-spectrum antibiotic directed at the most likely pathogen and given for a short period (not more than one day) is all that is required to give a high probability of infection prevention.

With regard to preventing potential infection, when patients arrive for treatment with an open wound—in addition to selection of the most appropriate antibiotic based on the principles stated—the major therapeutic instrument is prompt institution of surgical toilet, commonly called debridement, with voluminous irrigation to physically dilute the bacterial inoculum, excision of any tissue of doubtful viability, and hemostasis to reduce the volume of clotted blood. If there is any doubt at all about the "cleanliness" of the open wound, then it should be left open and no attempt made at suture. The best policy is to perform repeated surgical toilet, as many times as is necessary and at daily intervals, until it appears safe to close the wound by delayed primary suture or tissue transplantation of skin or muscle. This decision can be made by clinical inspection and does not need microbiological laboratory confirmation. Only frankly infected wounds require identification of causative organisms so that the appropriate antibiotic can be administered.

Such principles do not evoke a great deal of controversy, although there is a reluctance by some to follow them for emotional or logistical reasons. Controversy occurs in the management of infections that arise by the hematogenous route. Management means both diagnosis and treatment. Although the precise details of both are addressed in succeeding chapters, a general method of approach is considered. It must always be remembered that "infection must be considered as a struggle between two organisms . . . the parasite and its host. This brings about adaptations on both sides" (Elie Metchnikoff, 1891). The aim of treating physicians is obviously to cure the disease, but in general this is done by tipping the balance of the struggle in favor of the host.

A second principle is that the destructive changes evoked by the infective process must be minimized so that there is little irreversible change to bone or cartilage, particularly in infants and children. In this regard, the rate of destruction is different in those infections labeled chronic and acute.

The first thing physicians must do is a clinical evaluation of the patient and decide whether the problem is an acute or chronic infection. If the infection is acute, then treatment should commence without delay on a provisional basis with respect to choice of antibiotic and restoration of homeostasis disturbed by the acute illness. If the infection is chronic, then there is no urgency in treatment and there is time to confirm a precise diagnosis.

Apart from the decision to begin antibiotic medication without absolute laboratory proof of diagnosis (the growth and identification of organisms cultured from the site of presumed infection), all subsequent management of acute and chronic musculoskeletal infection follows an identical path. The therapeutic decisions that must be made will be determined by several factors, some for which there is strong evidence and others for which clinical experience is the principal advocate.

Following clinical evaluation, diagnosis must be established, which requires location of the site of infection and identification of the organism. Location of site is essential in the decision-making process about the requirement for surgical intervention, whereas identification of organism determines the correct antibiotic choice.

Antibiotics and surgery must be considered in the treatment of all cases of musculoskeletal infection. There is an abundance of historical evidence about the morbidity and mortality of such infections in the preantibiotic era, which underlies the surgical principles of treatment. There is no doubt that antibiotics have changed the natural history of these diseases. However, in some parts of the world, there is not ready availability of these drugs and surgery remains a mainstay of treatment.

The questions the treating physician must answer regarding surgery are:

1. Is surgery necessary for this patient?
2. When should the surgery be performed?
3. What operative procedure is indicated?

The questions regarding antibiotics are:

1. Which antibiotics should be used for provisional treatment?
2. Which antibiotics should be used for specific treatment?
3. By what route should the antibiotic be administered and in what dose?
4. For how long should the antibiotic be given?

As indicated, the prime aim in achieving a cure, if possible, is to prevent structural changes in bone or cartilage, which is the prime cause of crippling morbidity in the longer term.

Antibiotics achieve this prevention by sterilization (i.e., killing bacteria or other organisms, and preventing their invasive spread). Surgery aims at removing pus, necrotic tissue, foreign materials, glycocalyx and bacterial slime, and the infection source, and restoring blood supply, phagocytosis, mechanical strength, and function. The prime aim of the whole treatment process is to help tip the balance by improving the general state of the patient as well as the infected site either to achieve a cure or to avoid or minimize recurrence of infection.

Controversies arise because patients present with infections to different types of medical practitioners—internists, surgeons, pediatricians, rheumatologists, infectious disease specialists, or family general practitioners. The greatest controversy arises about surgical operation because some of these practitioners are not as disposed to recommend invasive treatment as others. It is the aim of the chapters that follow to indicate the rational basis for treatment of musculoskeletal infections and the way in which decisions are made about the surgical and antibiotic modes.

Will there be a new era, such as that launched by antibiotics? Will we produce vaccines against musculoskeletal infections? Will we find new ways of "stimulating the phagocytes"? By reading this book, some may be stimulated to think about other potential treatment strategies, particularly if the time might come when bacteria become resistant to all or most antibiotics or if the immune competence of patients drops to a low level (e.g., as a result of human immunodeficiency virus infection or iatrogenic immunosuppression), so that the balance is not as easily tipped as it currently is in favor of the host.

CHAPTER 8

Antimicrobial Agents and Other Forms of Therapy Used in the Treatment of Bone Infections

Overview

The principles of the management of osteomyelitis and septic arthritis have been stated in Chapter 7. The modes of treatment used in the management of osteomyelitis vary depending on the type and location of osteomyelitis, the host, the need for and extent of surgery, and the etiological micro-organism (1). Classification schemes based on localization and type of osteomyelitis, as well as the immune status of the host, are reviewed in Chapter 1. In this chapter, we concentrate primarily on the use of antimicrobial therapy as well as other nonsurgical modalities.

Classes of Agents Used

Three major considerations are critical in the antimicrobial management of osteomyelitis. First is the spectrum of activity of the agent chosen. The drug selected must be active against the specific pathogen recovered from bone or blood of the infected patient; if, for any reason, an organism cannot be isolated, then the spectrum of activity of the agent chosen must be such that it encompasses those organisms most frequently found in the specific type of osteomyelitis and host. Second is the ability of the antimicrobial agent to reach the site of infection. In general, most antimicrobial agents penetrate adequately into bone and there appears to be no compelling reason to choose one antimicrobial agent over another because of this variable. Third is the duration of therapy. There is a paucity of controlled data to determine both the optimal and the minimal period of time required for administration of antimicrobial agents in the management of osteomyelitis or septic arthritis. Because micro-organisms are frequently sequestered in areas of bone relatively inaccessible to antimicrobial agents, because local factors such as glycocalyx impede penetration of antimicrobial agents, and because the organisms are frequently in a relatively dormant state, it has been argued that high levels of antimicrobial agents should be administered for prolonged periods. In reality, there are little data to support specific recommendations for the actual dose of antimicrobial agent or for the duration for which it is given.

A detailed review of all the antimicrobial agents that may be useful in treating osteomyelitis is beyond the scope of this text. For more details regarding antimicrobial agents, the reader is referred to either Kucers and Bennett *The Use of Antibiotics* or Mandel and colleagues *Anti-infective Therapy*. Table 8-1 summarizes our recommendations for preferred and alternative antimicrobial therapy for the major bacterial pathogens causing bone and joint infections.

Penetration of Antimicrobial Agents into Bone and "Bone Levels"

Measurement of "antibiotic levels" in normal or diseased bone is usually performed by bioassay using one of three techniques: (a) assay of a solution produced by agitating pieces of bone in an appropriate buffer; (b) assay of a slurry created by adding bone to a buffer; and (c) assay of specimens of bone placed directly on bacterially impregnated plates (2). There are several concerns about the methods used. First, it is unclear whether these procedures measure the total amount of antibiotic in bone or if bound drug is assayable. Second, it is possible that enzymatic reactions, pH changes, among other factors, may affect the antibiotic concentration in vivo before the samples can be processed in vitro. Finally, hydrolysis of the drugs, in the bioassay process, may measure concentrations of unbound and antimicrobially active drug in bone (3). Despite these concerns with methodology, many studies have been done measuring antibiotic concentrations in bone.

The majority of studies measuring "penetration characteristics" of antimicrobial agents in bone have been performed in patients having arthroplasty of the hip who received prophylactic antibiotics prior to surgery. Although assay techniques varied from center to center, in

Table 8-1. Antimicrobial Therapy for Infections of Bone and Joints

ORGANISM	ANTIMICROBIAL AGENT OF CHOICE	ALTERNATIVE AGENTS
Staphylococcus aureus (methicillin-sensitive)	Nafcillin or oxacillin (2 gm q6h IV)	Cefazolin, vancomycin, clindamycin
Staphylococcus aureus (methicillin-resistant)	Vancomycin (1 gm q12h IV)	TMP/SMX plus rifampin
Streptococcus pneumoniae	Penicillin G (5×10^6 U q6h IV)	Cefazolin, vancomycin, clindamycin
GpA beta-hemolytic streptococci	Penicillin G (5×10^6 U q8h IV)	Cefazolin, vancomycin, clindamycin
Enterococci	Ampicillin (2 gm q4h IV)	Vancomycin
Hemophilus influenzae (beta-lactamase–negative)	Ampicillin (2 gm q4h IV)	TMP/SMX, ceftriaxone
Hemophilus influenzae (beta-lactamase–positive)	Ceftriaxone (1 gm q12h IV)	TMP/SMX
Klebsiella pneumoniae	Ceftriaxone (1 gm q12h IV)	Ciprofloxacin, piperacillin, Imipenem
Escherichia coli	Cefazolin (1 gm q8h IV)	Ciprofloxacin, ceftriaxone, Imipenem
Pseudomonas aeruginosa	Ciprofloxacin (400 mg q12h IV)	Piperacillin plus aminoglycoside, Aztreonam
Serratia marcescens	Ceftriaxone (1 gm q12h IV)	Imipenem, TMP/SMX, Ciprofloxacin
Salmonella	Depends on sensitivity test; choose between ampicillin, ceftriaxone, imipenem, ciprofloxacin	
Bacteroides species	Clindamycin (600 mg q8h)	Imipenem, metronidazole

general, the type of bone assayed is similar and the results appear reasonably constant.

Table 8-2 shows different agents administered, the dosage and route of administration, the time of sampling, serum levels, and level of antimicrobial agent in bone (4–22).

Despite all this available data on concentrations of these agents in

Table 8-2. Bone and Serum Concentrations of Antimicrobial Agents Administered to Humans

DRUG AND REFERENCE	DOSE AND ROUTE OF ADMINISTRATION	SAMPLING TIME (MIN)	SERUM LEVEL (μg/mL)	BONE LEVEL CORTICAL (μg/gm)	BONE LEVEL CANCELLOUS (μg/gm)
Cephalothin					
4	2 gm IV	Variable	6.2		0
5	1 gm IV	60	13		2.5
6	1 gm IV	60	11.9		3.9
7	2 gm IV bolus	Variable	12		ND
7	2 gm IV infusion	Variable	30		35
8	20 mg/kg/IV	31	107		1.4
8	20 mg/kg IV	32	89		1.4
9	10 mg/kg IM	Variable	4.3		1.3
Cefazolin					
10	2 gm IV	52	41.6		2.5
11	1 gm IV	Variable	22.5		7.5
12	50 mg/kg IV	30	59.9		6.0*
5	1 gm IV	60	60		30
4	1 gm IV	Variable	36.4		2.6†
9	10 mg/kg IM	Variable	4.2		2.0
13	1 gm IV	Variable	43.3	12‡	
Cefamandole					
7	2 gm IV	Variable	20		8.5
14	2 gm IV	51	73.6	9.4	
15	1.5 gm IM and IV	Variable	75.2	10.3	13.1
Cephradine					
5	1 gm IV	60	30		15
16	1 gm IV	Variable	167.9		11.1
Cephapirin					
17	1–2 gm IV	Variable			9.2
Clindamycin					
4	600 mg IV	Variable	8.6		8.4§
18	300 mg IM	60	7.3		2.6
19	600 mg IM	120	8.5	3.7	3.8
Oxacillin					
20	2 gm IV	Variable	86	4.2	7.7
21	1 gm IV	60	19	2.1	

Table 8-2, continued

DRUG AND REFERENCE	DOSE AND ROUTE OF ADMINISTRATION	SAMPLING TIME (MIN)	SERUM LEVEL (μg/mL)	BONE LEVEL CORTICAL (μg/gm)	BONE LEVEL CANCELLOUS (μg/gm)
Rifampin					
22	300 mg IV	150–210	18.8		4.0

*Undetectable concentrations in 1 of 5 patients.
†Undetectable concentrations in 3 of 4 patients.
‡Undetectable concentrations in 6 of 7 patients.
§Undetectable concentration in 1 of 3 patients.
ND = none detected.
Modified from Fitzgerald R. Antibiotic distribution in normal and osteomyelitic bone. Orthop Clin North Am 1984;15:537–546.

bone, it is difficult to be certain that one agent is superior to another. Furthermore, experimental studies show no correlation between the "penetration" of antimicrobial agents into bone tissue and success of therapy in eradicating infection (23).

The arguments that bone tissue may inhibit penetration of antibiotics are not supported by most available data (2). Any barrier to passage of antimicrobial agents through capillaries in bone would have to be either anatomical or physiological. Evidence for an anatomical barrier is lacking, and electronmicroscopic studies showed a discontinuous endothelial lining for the bony capillary network (24). It was suggested that there may be physiological mechanisms in bone tissue to control the movement of calcium ions; were such a barrier to exist, it is theoretically possible that it would affect movement of antimicrobial agents as well (25). In a series of experiments critically reviewing the ability of various antibiotics to cross capillary membranes and enter different fluid spaces of bone in normal dogs and in an osteomyelitic model, the following conclusions, which seem well supported, were drawn. (a) Both beta-lactam antimicrobial agents and aminoglycosides can traverse the capillary membranes of normal and osteomyelitic bone; it seems likely that there is no physiological barrier to the passage of antibiotics into the interstitial fluid. (b) These agents distributed within the two extracellular fluid compartments of bone (i.e., plasma and interstitial fluid space). (c) Interstitial fluid concentration of beta-lactam antimicrobial agents and aminoglycosides generally agreed with serum concentrations, and the variations observed are within the errors of the method. (d) Under steady-state conditions, serum concentrations of antimicrobial agents appeared to predict bone interstitial fluid concentration (2). This last conclusion strongly suggests that measurement of "bone levels" of antimicrobial agents is not necessary and can be predicted by determination of serum concentrations.

Serum Bactericidal Levels

A general tenet of therapy for osteomyelitis has been the need to deliver high concentrations of antimicrobial agents in serum to achieve adequate levels in bone. One measure of serum levels is to determine the serum bactericidal titer (SBT), either peak or trough. In the pediatric literature, SBT in patients receiving oral therapy has been examined (26,27). It was suggested that a peak SBT of 1:16 or greater and a trough of 1:2 or greater would reflect adequate levels for the treatment of osteomyelitis. The SBT was basically used as a means of assuring that oral therapy was equivalent in intensity to parenteral therapy.

Others have attempted to determine whether a standardized SBT would help predict the outcome of treatment of osteomyelitis. In a study of 30 episodes of acute osteomyelitis and 18 chronic, the following conclusions were drawn. (a) In patients with acute osteomyelitis, peak SBT was not predictive, whereas trough SBT of 1:2 or greater predicted cure. (b) In chronic osteomyelitis, a peak SBT of 1:16 or greater and a trough of 1:4 or greater predicted cure. (c) SBT appears to be useful in the management of patients with osteomyelitis. (d) Patients with acute osteomyelitis should have serum bactericidal titers of 1:2 or greater at all times, and patients with chronic osteomyelitis should have serum bactericidal titers of 1:4 or greater at all times (28) (Figure 8-1).

Several questions can be raised regarding these conclusions. (a) It is possible that measurement of the ability of serum to inhibit bacterial growth (rather than to kill organisms) would be equally predictive because there is no evidence to suggest that bactericidal antimicrobial agents are superior to nonbactericidal agents in the treatment of osteomyelitis. (b) Regarding the conclusion that patients with acute osteomyelitis should have an SBT of 1:2 or greater at all times—of

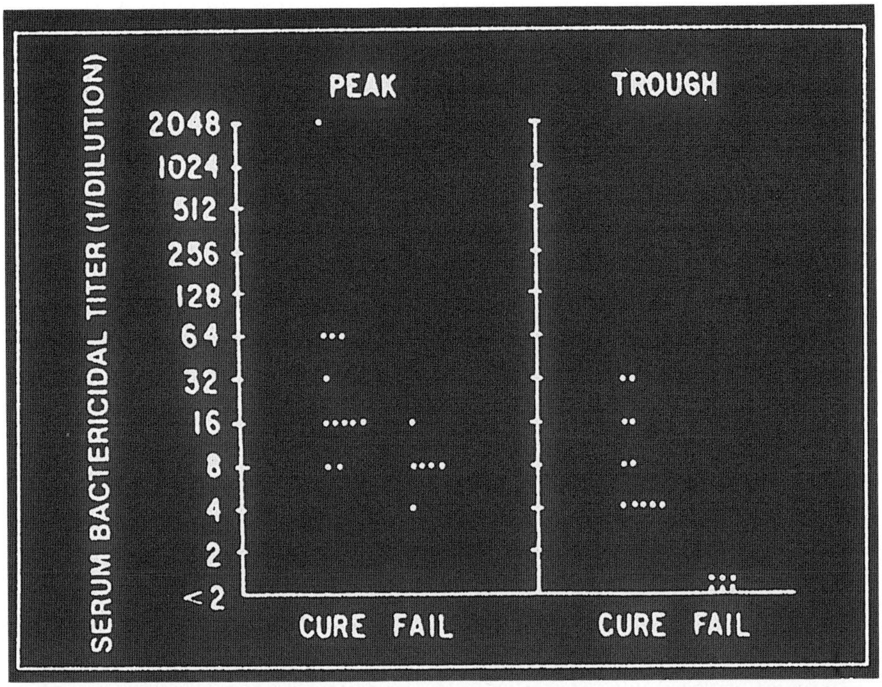

Figure 8-1. *Relationship of outcome of chronic osteomyelitis to serum bactericidal tests.* (Reproduced with permission from Weinstein M, Stratton C, Hawley H, et al. Multicenter collaborative evaluation of a standardized serum bactericidal test as a predictor of therapeutic efficacy in acute and chronic osteomyelitis. Am J Med 1987;83:218–222.)

seven patients who had trough levels of less than 2, two were cured and five represented failures. (c) The number of patients with chronic osteomyelitis is small (total, 18), and the predictive value of a trough titer of less than 2 might change if more patients were studied.

We believe use of the SBT in the management of osteomyelitis has some value and that one should aim for trough values of 1:2 or greater whenever possible. However, one should not draw rigid lines such that potentially toxic concentrations of antimicrobial agents will be achieved to attain an SBT trough level of 1:2 or greater at all times. If a patient appears to be doing clinically well and the erythrocyte sedimentation rate (ESR) is decreasing but the SBT trough is not 1:2 or greater, we would not attempt to push the serum concentration higher, but would rather be guided by clinical parameters and not alter dosage if the patient is improving.

Results of Treatment with Different Antimicrobial Agents

Table 8-3 summarizes the results of several clinical trials using different classes of newer antimicrobial agents to treat chronic osteomyelitis. The table is selective rather than inclusive and represents trials that adhered to a reasonable set of standards for conduct and analysis. Most agents achieved results comparable to those of others tested; however, interpretation of many of these trials is difficult because of lack of comparison with concurrent randomly assigned treatment with comparative agents.

Currently, through a contract between the Infectious Disease Society of America and the Food and Drug Administration, guidelines have been drafted for controlled clinical trials of many infections, including those of bones and joints (29). Among the criteria considered important in calling a trial "well conducted" are the following: (a) clear inclusion and exclusion criteria for patients; (b) clear definitions of "acute" and "chronic" osteomyelitis; (c) appropriate diagnostic techniques, including cultures; (d) appropriate identification and susceptibility testing of bacteria; (e) a defined antimicrobial regimen with exceptions from that regimen noted; (f) appropriate adjunctive surgical drainage or debridement; and (g) defined critieria for both clinical and microbiological responses, recognizing that chronic osteomyelitis may well be a life-long disease (i.e., the potential for reactivation exists for the life of the patient).

Table 8-3. Clinical Trials—Newer Agents in Osteomyelitis

AGENT	NO. PATIENTS	CLINICAL SUCCESS (%)
Cefotaxime	84	87
Ceftriaxone	104	79
Ceftazidime	122	84
Aztreonam	69	78
Imipenem/cilastatin	58	79
Ticarcillin/clavulanic acid	75	81
Ciprofloxacin	235	78

Adapted from Gentry LO. Antibiotic therapy for osteomyelitis. Infect Dis Clin North Am 1990;4:485–499.

Management of Osteomyelitis Outside the Hospital

Patients receiving antimicrobial therapy for osteomyelitis are frequently ambulatory and, with the exception of the local bone infections, are generally quite well. In such patients, home health care is a strong consideration if the patient, with the assistance of family members, can self-administer the antibiotics through a vascular access catheter. Such a catheter (Broviac or Hickman) is surgically inserted while the patient is in the hospital and remains in place throughout the course of home therapy. The advantages of home care include the preference of patients for life with family and a decreased risk of superinfection.

Out-patient therapy of osteomyelitis with intravenous antibiotics has been shown to be highly effective (30–33). Although none of these studies compared home intravenous antimicrobial therapy with treatment received entirely in the hospital, the results with home intravenous (IV) antibiotic therapy seem comparable in terms of efficacy to those previously reported in other controlled trials. One alternative to the use of home IV antimicrobial therapy is the use of intramuscular agents, such as ceftriaxone, which can be given once daily (34). Intramuscular therapy has been well tolerated, and the use of lidocaine appeared to reduce pain from the injection. The advantage of the intramuscular route, used once daily, is avoidance of an intravascular catheter and more frequent injection of antimicrobial agents. Out-patient therapy with orally administered agents is an alternative form of therapy that obviates the need for an intravascular access device.

Authors of several studies (35–37) reviewed the economic advantages of out-patient IV antibiotic therapy in the management of osteomyelitis. Estimated savings per patient ranged from \$500 to \$2,200, which demonstrates a wide difference if different sources of data on hospital costs are employed (35). The large decreases in in-patient cost are often shifted to an increased out-patient cost. Therefore, because out-patient costs are more often borne by patients than in-patient costs, out-patient therapy could be more expensive to individual patients despite the savings to the hospital and to society as a whole.

Oral Antimicrobial Therapy

Use of oral antimicrobial therapy for osteomyelitis is highly desirable, both from an economic point of view and from avoidance of intravascular catheterization. Administration of oral antimicrobial agents, following IV therapy, became widely accepted as a means of treating acute bone and joint infections in children (38,39). These observations were extended by comparing children with osteomyelitis or septic arthritis who were switched to oral antibiotics within 72 hours of IV therapy with another group continuing on IV therapy for 4 weeks (40). A similar clinical course and outcome in both groups and no treatment failures were observed. We believe that antibiotic therapy can be safely changed to an oral route as soon as an organism is isolated and antimicrobial susceptibility is determined. Children treated in this manner should have absorption of oral agents monitored by measurement of serum bactericidal titers and by frequent discussions with the parents that the child is taking the medication and is clinically improving.

In adults, use of oral antimicrobial therapy for chronic osteomyelitis has lagged behind that in children. Excellent results were reported from Australia, with follow-up periods of up to nine years, for treatment of adults with chronic staphylococcal osteomyelitis with oral doses of cloxacillin or phenoxymethylpenicillin (41). All patients received at least six months of therapy, and, for some patients who were apparently well, therapy was maintained at a lower dose for periods as long as seven years. In all patients, probenecid was given in addition to the penicillin. These reports were not given wide credence because of the objections raised that the doses seemed extremely high and that continued maintenance therapy did not allow for determination of relapse or failure. In general, we do not support this approach of "long-term suppression" without better evidence that the benefits outweigh the potential complications and costs of prolonged administration.

More recently, a retrospective review of 21 adults with osteomyelitis or septic arthritis who received oral antimicrobial agents following an initial course of IV therapy (mean duration of IV therapy, 3.6 days) was conducted (42). Oral therapy lasted a mean of 43 days, and trough serum bactericidal titers were adjusted to be 1:8 greater. Eighteen of 21 patients had no clinical signs of recurrence; the follow-up period ranged from six to 66 months, with a mean of 42 months. The oral agents used included cloxicillin, trimethoprim-sulfamethoxazole, and cephalexin. The preference for maintaining a trough SBT of 1:8 or greater was empirical, and there was no data to indicate that such measurements or adjustments of dosage improved efficacy.

A recent comparison of oral ciprofloxacin with parenteral therapy (a cephalosporin or nafcillin combined with an aminoglycoside) for the treatment of biopsy-proven osteomyelitis was performed (43). Mean durations of therapy were 56 days in the oral group and 47 in the IV group. The clinical success rates were 77% for the ciprofloxacin group and 79% for the parenteral therapy group. In each group, the majority of failures were due to relapse of the infection within one year of therapy. Of interest, and not totally explained, is the fact that infection with *Pseudomonas aeruginosa* as a single pathogen was successfully treated by both regimens, whereas polymicrobial infection, in which *P. aeruginosa* was one pathogen, failed in almost every instance despite the regimen chosen. Emergence of resistance to ciprofloxacin did not occur except in a single strain of *P. aeruginosa,* which was resistant at the time of relapse. Superinfection with *Staphylococcus aureus* occurred in a few patients receiving ciprofloxacin despite in vitro susceptibility of these strains to ciprofloxacin. Oral ofloxacin has also been compared with parenteral therapy with either cefazolin or ceftazidime in biopsy-confirmed osteomyelitis (44). The outcomes were generally similar, with long-term response rates of 14 of 19 patients (74%) receiving ofloxacin and 12 of 14 (86%) receiving parenteral antibiotics. In the group treated with ofloxacin, one patient had persistent *P. aeruginosa* infection in which the organism had acquired resistance; four other subjects whose initial response to therapy was successful with ofloxacin treatment suffered relapses, three due to *S. aureus* and one due to *P. aeruginosa*. In contrast, only one patient treated with parenteral therapy suffered relapse (44).

We believe that oral therapy may be as effective as parenteral therapy in patients with chronic osteomyelitis caused by susceptible organisms. However, therapy with quinolones may be problematic given the rapid rate of emergence of resistance of *S. aureus* and the potential for development of resistance of *P. aeruginosa*. The choice of oral agents for the treatment of chronic osteomyelitis will be critical because it seems plausible that if adequate levels of active drug can be achieved at the site of infection with oral administration of agents, such therapy should be effective. It is clear that further trials with larger populations comparing oral and parenteral therapy need to be performed.

Hyperbaric Oxygen

The principal effect of hyperbaric oxygen (HBO) is enhancement of host defenses and repair. Its use in treatment of chronic osteomyelitis was first reported in 1965 (45). Hamblen (46) was the first to describe an experimental evaluation of its use. In his model, approximately 25% of control animals healed spontaneously; intermittent HBO increased healing to 66%. Studies of inhibition of growth in vitro of many aerobic bacteria and fungi by HBO have produced conflicting results (47,48), but there is general agreement that increasing oxygen tension is lethal to anaerobes. Subsequent experimental studies of HBO have contributed significantly to understanding of its effects (49–52). The killing capacity of normal leukocytes is seriously inhibited at oxygen tensions of less than 10 mm Hg (53). Fibroblastic activity, collagen formation, and capillary proliferation are depressed in hypoxic tissue. Intramedullary oxygen tension is depressed in infected bone but can be raised to normal levels by breathing 100% oxygen at one atmosphere pressure (50). HBO, although it does not benefit tissues with normal vasculature and cannot affect avascular tissue, will raise tissue Po_2 in areas of marginal vascularity.

Hyperbaric oxygen is being used with increasing frequency as adjunctive therapy for osteomyelitis. The difficulties of evaluating the effects of HBO in the treatment of osteomyelitis given the multiple clinical variables in this disease have been reviewed (54). There are several open clinical trials that suggest adjunctive HBO therapy is useful in the management of chronic osteomyelitis (55–59). In two studies (58,59), patients were used as their own controls, and the patients appeared to have significant improvement as noted by arrest of the disease and clinical freedom from disease following HBO therapy. In the only randomized study of HBO therapy in chronic osteomyelitis, the four failures (one in the conventional group and three in the HBO group) unfortunately refused further surgery or had such extensive osteomyelitis that amputation was required (60). It was concluded that all four treatment failures would have failed regardless of whatever therapy they received. Thus, the problem in this series was patient compliance with regard to surgical management. The value of adjunctive HBO in the management of chronic osteomyelitis can probably only be judged accurately through further efforts at such controlled clinical trials.

In summary, the jury is still out on the value of HBO in the management of chronic osteomyelitis. However, we believe that the potential uses of HBO include adjunctive therapy to conventional management in chronic osteomyelitis in special situations such as chronic hypoxia, arteritis, extreme scarring, radiation fibrosis, or as suppressive treatment with antibiotics when surgical management is inappropriate.

References

1. Cierney G, Mader J. Approach to adult osteomyelitis. Orthop Rev 1987;16:95–106.
2. Fitzgerald R. Antibiotic distribution in normal and osteomyelitic bone. Orthop Clin North Am 1984;15:537–546.
3. Tetzlaff TR, Howard G, McCracken G, Calderon E, Larrondo J. Antibiotic concentrations in pus and bone of children with osteomyelitis. J Pediatr 1978;92:135–140.
4. Smilack JD, Flittie H, Williams TW Jr. Bone concentrations of antimicrobial agents after parenteral administration. Antimicrob Agents Chemother 1976;9:169–171.
5. Cunha BA, Gossling HR, Pasternak HS, Nightingale CH, Quintiliani R. The penetration characteristics of cefazolin, cephalothin, and cephradine into bone in patients undergoing total hip replacement. J Bone Joint Surg [Am] 1977;59:856–859.
6. Fitzgerald RH Jr, Kelly PJ, Snyder RJ, Washington JA II. Penetration of methicillin, oxacillin and cephalothin into bone and synovial tissues. Antimicrob Agents Chemother 1978;14:723–726.
7. Quinn EL, Madhaven T, Wixson R, et al. Cefamandole: observations on its spectrum concentration in bone and bile excretion in renal failure and clinical efficacy. Curr Chemother 1978;2:803–804.
8. Patel D, Moellering RC Jr, Thrasher K, et al. The effect of hypotensive anesthesia on cephalothin concentrations, in bone and muscle of patients undergoing total hip replacement. J Bone Joint Surg [Am] 1979;61:531–538.
9. Kondo S, Marumo M, Takeda K, et al. Experimental studies on the chemotherapy of open fractures. 9. Clinical studies on the distribution of cephalosporin C antibiotics and penicillin G concentrations into human bone marrow and bone marrow bleeding. Bull Osaka Med School 1973;19: 32–44.
10. Schurman DJ, Hirshman HP, Kajiyama G, et al. Cefazolin concentrations in bone and synovial fluid. J Bone Joint Surg [Am] 1978;60:359–362.
11. Rosdahl VT, Serensen TS, Colding H. Determination of antibiotic concentrations in bone. J Antimicrob Chemother 1979;5:275–280.
12. Tetzlaff TR, Howard JB, McCracken GH Jr, et al. Antibiotic concentra-

tions in pus and bone of children with osteomyelitis. J Pediatr 1978;92: 135–140.
13. Sorensen TS, Colding H, Schroeder E, Rosdahl VT. The penetration of cefazolin, erythromycin and methicillin into human bone tissue. Acta Orthop Scand 1978;49:549–553.
14. Schurman DJ, Hirshman HP, Burton DS. Cephalothin and cefamandole penetration into bone, synovial fluid and wound drainage fluid. J Bone Joint Surg [Am] 1960;62:961–965.
15. Roncoroni AJ, Manuel C, Nedjar C, Bauchet J, Mariani D. Cefamandole bone diffusion in patients undergoing total hip replacement. Chemotherapy 1981;27:166–172.
16. Parsons RL, Beavis JP, Paddock GM, et al. Cephradine bone concentrations during total hip replacement. In: Williams JD, Geddes AM, eds. Chemotherapy, vol. 1. Clinical aspects of infections. New York: Plenum, 1976:201–211.
17. Schurman DJ, Burton DS, Kajiyama G, Moser K, Nagel DA. Sodium cephapirin disposition and distribution into human bone. Curr Ther Res 1976;20:194–203.
18. Nicholas P, Meyers B, Levy R, Hirschman S. Concentration of clindamycin in human bone. Antimicrob Agents Chemother 1975;8:220–221.
19. Schurman D, Johnson B, Finerman G, Amstutz H. Antibiotic bone penetration. Clin Orthop 1975;111:142–146.
20. Kolczun MC, Nelson CL, McHenry MC, Gavan TL, Pinovich P. Antibiotic concentrations in bone. J Bone Joint Surg [Am] 1974;56:305–310.
21. Fitzgerald R, Kelly P, Snyder R, Washington J. Penetration of methicillin, oxacillin and cephalothin into bone and synovial tissues. Antimicrob Agents Chemother 1978;14:723–726.
22. Roth B. Penetration of parenterally administered rifampicin into bone tissue. Chemotherapy 1984;30:358–365.
23. Norden C. Lessons learned from animal models of osteomyelitis. Rev Infect Dis 1988;10:103–110.
24. Cooper RR, Milgram JW, Robinson RA. Morphology of the osteon: an electron microscopic study. J Bone Joint Surg [Am] 1966;48:1239–1271.
25. Talmage RV, Grubb SA. A laboratory model demonstrating osteocyte-osteoblast control of plasma calcium concentrations: table model for plasma calcium control. Clin Orthop 1977;122:299–306.
26. Tetzlaff TR, McCracken GH, Nelson JD. Oral antibiotic therapy for skeletal infections of children. II. Therapy of osteomyelitis and suppurative arthritis. J Pediatr 1978;92:485–490.
27. Prober C, Yaeger A. Use of the serum bactericidal titer to assess the adequacy of oral antibiotic therapy in the treatment of acute hematogenous osteomyelitis. J Pediatr 1979;95:131–135.
28. Weinstein M, Stratton C, Hawley H, Ackley A, Reller LB. Multicenter collaborative evaluation of a standardized serum bactericidal test as a predictor of therapeutic efficacy in acute and chronic osteomyelitis. Am J Med 1987;83:218–222.

29. Norden C, Mader J, Nelson J, Calandra G. Guidelines for evaluation of new anti-infective drugs for treatment of skin, skin structure, bone and joint infections. Clin Infect Dis 1992;15:S148–S181.
30. Couch L, Cierny G, Mader J. Inpatient and outpatient use of the hickman catheter for adults with osteomyelitis. Clin Orthop Related Res 1987;219:226–235.
31. Wagner D, Collier B, Rytel M. Long term intravenous antibiotic therapy in chronic osteomyelitis. Arch Intern Med 1985;145:1073–1078.
32. Ingram C, Eron L, Goldenberg R, et al. Antibiotic therapy of osteomyelitis in adults. Med Clin North Am 1988;72:723–738.
33. Merar J, Bower T, Neri C. Long term outpatient intravenous antibiotic therapy for orthopedic patients. Orthopedics 1984;7:1280–1283.
34. Eron LJ, Park CH, Hixon D, Goldenberg RI, Poretz DM. Ceftriaxone therapy of bone and soft tissue infections in hospital and outpatient settings. Antimicrob Agents Chemother 1983;23:731–737.
35. Eisenberg J, Kitz D. Savings from outpatient antibiotic therapy for osteomyelitis. JAMA 1986;255:1584–1588.
36. Chamberlain TM, Lehman ME, Groh MJ, Munroe WP, Reinders TP. Cost analysis of a home intravenous antibiotic program. Am J Hosp Pharm 1988;45:2341–2345.
37. Balinsky W, Nesbitt S. Cost effectiveness of outpatient parenteral antibiotics—a review of the literature. Am J Med 1989;87:301–305.
38. Cole W, Dalziel R, Leitl S. Treatment of acute osteomyelitis in childhood. J Bone Joint Surg [Br] 1982;64:218–223.
39. Bryson Y, Connor J, LeClarc M, Giammona S. Brief clinical and laboratory observation. High dose oral cloxacillin treatment of acute staphylococcal osteomyelitis in children. J Pediatr 1979;94:673–675.
40. Kolyvas E, Ahronheim G, Marks M, Gledhill R, Owen H, Rosenthall L. Oral antibiotic therapy of skeletal infections in children. Pediatrics 1980;65:867–871.
41. Bell S. Further observations on the value of oral penicillins in chronic staphylococcal osteomyelitis. Med J Aust 1976;2:591–593.
42. Black J, Hunt TL, Godley PJ, Matthew E. Oral antimicrobial therapy for adults with osteomyelitis or septic arthritis. J Infect Dis 1987;155:968–972.
43. Gentry L, Rodriguez-Gomez G. Oral ciprofloxacin compared with parenteral antibiotics in the treatment of osteomyelitis. Antimicrob Agents Chemother 1990;34:40–43.
44. Gentry L, Rodriguez-Gomez G. Ofloxacin versus parenteral therapy for chronic osteomyelitis. Antimicrob Agents Chemother 1991;35:538–541.
45. Slack WK, Thomas DA, Perrins D. Hyperbaric oxygen in chronic osteomyelitis. Lancet 1965;1:1093–1094.
46. Hamblen DL. Hyperbaric oxygenation: its effect on experimental staphylococcal osteomyelitis in rats. J Bone Joint Surg [Am] 1968;50:1129–1141.
47. Hopkinson WI, Towers AG. Effects of hyperbaric oxygen on some common pathogenic bacteria. Lancet 1963;2:1361–1362.

48. McAllister TA, Stark JM, Norman JN. Inhibiting effects of hyperbaric oxygen on bacteria and fungi. Lancet 1963;2:1040–1042.
49. Mader JT, Brown GL, Guckian JC, Wells CH, Reinarz JA. A mechanism for the amelioration by hyperbaric oxygen of experimental staphylococcal osteomyelitis in rabbits. J Infect Dis 1980;142:915–922.
50. Mader JT, Adams KR, Wallace WR, Calhoun JH. Hyperbaric oxygen as adjunctive therapy for osteomyelitis. Infect Dis Clin North Am 1990;4:433–440.
51. Esterhai JL, Clark JM, Morton HE, Smith DW, Steinbach A, Richter SD. Effect of hyperbaric oxygen tension within the medullary canal in the rabbit tibial osteomyelitis model. J Orthop Res 1986;4:330–336.
52. Esterhai JL, Clark JM, Morton HE, Smith DW, Steinbach A, Richter SD. Effect of hyperbaric oxygen exposure on oxygen tension within the medullary canal in the rabbit tibial osteomyelitis model. J Orthop Res 1986;4:330–336.
53. Mandell GL. Bactericidal activity of aerobic and anaerobic polymorphonuclear neutrophils. Infect Immun 1974;9:337–341.
54. Mader J, Adams K, Wallace W, Calhoun J. Hyperbaric oxygen as adjunctive therapy for osteomyelitis. Inf Dis Clin North Am 1990;4:433–440.
55. Slack WK, Thomas DA, Perrins DJD. Hyperbaric oxygenation in chronic osteomyelitis. Lancet 1965;1:1093–1094.
56. Perrins JD, Maudsley RH, Colwill MW, et al. OHP in the management of chronic osteomyelitis. In: Brown IW, Cox BG, eds. Proceedings of the Third International Conference on Hyperbaric Medicine. Washington, DC: National Academy of Sciences, National Research Council, 1966:578–584.
57. Depenbusch FI, Thompson RE, Hart GB. Use of hyperbaric oxygen in the treatment of refractory osteomyelitis: a preliminary report. J Trauma 1972;12:807–812.
58. Morrey BF, Dunn JM, Heimbach RD, Davis J. Hyperbaric oxygen and chronic osteomyelitis. Clin Orthop 1979;144:121–127.
59. Davis JC, Heckman JD, DeLee JC, Buckwold FJ. Chronic non-hematogenous osteomyelitis treated with adjuvant hyperbaric oxygen. J Bone Joint Surg [Am] 1986;68:1210–1217.
60. Esterhai JL, Pisarello J, Brighton CT, Heppenstall RB, Gellman H, Goldstein G. Adjunctive hyperbaric oxygen therapy in the treatment of chronic refractory osteomyelitis. J Trauma 1987;27:763–768.

PART THREE

Clinical Syndromes

CHAPTER 9

Hematogenous Osteomyelitis

Introduction

Hematogenous osteomyelitis (HO) is characteristically a disease of children. It may, of course, occur at any time throughout life and may involve any bone in the body, but the typical infection is juxtaphyseal in the metaphysis of a growing long bone. In adults, the majority of hematogenous infections occur in the spine. These infections are covered in Chapter 14. Herein, we concentrate on HO in the pelvis and the appendicular skeleton. Contemporary views of natural history and pathophysiology were largely elaborated in the nineteenth century (1,2). The bacterial etiology was established in the late 1870s and the early 1880s by a number of researchers, including Pasteur (3), who isolated *Staphylococcus aureus* from a typical patient. Subsequent studies confirmed that most cases of HO are caused by this organism (4–7). Recent studies have confirmed the ability of *S. aureus* to bind to a range of structural and nonstructural proteins in bone and cartilage matrix (see Chapter 2), some of which at least appear important in osteomyelitis (8).

Prior to the introduction of antibiotics, HO was an urgent and serious disease with a mortality of approximately 20% and a morbidity three times that (9). In the developing world, and in its acute presentation in the developed world, it remains a dramatic and potentially dangerous disease (10). When prompt diagnosis and treatment are available, however, the outcome has changed radically. Mortality in the developed world is now negligible, and the complication rate is approximately 5% (6). Subacute presentations may be becoming more common, perhaps reflecting increased empirical use of antibiotics in the community (11).

Historical Review

Although it has been held that HO was rarely recognized until the latter part of the nineteenth century (12), careful examination of the literature shows that the disease is old and that changing terminology obscured the record. There is paleontologic evidence from a number of early civilizations (13), and probable descriptions of acute osteoarticular sepsis have been identified from classic Mediterranean and Indian literature (14,15). The medieval Latin term *spina ventosa,* now confined to use in tuberculous dactylitis, was derived from Arabic descriptions of articular or periarticular infection (16). Severinus ("De recondita abscessuum natura," 1632 [17]) recorded the typical acute presentation in childhood. Cheselden (1756 [18]) and Smith (1827 [1]) described the natural history and anatomical pathology of HO in detail, calling the disease "necrosis." Chassaignac (19), in 1854, first used the term *osteomyelitis* to describe HO. His example was rapidly and widely adopted, and older terms, including *necrosis, fever sore, adolescent growth fever, malignant periostitis,* and *juxtaepiphyseal osteitis,* were abandoned.

The seminal nineteenth century monograph is Lannelongue's *De l'osteomyelite aigue pendant la croissance* (1879 [2]). Although he did not discuss a bacterial etiology for HO, his description of the natural history and pathology is essentially modern. Within one year of its publication, Pasteur isolated *S. aureus* from one of his patients. In the ensuing 20 years, despite initial reluctance on the part of established figures in European surgery, such as Billroth (20) and Lister (21), the bacterial hypothesis was soundly established by observational studies, as well as in a series of animal experiments by Rosenbach (22), Becker (23), Rodet (24), Lexer (25), and others (see Chapter 3).

In the twentieth century, until the introduction of chemotherapy, many different treatments were tried as adjuvants to surgery. They included a variety of topical dressing regimens applied to discharging sinuses (26) and attempts to control infection with bacteriophage (27). Trials of immunization with Staphylococcal toxoid were unsuccessful (28).

Crossan (26) reviewed the management of HO in the preantibiotic era. Surgical opinion on the management of HO was divided; arguments focused on whether surgery should be early, late, conservative, or radical. Echoes of these controversies are only now fading, some 50 years after the first antibiotics began to change the outlook in osteoarticular infections.

Terminology

Osteomyelitis has been classified in many different ways, based on the route of infection (29), histological appearance (30), and the anatomy of the infection within the bone (31). In HO, recognition and management critically depend on the clinical context of the infection, which may range from a fulminating acute illness, through a subtle and sometimes obscure presentation emphasizing pain, to established chronic infection. Lack of rigorous classification and the generally poor quality of available outcome studies leave a number of unanswered dilemmas in management. Most published data have failed not only to distinguish clearly between positive, probable, and possible bacterial infection (32), but also to stratify patients by stage at presentation. Future studies need to take these factors into account.

Epidemiology

Until the early 1950s, data on HO were confined to collected institutional series, some of which were impressively large (9). A prospective study in Northern England (33) reported the incidence of staphylococcal infections, including osteoarticular sepsis, in a cohort of children born in 1947 and followed to the age of 15 years.

Incidence has also been estimated from national and state hospital morbidity data (34). These data confirm the clinical impression that HO is predominantly a disease of childhood and is more common in boys. The male/female ratio appears to increase during childhood and is greatest in adolescence. Apparently comparable groups of children in different societies have different incidences. In general, incidence appears higher in lower latitudes, suggesting a role for environment in determining attack rate. Correlation has also been shown between incidence and some climatic variables. A seasonal variation of presentation with a peak in late summer and early autumn has been identified in three separate studies from different parts of the world (34–

36). These observations are also compatible with an environmental effect, perhaps mediated through seasonal variation in skin sepsis. Clear evidence of racial differences in incidence within national communities is evident and may indicate an increased risk in poorer socioeconomic groups. Children presenting with HO may be suboptimally nourished (37). The incidence of HO in developed societies is generally considered to have decreased, and a significant decline has been confirmed for acute HO in New Zealand (33), Scotland (38), and Denmark (39). Subacute HO, in contrast, may have become more common, although no trend data exist to confirm this view.

Natural History

The clinical observations of Pasteur (3), and the experimental studies of Rodet (24), Lexer (25), and others, indicated that the septic focus in bone arose from the lodging of blood-borne bacteria, or septic emboli, in the metaphyseal blood vessels. Starr (1922 [4]) adopted this view and postulated that the infection might be confined as a small local abscess or extend widely within the medulla, particularly along the metaphyseal aspect of the growth plate. In neglected infections, the infection might spread through cortical Haversian canals into the subperiosteal space, or, if the metaphysis were intracapsular, into a joint cavity. If a subperiosteal abscess were to become very large, it might elevate the periosteum completely from the shaft of the bone, causing occlusion of the main nutrient vessels and death of the cortex (sequestrum). In such a situation, the stripped periosteum, provided with its own blood supply from muscle attachments, would lay down new bone in a shell around the old shaft (involucrum; Figure 9-1). Ultimately, cellulitis, soft-tissue abscesses, and sinus formation might occur.

Starr's proposal seemed plausible and has been widely accepted. Leveuf (40) argued that the primary lesion may not be confined to the metaphyseal spongiosa, but may also involve cortex, and, indeed, sometimes the cortex alone. This localization is certainly true of the distinct diaphyseal presentation of HO that comprise most of Leveuf's cases. But it may also be true for metaphyseal HO: Independent discrete subperiosteal abscesses, separated from a typical juxtaphyseal focus, have been observed in an avian experimental model of metaphyseal HO (41).

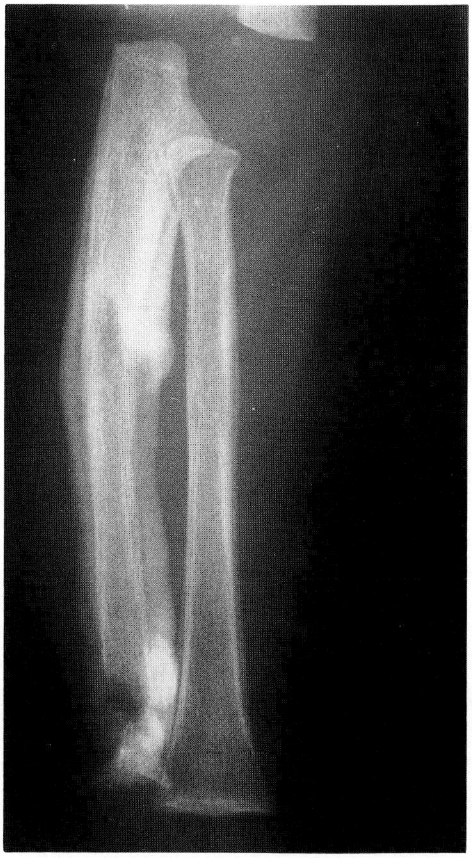

Figure 9-1. *A thick involucrum formed around the shaft of the ulna following osteomyelitis. Destructive changes are greatest in the distal metaphysis. Some reactive new bone formed on the periosteal surface of the uninvolved radius.*

Microbiology

S. aureus has been the most common isolate in almost every clinical report of HO since its first isolation from bone by Pasteur. *S. aureus* bacteremia in the community, however, has been relatively uncommon compared, for example, with that from *Streptococcus pneumoniae* or *Hemophilus influenzae* (42,43). The majority of patients with confirmed staphylococcal bacteremia in childhood (except in immunosuppressed hosts) have bone or joint infections (39).

The source of the bacteremia may be an identified septic focus elsewhere in the body. Reported sites include venous catheterization (44), omphalitis (45), other skin infections (46), tonsilitis, and otitis media (47). The seasonal peak of HO corresponds with that of staphylococcal impetigo (34,48). However, approximately half the reported patients with HO lack an identified source for bacteremia (49). In these individuals, it is assumed that normal mucocutaneous defense mechanisms in the nose and elsewhere are penetrated, without local signs. Nasal and skin carriage of *S. aureus* is common (50), and high rates and more persistent carriage are reported in children (51). Viral infections may enhance mucocutaneous susceptibility (52). Children with a history of cured HO have a higher incidence of nasal carriage of *S. aureus* than age- and sex-matched control subjects (53). In neonates, there is evidence for a relative immune deficiency (54,55). A number of groups have investigated the possibility of a general disorder of immune function in osteoarticular infection (53,56,57). Although the immunosuppressed individuals are clearly at risk, no pattern has emerged in studies of previously healthy individuals.

Mechanism of Bacterial Deposition

Except in neonates and immunosuppressed patients, HO is rarely associated with miliary deep infection (6). This observation, and the preponderance of metaphyseal infections in childhood HO, encouraged speculation on the apparent tropism of *S. aureus*. Lexer (25) believed that the local vascular anatomy in the metaphysis encouraged the mechanical trapping of septic emboli. Koch (58) confirmed that bacteria could indeed be found close to the epiphyseal plate at necropsy in children dying of septicemia, but postulated favorable local conditions for survival and growth, rather than mechanical factors. Starr (4) accepted both these ideas. Hobo (59) pointed out that if septic embolization from distant foci were to occur, then pulmonary abscesses should be expected frequently; in fact, they are reported only rarely (60). Exploring the issue experimentally, Hobo showed that the normal ability of endothelial cells to phagocytose Indian ink particles seemed to be deficient in the metaphyseal capillary loops. Trueta (61), whose work has since been widely quoted, offered a synthesis of the views of Starr and Hobo. Slow flow and phagocytic deficiency, he believed, combined to increase the probability of bacterial deposition. We now know that metaphyseal blood flow rates are high (62), compared, for example, with cortex, diaphyseal marrow, and epiphyseal spongiosa. It is clear that acute HO occurs more commonly in the knee and the hip than in other sites (4–6,49). Ogden (63) revived the old idea of Park (64) that the incidence of infection in different metaphyses is proportional to the size and relative growth contribution of the adjacent physis.

More recent studies offer other possible explanations. There is steady formation of new metaphyseal capillaries during growth, and ultrastructural studies suggest that these capillaries may be fenestrated (65), allowing escape of red blood cells and other blood elements, and presumably smaller structures, into the extravascular space. *S. aureus* has been found adhering to the cartilage of the growth plate at the physometaphyseal junction in experimental avian HO (66). This zone of great metabolic activity may offer opportunities for specific bacterium-substrate adhesion (67). A number of such interactions have now been identified, and the molecular architecture of surface receptors on some strains of *S. aureus* for a number of structural proteins, including vitronectin, fibronectin, type II collagen (7), and bone sialoprotein (8), have been characterized (see Chapter 2).

The etiological role of blunt trauma has been widely accepted based on both observation of the clinical association (1) and on late nineteenth century (22,23,25) and recent (68) experiments, which require local trauma to the metaphysis. Although reliable models have been reported (24,41), it has been difficult to reproduce HO in a mammalian model by injection of bacteria alone. The increased frequency of facial and shoulder girdle HO in infants has also been associated with birth trauma (44). Observational precedent and the bulk of the mammalian experiments support blunt trauma as a significant etiological cofactor, but there are difficulties. The pattern of epiphyseal fractures in childhood is dominated by the lower radius, a less common site in HO (69). Also, there is no firm evidence that local trauma occurs more frequently preceding HO than in the community at large, or that it is more common in boys than girls (70).

Spread of Infection and Complications

The initial abscess in the metaphysis may, as was briefly described earlier, remain contained by host defense mechanisms within the metaphysis and resolve. It may, alternatively, persist as a subacute or chronic localized abscess or spread to involve adjacent structures. The mechanisms of bone death and structural degradation are discussed in Chapter 2. Briefly, these findings appear to confirm that extent and

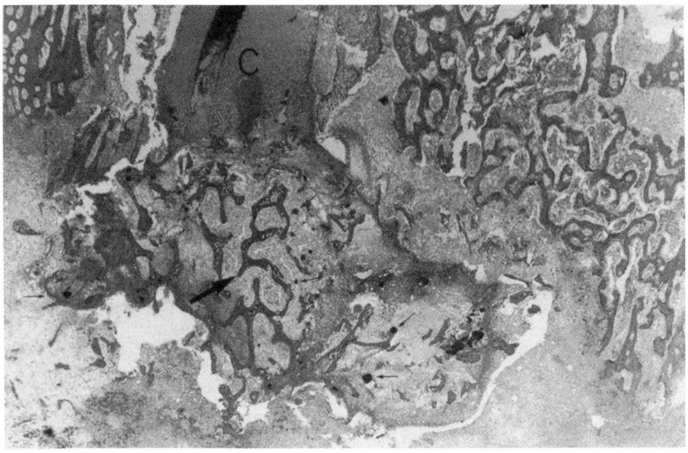

Figure 9-2. *Experimental osteomyelitis in a chicken; surgical drilling was performed 4 days after onset of infection. The drilled zone is shown in the lower half. A sequestrum formed, consisting of the original abscess and surrounding cartilage (C), together with a portion of the drilled region containing bacteria* (small arrows) *and spicules of necrotic bone* (large arrow) *(Hematoxylin and eosin, original magnification × 5.5).*

duration of the inflammatory response determine the degree of local bone destruction. The routes of spread are a matter of controversy. Starr (4) and Trueta (61) proposed that infection could spread from the metaphyseal medulla to the subperiosteal space via Volkmann's canals. If the metaphysis were intracapsular, such spread could enter a joint. The physis was considered in general as a barrier to the spread of infection. The presence in neonates and infants of transphyseal vessels has been demonstrated by Trueta (61) and others (63). It was proposed that this finding might explain both the occasional spread of infection into the epiphysis and the increased frequency of intra-articular spread in infants. Transphyseal spread, however, does occur in older children (71) and has been demonstrated also in the avian experimental model (41). We conclude that the physis is a relative but certainly not an absolute barrier to spread of infection, regardless of whether transphyseal vessels are present.

Can we accept the rather mechanistic idea of escape of pus through Volkmann's canals? Discrete subperiosteal abscesses have been seen both in clinical (40) and experimental (41) situations associated with small and well-localized metaphyseal abscesses, early in the natural history of infection. Is it possible that Leveuf's concept of independent cortical and subperiosteal abscesses is correct? Currently, the evidence is inconclusive. Subperiosteal abscesses certainly occur and are a significant cause of pain and morbidity. In contemporary practice, it is agreed that they should be recognized and drained, unless very small.

Should the metaphysis also be debrided? "Decompression" still receives support, based on the concept of an abscess under tension within the metaphysis awaiting relief (72). Others have argued that once a subperiosteal abscess is present, decompression of bone is redundant (73). The question has recently been studied experimentally (74). In the avian model, bone debridement is associated with significant extension of the area of bone necrosis (Figure 9-2). Furthermore, there is a risk of fracture, through drillholes (Figure 9-3). We believe that there is currently insufficient evidence to justify routine

A B

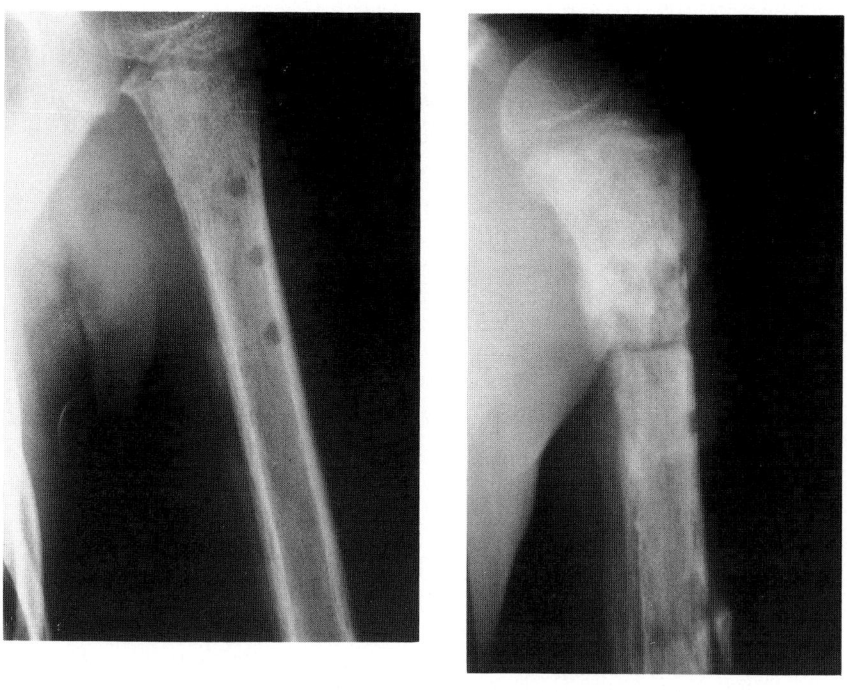

Figure 9-3. *(A) Drilling performed in osteomyelitis of the proximal humerus. (B) A fracture occurred through the weakened area.*

decompression of bone, provided that soft tissue and subperiosteal abscesses have been identified and drained.

Acute Hematogenous Osteomyelitis

Clinical Staging

The pathology of metaphyseal HO is reflected in the three clinical stages described by Trueta (61). In stage I, bone pain and dramatic local tenderness are present without any sign of soft-tissue inflammation. In stage II, as the infection spreads into the subperiosteal space, local signs become more marked. Systemic symptoms and signs appear and may dominate the clinical picture. In stage III, pus is present in the soft tissues, with erythema, swelling, and tenderness.

Recognition

Acute osteoarticular sepsis may usually be diagnosed by history and clinical examination alone, although it may be difficult to distinguish HO from pyogenic arthritis. The typical presentation is an infant, child, or adolescent with fever, some dehydration, pain, and loss of function around a major joint of 12 to 48 hours' duration. Inquiry may indicate a source of infection or predisposing factors. The presence of a painful, tense joint effusion usually indicates septic arthritis, but it is important to remember that metaphyseal or epiphyseal osteomyelitis can cause a sterile "sympathetic effusion." Acute local bone tenderness is the cardinal physical sign of osteomyelitis. This symptom alone should be sufficient in the presence of systemic signs and a fever to make a provisional diagnosis. However, in stage III disease, local swelling and erythema in the soft tissues may give rise to difficulty in distinguishing between osteomyelitis and cellulitis. In the presence of clinical features suggesting HO, a needle aspirate should be performed at the site of maximum tenderness. If there is uncertainty about the presence or location of an abscess, imaging (ultrasound [75] or computerized tomography (CT) [76]) can be helpful in guiding aspiration. Lavage of the site with 5 mL saline is recommended if there is no initial yield. Bacteria may be isolated from this local aspiration in up to 70% of patients (77). Modern techniques for identification of bacterial antigen fragments seem likely to increase the utility of aspiration (78). Blood culture, full blood count, C-reactive protein (CRP), and erythrocyte sedimentation rate (ESR) should also be carried out. In acute HO, white cell count, ESR, and CRP are normally increased. In children with sickle-cell disease, distinction between an infarct and an osteomyelitis may be very difficult clinically. In such circumstances, identification of a subperiosteal abscess by imaging is in favor of infection (79).

Imaging Assessment

Conventional radiology in stage I lesions shows no changes. Nevertheless, radiographs are always performed at presentation, both to exclude other lesions (e.g., Ewing's tumor or leukemia) and to establish a baseline for interpretation of subsequent changes. In stage II lesions, loss of definition of soft-tissue planes can usually be readily identified by conventional radiography and by ultrasound. Both CT and magnetic resonance imaging (MRI) effectively identify the changes that follow development of an inflammatory lesion. CT readily demonstrates a subperiosteal abscess (79); MRI may be particularly useful while the lesion remains confined to bone (80).

Radiological changes of periostitis and bone destruction usually become apparent approximately 10 to 14 days from the onset of the illness. These changes appear more quickly in neonates. The appearance of reactive bony changes at presentation indicates the presence of established disease. In this circumstance, biopsy should be considered unless the appearances are entirely typical of subacute HO.

Although both radionuclide bone and leukocyte scans may be positive early in acute HO, the objective in management is to determine the organism, to select an appropriate antibiotic, and to drain any abscess present. CT or ultrasound readily aid that objective by locating an abscess. Scintigraphy, although it may demonstrate a central photopenic area overlying a zone of increased uptake in a three-phase bone scan (81), lacks the precision to guide aspiration and has only limited indications in acute HO. Its use, we believe, should be reserved for those patients in whom the exact site of the disease is obscure on clinical examination (e.g., pelvis or spine). In such circumstances, it may provide sufficient information for a localized examination by ultrasound or CT.

Initial Management

Systemic fluid support, elevation, and splintage of the affected limb should be instituted immediately. Results of initial examination of the aspirate should be obtained promptly. Once known, antibiotic therapy should be started. If organisms have been identified, the choice of antibiotic, although not definitive until sensitivities become available, can be fairly precise. If organisms are not identified, the infection should be treated on the basis of probability, depending on age. The choice of agent for provisional therapy depends on availability and on the usual sensitivity of likely pathogens, based on local experience. Typically, in infants, provisional therapy should be effective against both gram-positive cocci and enterobacteria. In preschool children, *H. influenzae* type B is a cause of septic arthritis and, increasingly, osteomyelitis (10); until the organism is identified, an agent effective against *H. influenzae* and *S. aureus* (e.g., ceftriaxone) should be used, particularly if there is any suspicion of joint involvement. It is conceivable that with increasing availability of immunization against *H. influenzae* type B, infection with this organism will be less common in the future. In older children, coverage against gram-positive cocci is likely to be adequate.

If a significant abscess, either subperiosteal or in the overlying soft tissues, is identified, it should be drained by surgery or, if readily accessible, by aspiration through a wide-bore needle. In stage I and in some stage II lesions, however, an abscess may not be identified. In these circumstances, a program of antibiotics and supportive therapy should be followed by regular critical review at frequent intervals, and certainly within 24 hours. Stage I and many stage II lesions resolve on this conservative program alone, demonstrating dramatic clinical improvement with lysis of fever within 12 to 24 hours. Persisting systemic signs indicate the high probability of an abscess, for which a vigorous search should be made so that it may be drained.

Another explanation for continuing fever and systemic illness might be that the provisional antibiotic therapy has been inappropriate. In our experience, if the choice has been made as described above, that is unlikely. Once an organism is isolated and its sensitivity known, definitive antibiotic therapy can be determined and administered. In most patients, this means continuation of the "provisional" drug.

Duration and Route of Antibiotic Management

The duration of antibiotic treatment remains controversial. Optimal management involves the shortest antibiotic program compatible with an acceptable cure rate. In contemporary practice, complete resolution of the disease should be expected in more than 95% of patients (6,82). Surprisingly, but unfortunately, no controlled studies have thus far addressed the problem of duration of therapy. Periods as short as 10 days and as long as 6 weeks have been proposed on an empirical basis (6,74,82,83). Practicing clinicians with extensive experience with HO suspect that in stage I and stage II disease at least, quite short courses of 7 to 10 days' therapy suffice. In extensive or neglected disease, where a large volume of infarcted bone is present, it is possible that antibiotics might have a useful adjuvant role for a substantial period until revascularization and repair of the lesion are complete. In view of the costs and potential hazards of prolonged antibiotic therapy, careful clinical trials are indicated; however, until these trials are done, we recommend 3 to 4 weeks of antimicrobial therapy.

The route of antibiotic administration is also controversial. In the English-speaking world outside North America, intravenous antibiotics have generally been given only until control of septicemia seemed secure and the fever abated (6,74,82,83). Antibiotics have then been administered orally. For the most part, this experience has been with semisynthetic penicillins, erythromycin, and fusidic acid. Although oral therapy with such agents was used successfully (84,85), the North American literature has placed a strong emphasis on intravenous administration (49). Interest in oral therapy has increased with the introduction of quinolone antibiotics, but their use has been mainly in patients with chronic osteomyelitis (86). Intravenous programs may be successfully administered at home by regular injection (87). Oral treatment is also successful at home, provided that careful attention is paid to the education of patients and relatives (82,84).

Surgical Management

Whether and when surgical intervention is indicated may be a difficult decision. Modern practice still reflects the teaching of Starr and others from the preantibiotic era, who advocated routine early surgical drainage with incision of the periosteum and drilling or removal of a window of cortical bone to allow drainage from the medulla. A number of studies, however, have cast doubt on the value of indiscriminate surgery. In one large series (6), among the failures of primary treatment was a significantly higher number treated by antibiotics and surgery than by antibiotics alone. In another series (82), nonoperative treatment produced a cure in 78% of patients. In these studies, decision-making was empiric, and patients with a wide range of duration, extent, and clinical severity were included. The place of surgery, therefore, remains to be precisely defined by controlled studies. However, the balance of available evidence supports the policy of selective surgical intervention. Recommended indications for surgery include (a) presence of a significant soft-tissue or subperiosteal abscess, identified either clinically or by imaging techniques (ultrasound or CT) at the time of presentation; and (b) development of such an abscess following initial conservative therapy.

Surgery should be carried out with a pneumatic tourniquet if a distal limb site is involved, but compressive exsanguination is best avoided. The incision, centered over the point of maximum tenderness or the ultrasound detected site, is deepened through the periosteum to release the abscess. Routine drilling or windowing of bone is not recommended, because it is likely that this procedure increases the volume of necrotic bone (75). Necrotic soft tissues, however, should be excised, and copious irrigation should be carried out to wash out or dilute remaining bacteria.

Outcome of Treatment

Recurrence of infection for the first time may occur years or decades after HO (88). Reported cure rates should be interpreted with this fact in mind. However, the majority of failures of primary treatment appear to manifest within one year (6). The fundamental importance of effective antibiotic management in this disease is supported by the observation that recurrence rates, after decreasing dramatically with the introduction of penicillin, increased again in the 1950s to levels approaching those of the preantibiotic era, as penicillin resistance became apparent (6). Introduction of new antibiotic agents has been associated with a reduction in the incidence of failure of primary treatment to approximately 5%.

Complications

The important complications of HO are (a) recurrent or chronic infection; (b) involvement of an adjacent joint; (c) pathological fracture; and (d) disturbance of growth.

Chronic osteomyelitis is considered in Chapter 15. In joints such as the hip and the shoulder, in which the metaphysis is intracapsular, infection spreads readily into the joint. The persistence of transphyseal vessels in infants may facilitate extension into the epiphysis, resulting both in its necrosis and in widespread infection of the joint. Regardless of the route of spread to the joint, the risk of necrosis of the femoral head appears from clinical experience to be substantial. For this reason, urgent decompression is indicated in involvement of the hip joint (see Chapter 18).

Pathological fracture is rare; it occurs in approximately 2% of patients (6). Many pathological fractures occur where the bone has been additionally weakened by windowing or drilling of the cortex (see Figure 9-3). Pathological fractures will usually heal with cast support and antibiotic control of the disease.

The effect of metaphyseal infection on the growth plate depends on the degree of damage. Destruction of the germinal layer of the physis may cause arrest or retardation of growth. In one series (89), limb shortening was found in every patient in a series of children who had osteomyelitis in infancy. Partial destruction of the growth plate may produce an angulatory deformity (90–92). In the leg and the forearm, major ankle or wrist deformity may be a consequence of growth retardation of one bone. If, however, the growth plate itself is undamaged, a period of overgrowth appears to be a normal sequelae of acute osteomyelitis (93). The incidence of growth retardation or deformity as a result of epiphyseal damage has been estimated at approximately 3% (90), but it may be higher in patients with neonatal osteomyelitis (94).

Diaphyseal Osteomyelitis

In neglected typical metaphyseal disease, the infection may spread to involve the diaphysis of long bones. Disease localized to the diaphysis also occurs, most commonly in adults, in whom it may constitute up to half of all cases (72). Both acute and subacute presentations occur, and chronic osteomyelitis may ensue in up to one third of severe diaphyseal infections (94).

Although isolated diaphyseal lesions may be confined to trabecular bone and marrow, many appear to involve the cortex primarily. The pathological anatomy of diaphyseal cortical osteomyelitis was described by Leveuf (40). Distinct intracortical abscesses form, and some Haversian canals contain pus, which results in a characteristic streaky destructive lesion of the cortex (Figure 9-4). Occasionally, a cortical sequestrum may occur (Figure 9-5), necessitating removal.

A B

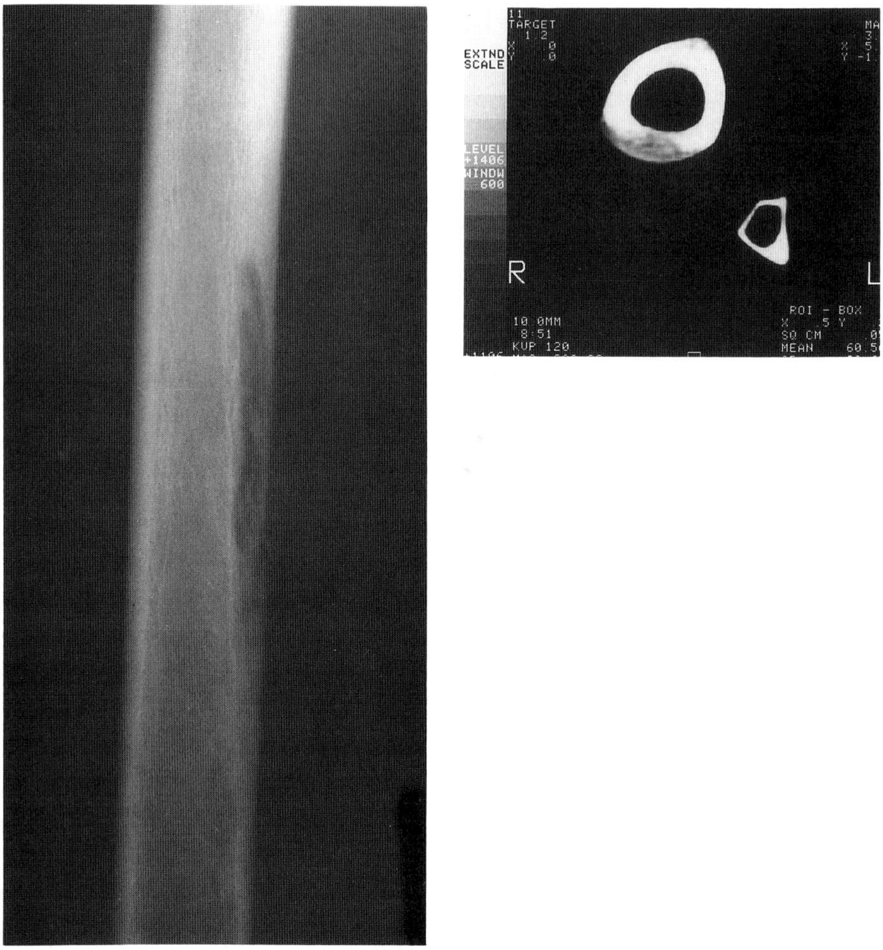

Figure 9-4. *(A) The characteristic streaky or "vermiform" appearance of cortical osteomyelitis. (B) Computerized tomography of cortical osteomyelitis.*

The principles of management of diaphyseal disease are the same as in typical metaphyseal disease.

Subacute Osteomyelitis

Subacute osteomyelitis in the appendicular skeleton may be viewed as an episode of disease contained but not eradicated by the host

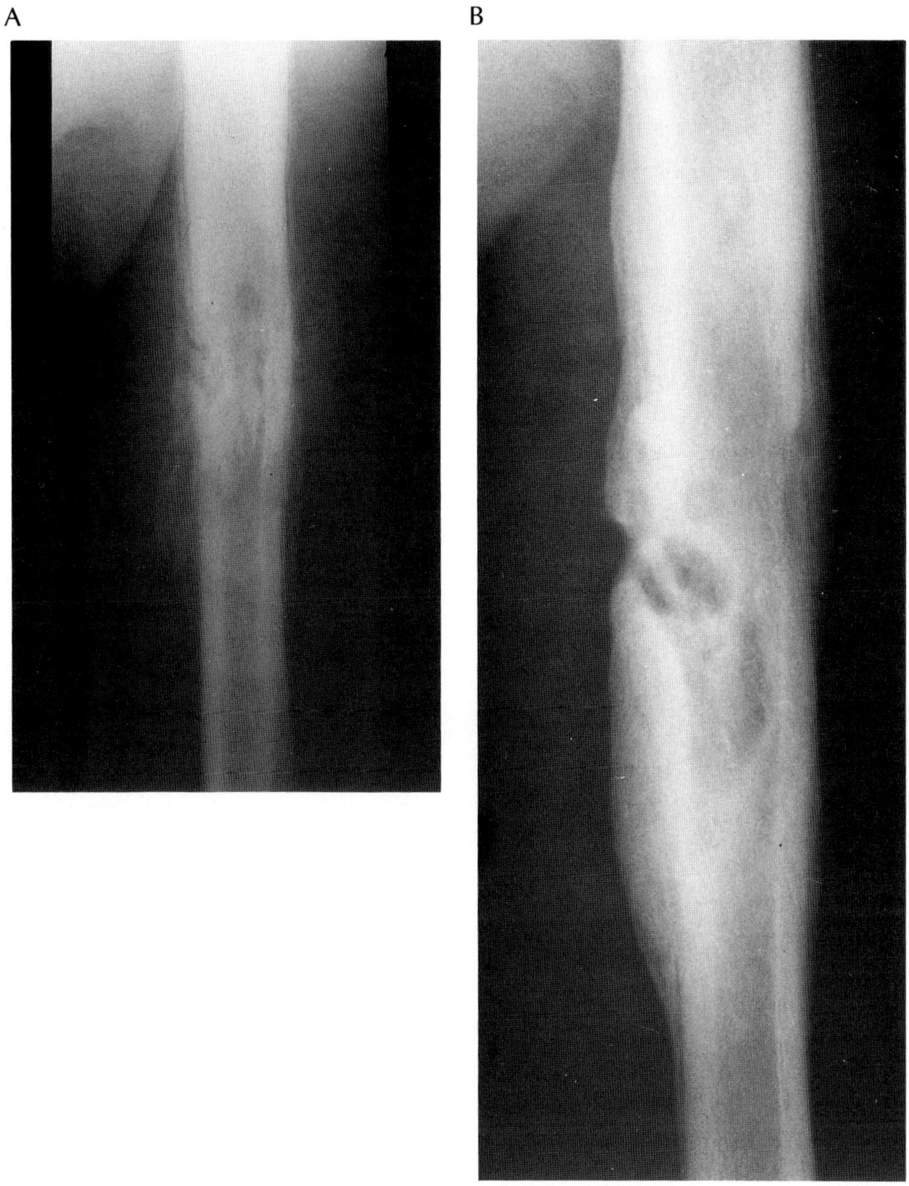

Figure 9-5. *(A) Cortical osteomyelitis around the nutrient foramen of the femur. (B) Eight months later, the periosteal new bone has matured: A small abscess surrounds a sequestrated cortical fragment.*

defenses, usually in stage I. Billroth, in 1881, appears to have introduced the term *subacute osteomyelitis* to describe those patients with osteomyelitis who lacked the typical acute presentation and systemic signs. Before antibiotics were introduced, the term was sometimes used to refer to the early recovery stage after an acute illness (95) or to presentations caused by less virulent organisms, such as *Salmonella typhi* and *S. pneumoniae* (96). In the last 25 years, classifications have evolved that emphasize the radiological appearances seen in primary infections of bone with subacute or indolent presentations (11,29). Common for many years in the European literature (97), the term *primary chronic osteomyelitis* is gaining wider acceptance (98).

Regardless of which nomenclature is favored, the dominant complaint at presentation of these patients is pain, present for at least 2 weeks, but sometimes for many months. Constitutional symptoms are usually absent. Fever, if present, is mild. Local signs of tenderness and loss of function are typically slight. In his original description, Brodie (99) stressed the fluctuant nature of the pain, with exacerbations superimposed on a constant, aching discomfort. Others have found the fluctuating history less impressive. It has been suggested that the pain is more commonly severe at night. Elevation of the ESR is present in less than 50% of patients, and white blood cell count is usually normal. Blood cultures are rarely positive, and subperiosteal abscesses are extremely unusual. Cultures obtained by aspiration, biopsy, or definitive surgery have been positive only in approximately 60% of patients (11). The majority of lesions occur in the tibia, but the tarsal bones are also well represented, particularly the calcaneum. Most patients are under 20 years of age, and males predominate by more than 2:1 (72).

In the classifications of Gledhill (100) and Roberts and colleagues (11), location and radiological nature of the lesion are important (Figures 9-6 to 9-11). However, many subacute presentations lack the specific radiological changes described, and some presentations with characteristic radiology are associated with an acute illness. In comparative studies of therapy, use of a more rigorous general classification in addition to the Gledhill-Roberts classification is desirable.

Microbiology and Pathology

In reports of patients from whom aspirates or surgical biopsy have been obtained, no growth was achieved on culture in 40% (72). The

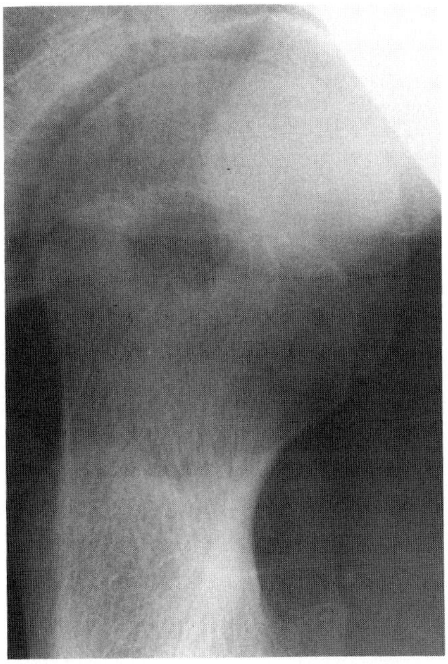

Figure 9-6. *Typical appearance of subacute osteomyelitis (type I).*

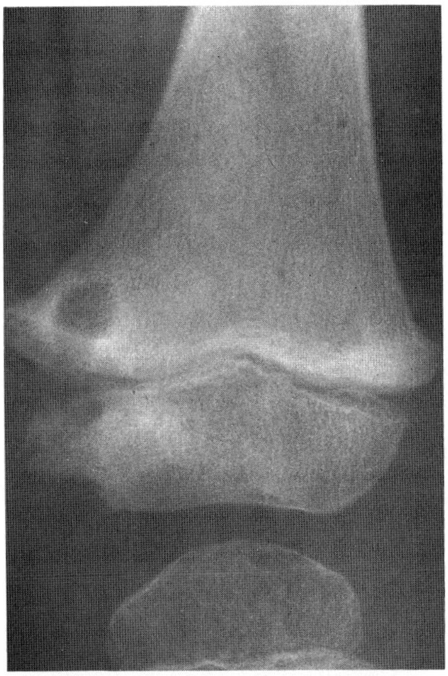

Figure 9-7. *A well-demarcated abscess crossing the physis (type I).*

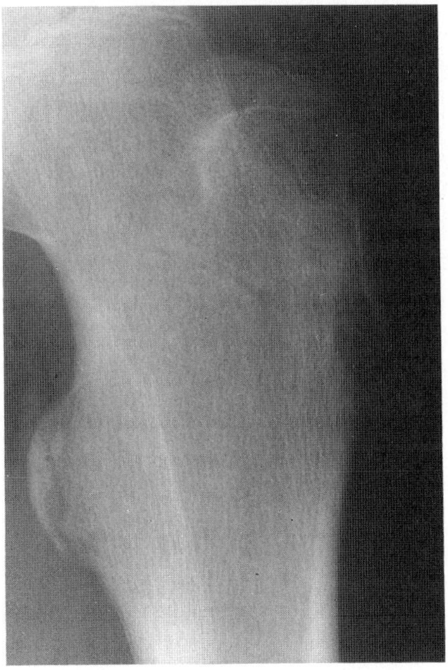

Figure 9-8. *An eccentrically placed metaphyseal infection eroding cortex (type II).*

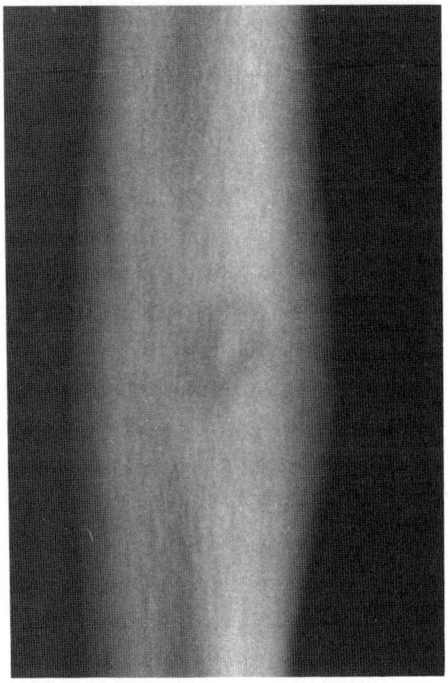

Figure 9-9. *Diaphyseal subacute osteomyelitis with a small sequestrum (type III).*

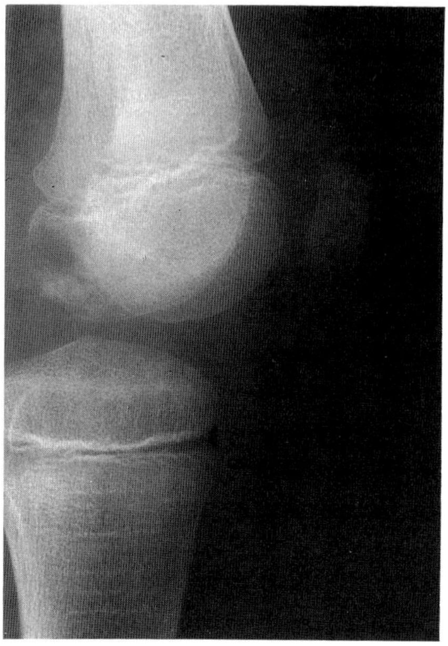

Figure 9-10. *Subacute osteomyelitis confined to the epiphysis (type V).*

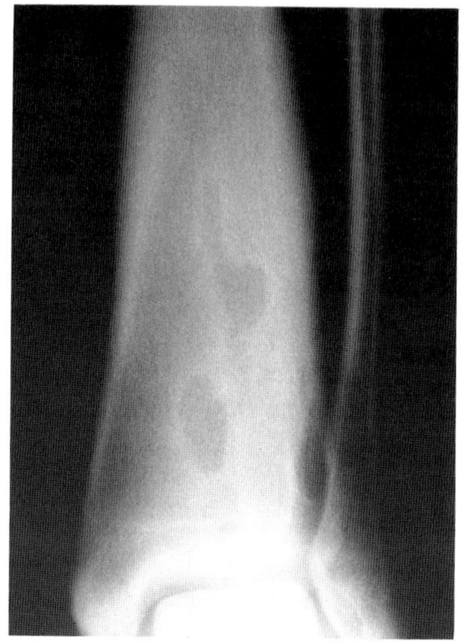

Figure 9-11. *Adolescent distal tibia with evidence of two episodes of infection. The proximal abscess has an elongated, spatulate appearance.*

most common isolate is *S. aureus*. The histopathology of the localized bone abscess has been described in detail (101). Around the abscess is coarse woven new bone with a variable amount of fibrous tissue. The abscess cavity presents a spectrum of histological appearances. Chronic round-cell infiltration is common; this presentation has given rise to the term *plasma-cell osteomyelitis* (30), particularly in the European literature. Foci of acute inflammation may also be seen. The new bone formation is not specific—it may occur around foci of tuberculosis, staphylococcal and other pyogenic infections, as well as in syphilis, typhoid, and fungal osteomyelitis.

Management

Radiological appearances of the typical metaphyseal lesion are sufficiently specific to allow confident and successful management with antibiotics alone, without biopsy. A large series (102) confirmed the efficacy of this practical approach. In most earlier reported series, curettage of the lesion had been carried out in association with antibiotic therapy. Trephine aspiration was reported by Brickner in 1923 (103), but this approach has not received recent attention.

Osteomyelitis in Neonates

Neonatal osteomyelitis deserves special attention because it differs in a number of ways from the typical pattern of HO in older children (104). Its incidence is between 0.1 and 0.3 per 1,000 live births (105). It is more common in low birth weight infants (106).

The pattern of bone involvement is distinct. Upper limb sites are more common than in older children (106); the humerus accounts for nearly 30% of sites in some series (105), which may be due to trauma to the shoulder during birth (107). Although the disseminating focus is often unknown, primary sources of infection are evident in approximately half the patients. Intravascular access sites account for more than half the patients in neonatal intensive care units (106). Other sources include omphalitis (49), purulent rhinitis (108), infected operative sites (109), intramuscular injections (110), and heel puncture (49).

A special feature of neonatal osteomyelitis is the ease and rapidity with which adjacent joints may be involved, perhaps due to the presence of transphyseal vascular connections. Serious joint disease, particularly in the hip, may therefore be a sequelae of neonatal infection (111,112).

Lancefield group B streptococcus, *S. aureus,* and coliform species are currently the main agents associated with neonatal septicemia and osteomyelitis. There is clear evidence of a shift in the pattern of isolates over the last 50 years (44,113–115). Prior to 1940, group A hemolytic streptococci were a common cause of both septicemia and neonatal osteomyelitis, accounting for more than 50% of infections, and in the period between 1950 and 1970, the great majority of neonatal osteomyelitis infections were caused by *S. aureus.*

Two distinct syndromes occur in neonatal osteomyelitis. In the severe form, which occurs in children who have not left hospital since birth, particularly in very young infants in neonatal intensive care areas, signs of septicemia predominate. Bone and visceral abscesses, often multiple, become apparent as the disease progresses. Pseudoparalysis or limb swelling are important signs (105).

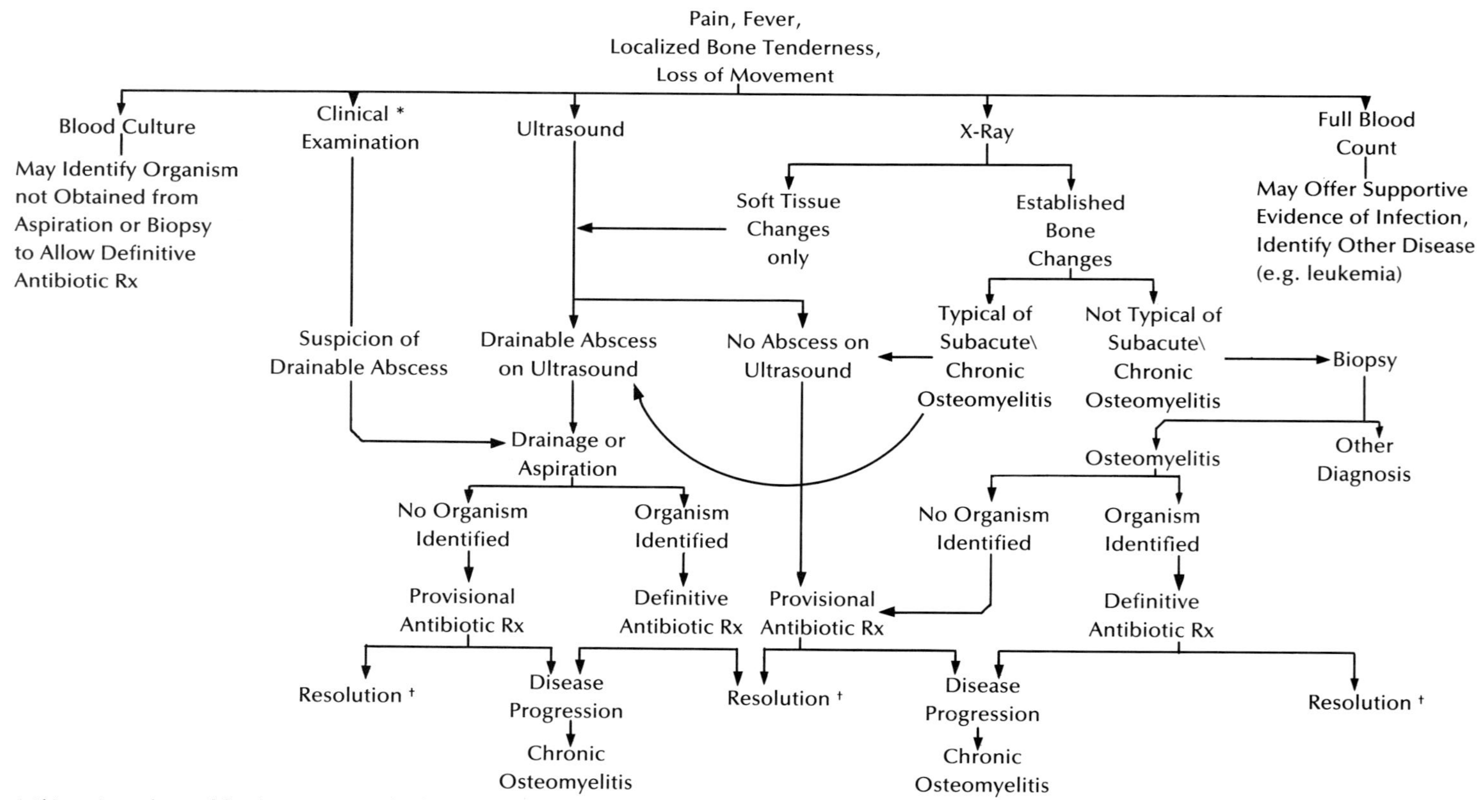

* If imaging of possible abscess unavailable, the decision on drainage must be made on clinical grounds.

† Overall, resolution occurs in around 95% of cases.

Figure 9-12. *Algorithm for investigation and management of acute or subacute hematogenous osteomyelitis*

In slightly older infants, usually in the fourth week of life or later, a subacute presentation is more common. This presentation is rarely recognized in the early stages and is more severe and destructive than the subacute presentations in older children (116). Systemic manifestations may be absent or slight, and temperature, white cell count, and sedimentation rate are normal or moderately increased. The infant may feed well and gain weight. Swelling of the limb and decreased movement, or "pseudoparalysis," are also the most pronounced signs. In this presentation, very large abscesses may be present, particularly around the shoulder.

Principles of management and indications for surgery are essentially the same in neonatal osteomyelitis as in other age groups. Once again, the importance of recognition and adequate drainage of an infected joint cannot be overemphasized. The incidence of permanent handicap, resulting particularly from infection around the hip, has been and remains high (108,111,112,117,118).

Conclusions

In the developed world, HO is becoming less common. In the developing world, there are probably between 10^5 and 10^6 new cases each year; experience in Australian Aboriginals (34), in Papua New Guinea (10), and in Africa (119), for example, shows that HO remains a serious crippling disease. Reports of experience from these areas read much like those from North America and Europe in the early days of antibiotic therapy nearly 50 years ago. Well-designed studies from centers in the developing world could examine some of the outstanding issues in the epidemiology and management of this disease, including the roles of nutritional deficiency, overcrowding, and socioeconomic status. The optimal length of antibiotic therapy remains unknown. Use of a more rigorous classification system should aid the design of studies to answer these and other questions. Sophisticated imaging devices certainly improve the precision of diagnosis and management, but their overall impact is slight compared with that which would follow universal application of simple, cost-effective diagnostic and management programs. An algorithm for investigation and management of HO offers an approach to this disease (Figure 9-12).

References

1. Smith N. Observations on the pathology and treatment of necrosis. Phil J Med Surg 1827;1:11–19; 66–75.
2. Lannelongue OM. De l'osteomyelite aigue pendant la croissance. Paris: Asselin, 1879.
3. Pasteur L. De l'extension de la theorie des germes a l'etiologie de quelques maladies communes. Bull Acad Med (Paris) 1880;9:435–447.
4. Starr C. Acute haematogenous osteomyelitis. Arch Surg 1922;4:567–587.
5. McHenry MC, Alfidi RJ, Wilde AH. Haematogenous osteomyelitis. A changing disease. Cleve Clin Q 1975;42:125–153.
6. Gillespie WJ, Mayo KM. The management of acute haematogenous osteomyelitis in the antibiotic era. A study of the outcome. J Bone Joint Surg [Br] 1981;63:126–131.
7. Faden H, Grossi M. Acute osteomyelitis in children. Reassessment of etiologic agents and their clinical characteristics. Am J Dis Child 1991;145: 65–69.
8. Ryden C, Yacoub AI, Maxe I, et al. Specific binding of bone sialoprotein to Staphylococcus aureus isolated from patients with osteomyelitis. Eur J Biochem 1989;184:331–336.
9. Wilensky AO. Osteomyelitis: its pathogenesis, symptomatology and treatment. New York: The MacMillan Company, 1934.
10. Van Gurp G, Kila R, Hutchison T. Management of childhood haematogenous osteomyelitis in a rural Papua New Guinea hospital. Papua New Guinea Med J 1989;32:117–122.
11. Roberts JM, Drummond DS, Breed AL. Subacute haematogenous osteomyelitis in children. J Pediatr Orthop 1982;2:249–254.
12. Pickett JC. A short historical sketch of osteomyelitis. Ann Med Hist 1935;7:183–191.
13. Roney JG. Palaeopathology of a Californian archeological site. Bull Hist Med 1959;33:97–109.
14. Aurelianus C. In: Drabkin IE, ed. On chronic diseases. 5. Sciatica and psoitis. Chicago: University of Chicago Press, 1950.
15. Singhal GD, Singh LM, Singh KF. Diagnostic considerations in ancient Indian surgery. In: Singhal GD, Singh LM, Singh KF, ed. The diagnosis of abscesses. India: Allahabad, 1972.
16. Augustin FL. De Spina Ventosa Ossium. Halle: 1797.
17. Severinus MA. De Recondita Abscessuum Natura. Naples: 1632.
18. Cheselden W. The anatomy of the human body. London: Hitch and Dabsby, 1756.
19. Chassaignac E. Memoire sur l'osteomyelite. Gazette Med 19 Aug, 9 Sept, 16 Sept, 1854.
20. Billroth T. Clinical surgery. London: The New Sydenham Society, 1881.
21. Lister J. Relation of microorganisms to inflammation. Lancet 1881;2:695.

22. Rosenbach J. Beitrage zur Kenntniss der Osteomyelitis. Dtsch Z Chir 1878;10:369–393.
23. Becker PF. Le microcoque specifique de l'osteomyelite aigue. Semin Med 1883;3:374.
24. Rodet A. Etude experimentale sur l'osteomyelite infectieuse. Compt Rend Acad Sci 1884;569–571.
25. Lexer E. Zur experimentellen erzeugung osteomyelitischer herde. Arch Klin Chir 1894;48:181–200.
26. Crossan ET. Haematogenous osteomyelitis: collective review of the literature from 1932–1937. Int Abstr Surg 1938;66:176–183.
27. Albee F. Treatment of osteomyelitis by bacteriophage. J Bone Joint Surg 1933;15:58–66.
28. Kleiger B, Blair JE. Correlation between clinical and experimental findings in cases showing invasion of the bloodstream by staphylococci. Surg Gynecol Obstet 1940;7:770–777.
29. Waldvogel FA, Medoff G, Swartz MN. Osteomyelitis: a review of clinical features, therapeutic considerations and unusual aspects. N Engl J Med 1970;282:198–206.
30. Exner GU. Die plasmacellulare osteomyelitis. Langenbecks Arch Klin Chir 1970;326:165–185.
31. Cierny G, Mader JT. Adult chronic osteomyelitis. Orthopedics 1984;7:1557–1564.
32. Peterson HA. Musculoskeletal infections in children. AAOS Instr Courst Lect 1984;33:33–37.
33. Miller FJW, Court SDM, Knox EG. The school years in Newcastle upon Tyne. London: Oxford University Press, 1974.
34. Gillespie WJ. The epidemiology of acute haematogenous osteomyelitis of childhood. Int J Epidemiol 1985;14:600–606.
35. Shandley B. Acute haematogenous osteomyelitis: a review of 300 cases. S Afr Med J 1960;34:520–524.
36. Trueta J. Studies in the development and decay of the human frame. Philadelphia: WB Saunders, 1968.
37. Chung SMK, Hardman J, Matsurro A. Protein calorie malnutrition in osteomyelitis and septic arthritis. Orthop Trans 1983;9:505.
38. Craigen MA, Watters J, Hackett JS. The changing epidemiology of osteomyelitis in children. J Bone Joint Surg [Br] 1992;74:541–545.
39. Espersen F, Frimodt-Moller N, Thamdrup Rosdahl V, Skinhoj P, Bentzon MW. Changing pattern of bone and joint infections due to Staphylococcus aureus: study of cases of bacteremia in Denmark, 1959–1988. Rev Infect Dis 1991;13:347–358.
40. Leveuf J. Les lesions initiales de l'osteomyelite aigue. Rev Orthop 1948;33:177–216.
41. Emslie KR, Nade S. Acute haematogenous staphylococcal osteomyelitis: a description of the natural history in an avian model. Am J Pathol 1983;110:333–345.

42. McCarthy PL, Grundy GW, Spiesel SZ, Dolan TF. Bacteremia in children: an outpatient clinical review. Pediatrics 1976;57:861–868.
43. Fleisher GR. Management of children with occult bacteremia who are treated in the emergency department. Rev Infect Dis 1991;13(suppl 2): S156–S159.
44. Edwards MS, Baker CJ, Wagner ML, Taber LH, Barrett FF. An etiologic shift in infantile osteomyelitis: the emergence of the group B streptococcus. J Pediatr 1978;93:578–583.
45. Dennison WM, McPherson DA. Haematogenous osteitis of infancy. Arch Dis Child 1952;27:375–381.
46. Thomson J, Lewis IC. Osteomyelitis in the newborn. Arch Dis Child 1950;25:273–279.
47. Robertson DE. Acute septic osteomyelitis. Med J Aust 1925;2:66–68.
48. Dillon HC. Impetigo contagiosa: suppurative and nonsuppurative complications. I. Clinical, bacteriologic and epidemiologic characteristics of impetigo. Am J Dis Child 1968;115:530–541.
49. Dich VQ, Nelson JD, Haltalin KC. Osteomyelitis in infants and children: a review of 163 cases. Am J Dis Child 1975;129:1273–1278.
50. Williams RED. Healthy carriage of Staphylococcus aureus: its prevalence and importance. Bacteriol Rev 1963;27:56–71.
51. Armstrong-Esther CA, Smith JE. Carriage patterns of staphylococcus aureus in a healthy non-hospital population of adults and children. Ann Hum Biol 1976;3:221–227.
52. Fainstein V, Husher DM. Bacterial adherence to pharyngeal cells during viral infection. J Infect Dis 1980;141:172–176.
53. Gillespie WJ, Haywood Farmer M, Fong R, Harding SM. Some aspects of the microbe-host relationship in staphylococcal haematogenous osteomyelitis. Orthopedics 1987;10:475–480.
54. Kuo KN, Lloyd Roberts GC, Orme IM, Soothill JF. Immunodeficiency and infantile bone and joint infection. Arch Dis Child 1975;50:51–56.
55. Klein RB, Fischer TJ, Gard SE, Biberstein M, Rich KC, Stiehm ER. Decreased mononuclear and polymorphonuclear chemotaxis in human newborns, infants and young children. Pediatrics 1977;60:467–472.
56. Williams RC, Dossett JH, Quie PG. Comparative studies of immunoglobulin opsonins in osteomyelitis and other established infections. Immunology 1969;17:249–265.
57. Veys EM, Gabriel PA, Priet JR, van-der-Jeught JD, van-Overschelde JL, Mastelinck CM. Humoral immunity in osteomyelitis and infectious arthritis. Acta Orthop Belg 1975;41:84–98.
58. Koch J. Untersuchungen uber die localisation der bakterien. Z Hyg Infect 1911;69:436–459.
59. Hobo T. Zur pathogenesis der akuten haematogen osteomyelitis. Acta Sch Med Univ Kioto 1921;4:1–29.
60. Felman AH, Shulman ST. Staphylococcal osteomyelitis, sepsis and pulmonary disease. Radiology 1975;117:649–655.

61. Trueta J. The three types of acute haematogenous osteomyelitis: a clinical and vascular study. J Bone Joint Surg [Br] 1959;41:671–680.
62. Light TR, McKinstry MR, Schnitzer J, Ogden JA. Bone blood flow: regional variation with skeletal maturation. In: Arlet J, Ficat RP, Hungerford DS, eds. Bone circulation. Baltimore: Williams & Wilkins, 1984.
63. Ogden JA. Pediatric osteomyelitis and septic arthritis. The pathology of neonatal disease. Yale J Biol Med 1979;52:423–448.
64. Park R. On the deformities and malformations resulting from acute infections in bone. Trans Am Orthop Assoc 1896;8:102–115.
65. Kalayjian DB, Cooper RR. Osteogenesis of the epiphysis. A light and electron microscopic study. Clin Orthop 1972;85:242–256.
66. Alderson M, Speers DJ, Emslie K, Nade S. Acute haematogenous osteomyelitis and septic arthritis: a single disease. J Bone Joint Surg [Br] 1986;68: 268–274.
67. Gristina AG, Oga M, Webb LX, Hobgood CD. Adherent bacterial colonization in the pathogenesis of osteomyelitis. Science 1985;228:990–993.
68. Whalen JL, Fitzgerald RH, Morrissy RT. A histological study of acute haematogenous osteomyelitis following epiphyseal injuries in rabbits. J Bone Joint Surg [Am] 1988;70:1383–1392.
69. Buhr AJ, Cooke AM. Fracture patterns. Lancet 1959;1:531–536.
70. Wald R. Risk factors for osteomyelitis. Am J Med 1985;78:206–212.
71. Gillespie WJ, Moore TE, Mayo KM. Subacute pyogenic osteomyelitis. Orthopedics 1986;9:1565–1570.
72. Goldschmidt RK, Hoffman EB. Osteomyelitis and septic arthritis in children. Curr Orthop 1991;5:248–255.
73. Blockey NJ, Watson JT. Acute osteomyelitis in children. J Bone Joint Surg [Br]1970;52:77–87.
74. Emslie KR, Nade SML. Acute haematogenous staphylococcal osteomyelitis: the effect of surgical drilling and curettage on an avian model. Pathology 1986;18:227–233.
75. Howard CB, Einhorn M, Dagan R, Nyska M. Ultrasound in diagnosis and management of acute haematogenous osteomyelitis in children. J Bone Joint Surg [Br] 1993;75:79–82.
76. Mueller PR, Ferruci JT, Wittenberg J, Simeone JF, Butch RJ. Iliopsoas abscess. Treatment by CT guided percutaneous catheter drainage. Am J Roentgenol 1984;142:359–362.
77. Aronoff SC, Scoles PV. Treatment of childhood skeletal infections. Pediatr Clin North Am 1983;3:271–280.
78. Ryden C, Yacoub A, Kvarnstrom A, et al. Detection of Staphylococcus aureus infection by enzyme-linked immunoabsorbent assay and immunoblotting, using high molecular weight staphylococcal proteins. FEMS Microbiol Immunol 1990;2:65–73.
79. Stark JE, Glasier CM, Blasier RD, Aronson J, Seibert JJ. Osteomyelitis in children with sickle cell disease: early diagnosis with contrast enhanced CT. Radiology 1991;179:731–733.

80. Hovi I, Hekali P, Korhola O, et al. Detection of soft tissue and skeletal infections with ultra-low field (0.02T) MR imaging. Acta Radiol 1989;30:495–499.
81. Allwright SJ, Miller JH, Gilsanz V. Subperiosteal abscess in children: scintigraphic appearance. Radiology 1991;179:731–733.
82. Cole WG, Dalziel RE, Leitl S. Treatment of acute osteomyelitis in childhood. J Bone Joint Surg [Br] 1982;64:218–223.
83. Editorial: Antibiotics for osteomyelitis. Lancet 1975:1:153–154.
84. Bryson YJ, Connor JD, Le Clerc M, Giammona ST. High dose oral dicloxacillin treatment of acute staphylococcal osteomyelitis in children. J Pediatr 1979;94:673–675.
85. Kolyvas E, Ahronheim G, Marks MI, Gledhill R, Owen H, Rosenthal L. Oral antibiotic therapy of skeletal infections in children. Pediatrics 1980;65:867–871.
86. Mader JT, Cantrill JS, Calhoun J. Oral ciprofloxacin compared with standard parenteral antibiotic therapy for chronic osteomyelitis in adults. J Bone Joint Surg [Am] 1990;72:104–110.
87. Grizzard MB, Harris G, Karns H. Use of outpatient parenteral antibiotic therapy in a health maintenance organization. Rev Infect Dis 1991;13(suppl 2):S174–S179.
88. Gallie WE. First recurrence of osteomyelitis eighty years after infection. J Bone Joint Surg [Br] 1951;33:110–111.
89. Roberts PH. Disturbed epiphyseal growth at the knee after osteomyelitis in infancy. J Bone Joint Surg [Br] 1970;52:692–703.
90. Macey HB. Epiphyseal changes resulting from acute infections of bone. Am J Surg 1940;50:239–248.
91. Langenskiold A. Growth disturbance after osteomyelitis of femoral condyles in infants. Acta Orthop Scand 1984;55:1–13.
92. Tudisco C, Farsetti P, Gatti S, Ippolito E. Influence of chronic osteomyelitis on skeletal growth: analysis at maturity of 26 cases affected during childhood. J Pediatr Orthop 1991;11:358–363.
93. Gilmour WN. Acute haematogenous osteomyelitis. J Bone Joint Surg [Br] 1962;44:841–853.
94. Bergdahl S, Ekengran K, Eriksson M. Neonatal hematogenous osteomyelitis: risk factors for long-term sequelae. J Pediatr Orthop 1985;5:564–568.
95. Nichols EH. Subacute and chronic infectious osteomyelitis: its pathology and treatment. JAMA 1904;42:439–466.
96. Knaggs RL. The inflammatory and toxic diseases of bone. Bristol: Wright and Sons, 1926.
97. Jani L, Remagen W. Primary chronic osteomyelitis. Int Orthop 1983;7: 79–83.
98. Cole WG. The management of chronic osteomyelitis. Clin Orthop 1991;264:84–89.
99. Brodie BC. An account of some cases of chronic abscess of the tibia. Trans Med Chir Soc 1832;17:238–249.

100. Gledhill RB. Subacute osteomyelitis in children. Clin Orthop 1973;96: 37–69.
101. Collins DH. Pathology of bone. London: Butterworths, 1966.
102. Ross ERS, Cole WG. Treatment of subacute osteomyelitis in childhood. J Bone Joint Surg [Br] 1985;67:443–448.
103. Brickner WM. The treatment of chronic bone abscesses by simple evacuation through a small drill hole. J Bone Joint Surg 1923;5:492–500.
104. Knudsen CJ, Hoffman EB. Neonatal osteomyelitis. J Bone Joint Surg [Br] 1990;72:846–851.
105. Klein JO, Marcy SM. Bacterial infections. In: Remington JS, Klein JO, eds. Infectious diseases of the fetus and newborn infant. Philadelphia: WB Saunders, 1976:747–891.
106. Ish Horowicz MR, McIntyre P, Nade S. Bone and joint infections caused by multiply resistant Staphylococcus aureus in a neonatal intensive care unit. Pediatr Infect Dis J 1992;11:82–87.
107. Ogden JA, Lister G. The pathology of neonatal osteomyelitis. Pediatrics 1975;55:474–478.
108. Lindblad B, Ekengren K, Aurelius G. The prognosis of acute haematogenous osteomyelitis and its complications during early infancy after the advent of antibiotics. Acta Paediatr Scand 1965;54:24–32.
109. Green N, Nyhan WL, Fousek MD. Acute haematogenous osteomyelitis. Pediatrics 1956;17:368–381.
110. Aractingi TR. Etude de 32 cas d'Osteomyelite du nouveaune. Rev Chir Orthop 1961;47:50–63.
111. Williamson JB, Galasko CS, Robinson MJ. Outcome after acute osteomyelitis in preterm infants. Arch Dis Child 1990;65:1060–1062.
112. Jackson MA, Burry VF, Olson LC. Pyogenic arthritis associated with adjacent osteomyelitis: identification of the sequela-prone child. Pediatr Infect Dis J 1992;11:9–13.
113. Vesikari T, Isolauri E, Tupparainen N, et al. Neonatal septicaemia in Finland 1980–85. Predominance of group B streptococcal infections with very early onset. Acta Paediatr Scand 1989;78:44–50.
114. Hanninen P, Terho P, Toivanen A. Septicaemia in a paediatric unit: a twenty-year study. Scand J Infect Dis 1971;3:201–208.
115. Crosson FJ, Fedcer HM, Bocchini JA, Hackell JM, Hackell JG. Neonatal sepsis at the Johns Hopkins Hospital 1969–1975. Johns Hopkins Med J 1977;140:37–41.
116. Dennison WM. Haematogenous osteitis in the newborn. Lancet 1955;269:474–476.
117. Betz RR, Cooperman DR, Wopperer JM, et al. Late sequence of septic arthritis of the hip in infancy and childhood. J Pediatr Orthop 1990;10:365–372.
118. Ho NK, Low YP, See HF. Septic arthritis in the newborn—a 17 years clinical experience. Singapore Med J 1989;30:356–358.

CHAPTER 10

Post-traumatic and Contiguous Osteomyelitis

Waldvogel and colleagues (1), in proposing a classification based on the route by which infecting organisms reached bone, distinguished between post-traumatic osteomyelitis and osteomyelitis arising from a contiguous soft-tissue infection. In practice, it is usually difficult to determine, in the context of an injured or operated limb in which the fascial planes have been disrupted, whether an infection has arisen in the bone or in the injured soft tissues. In some situations, such as penetrating injuries of the foot or the hand, involvement of two adjacent bones suggests a primary soft-tissue infection. Osteomyelitis arising in decubitus ulcers is an important example of contiguous spread. Contiguous infections associated with vascular insufficiency are considered in Chapter 11.

The principles of management of established chronic osteomyelitis, regardless of its source, are discussed in Chapter 15, and prevention and management of infection in total joint replacement are discussed in Chapter 17. In this chapter, we discuss risk factors for and prophylaxis against infection after injury or surgery; recognition of infection; and early management strategies that may prevent chronic complications. Some examples of infection in special sites are also considered.

Methodological Issues in Prophylaxis

In assessing the literature on prevention of infection in fracture management, a number of issues of nomenclature and methodology require attention. These issues include the desirability of using randomized, blinded methods in comparative studies, and, when these methods are not appropriate, ensuring that the quality of cohort and case-control studies meets contemporary standards. Specifically, the outcome measure—local infection—needs to be clearly defined (2). Categories recorded include "cellulitis," "superficial," "deep soft tissue," "deep," and "osteomyelitis," but the definitions of each, where described, have varied (3–6). Adequate follow-up is essential. Only 50% of infections are apparent by 3 weeks after injury (6); the remainder become apparent over many months. Stratification by known risk factors for nosocomial wound infection, which include sex and age (7), length of operation, preoperative hospital stay (7,8), preoperative serum albumin levels, and absolute lymphocyte count (8), is desirable. Because the site, size, and nature of the open fracture have been clearly established as important variables determining outcome (6,10; Table 10-1), com-

Table 10-1. Classification of open fractures

WOUND		FRACTURE	INFECTION RATES (%)
Type I:	< 1cm long; usually clean puncture; minimal soft-tissue damage.	Usually simple, transverse, or short oblique, with little comminution.	0–2
Type II:	> 1 cm long; moderate contamination; slight to moderate soft-tissue crusting.	Moderate comminution; moderate contamination.	2–7
Type III:	extensive damage to soft tissues.	Major comminution and instability.	
Type IIIA:	adequate soft-tissue coverage of fracture.	Fracture segmental or severely comminuted; includes any high-energy fracture, regardless of wound size.	7
Type IIIB:	extensive injury to or loss of soft tissue, periosteal stripping, exposure of bone.	Massive contamination; severe comminution.	10–50
Type IIIC:	associated with arterial injury regardless of degree of soft-tissue injury.		25–50

Adapted from Gustilo RB, Merkow RL, Templeman D. The management of open fractures. J Bone Joint Surg [Am] 1990;72:299–304.

parative studies that fail to match wound classification are also significantly confounded. Overall infection rates in cross-sectional studies depend arbitrarily on the proportion of different fracture grades and fracture sites involved. It is also difficult to control outcome studies for the quality of wound excision.

Prophylaxis for Closed Fracture Osteosynthesis

Use of internal fixation has become widely accepted in the last 20 years. Although the infection rate is higher following open fractures, the majority of osteosyntheses are carried out in closed fractures. Four placebo-controlled studies examined the effect of antibiotic prophylaxis compared with placebo in older patients with closed hip fractures (8,9,11,12). The two early studies indicated a sixfold reduction of risk of infection after 48 to 72 hours of antimicrobial administration. Surprisingly, this difference was not statistically significant at the chosen levels in either study, and in one (12), follow-up of 10 days was inadequate to identify the deep infection rate with any confidence. The two recent studies demonstrated a reduction in deep infection rate with antibiotic prophylaxis, but the 95% confidence intervals extend across unity in each. Thus, these studies failed to confirm the possibility of a modest protective effect of antibiotic prophylaxis in this group of patients. A fifth randomized study compared antibiotic with no prophylaxis in a similar population of elderly patients with hip fracture and found a significant reduction of infection rate in the treated group (13). However, the infection rate in the control group was extremely high by contemporary standards. Superficial or deep infections in elderly patients with hip fracture are a major source of morbidity. Perioperative antibiotic prophylaxis is widely accepted, and the published studies lack the power to refute its usefulness. Therefore, we recommend that perioperative antibiotic prophylaxis should be employed, but further studies need to be carried out.

For osteosynthesis of a range of closed fractures in a general trauma unit, only two placebo-controlled, randomized trials have been reported (14,15). Both lacked study power to confirm a reduction in deep infection rate. Both showed evidence of a reduction in superficial wound infection, but this reduction was significant in one study only (14). In the other, the authors concluded that because the reduction was not significant, there was no need for prophylactic antibiotics when internally fixing low-energy fractures (15). We do not consider this conclusion justified; rather, the need for further investigations is once more highlighted.

Although more powerful studies are desirable, it may be difficult to obtain ethical approval for further placebo-controlled investigations. Studies comparing single-dose prophylaxis with the longer regimens previously evaluated, however, may be acceptable and would be of value. Currently, we recommend that prophylaxis, introduced immediately prior to surgery and lasting 12 to 18 hours, should be offered to all patients with closed fractures undergoing operative fixation.

Prophylaxis for Open Fractures

Prior to the development of antiseptic and aseptic routines in surgery, the preferred initial management of significant open fractures was amputation. In contemporary practice, only a small number of very severe limb injuries, characterized by validated risk assessment protocols (16), are managed this way. Infection, however, remains a complication associated with considerable morbidity, including delayed and nonunion, poor functional outcome, and a small but significant incidence of late amputation (3,17). Prevention, therefore, has been a focus of attention.

Development and general adoption of wound management techniques directed toward thorough excision of dead and barely viable tissue (18) and early transfer of well vascularized soft-tissue flaps (19) have been and remain important elements in prevention. The importance of wound excision came to dominate surgical thought to the extent that many units in the late 1960s and early 1970s forbade the use of prophylactic antibiotics. In the last 20 years, evidence has emerged in favor of antibiotic prophylaxis, and it is now widely used, if not always in accordance with established principles. Indeed, so powerful has the reputation of antimicrobials become that the importance of adequate surgical toilet and excision of inadequately vascularized tissue (debridement) again requires emphasis.

The utility of quantitative biopsy to assist selection of antimicrobial prophylaxis has been studied. The degree of bacterial contamination of the wound during and at the end of surgical debridement has shown a strong correlation between the number of bacteria in standard samples at the end of debridement and subsequent infection

(20), but no significant correlation with those taken earlier. Essentially, quantitative biopsy is a proxy measure for the adequacy of surgical debridement, but results are not available at the time of surgery. Thus, because it is time-consuming and expensive, its routine use cannot be recommended.

Risk Factors for Infection in Open Fractures

Although surgeons have historically viewed the presence of implants in open fractures as a risk factor (in response to which the widespread use of external fixation ensued), recent studies suggest that the nature and management of open-fracture wounds are more important (6,21) than the method of fixation. A multicenter study (6) confirmed that a fracture grading of IIIb/IIIc; the need for, and the volume of, blood transfusion; and location of the injury below the knee significantly increase the relative risk. Surprisingly, in this study, age, injury severity score, and delay between injury and antibiotic or surgical treatment were not associated with increased risk of local infection around the fracture site. However, age, injury severity score, and blood transfusion were risk factors for distant site nosocomial infection.

Delayed primary closure or secondary closure after major open fractures, particularly gun shot wounds, are considered fundamental principles of wound management (9,17,20). In comparable wound circumstances, however, provided that adequate debridement has been achieved, primary closure may be as safe as delayed primary closure (22). The results of this study should not be interpreted as allowing primary closure to take precedence over adequate debridement; as its authors point out, delaying closure after adequate debridement, because it does not increase the infection rate, may be a prudent decision.

Experimental studies (23–25) established that antibiotics administered before or within 4 to 6 hours of the creation of an experimental skin wound significantly reduced the development of infection and increased the size of the inoculum necessary to create it. In open fractures, the great majority of wounds are contaminated by presentation and are likely to have been so for a number of hours. Therefore, administration of antibiotics as soon as possible after injury is a rational goal. However, delay in treatment may often mean that antibiotics, although potentially prophylactic against the spread of infection associated with the violation of tissue planes during surgical management of the fracture, will not prevent establishment and proliferation of micro-organisms in poorly vascularized areas, including bared bone surfaces. The levels of protection achieved in osteosynthesis of closed fractures or in joint replacement cannot be attained with antibiotic prophylaxis of open fractures (Table 10-2).

Two randomized studies demonstrated an advantage of antibiotic prophylaxis over placebo in open fracture management. In one in which the fractures were graded according to open fracture severity (3), the proportion of severe (grade III) fractures was higher in the antibiotic group, which could have been expected to reduce apparent effectiveness. The earlier study was influential in encouraging widespread adoption of antibiotic prophylaxis but is methodologically flawed in a number of aspects (26). However, the evidence for a protective effect is sufficiently strong for antibiotic prophylaxis to be advised and for further placebo-controlled studies to be ethically questionable.

In both studies, the duration of prophylaxis was 10 days. The principles established by experimental studies (23–25) and experience in prophylaxis in other clinical situations (27,28) suggests that much shorter programs should be effective. A recent study indicates that a single dose of cefonicid is as effective as 5 days of cefonicid or cefamandole if given within 6 hours of injury, shortly before surgical debridement and osteosynthesis (16).

Because appreciable numbers of gram-negative infections are now seen after open fracture, particularly in North America, broad-spectrum agents have been examined. Randomized trials reported thus far have shown no significant differences between antibiotic agents provided that their spectrum of activity includes *Staphylococcus aureus,* but these studies may have lacked power (17,29).

Table 10-2. Deep infection rates reported in fracture management with antibiotic prophylaxis

Closed fracture osteosynthesis	1.5% (13)
Proximal femoral fractures in the elderly	1% (8)
Grade I open fractures	2% (9)
Grade II open fractures	2%–7% (9)
Grade III open fractures	10%–25% (9)

We conclude that patients with open fractures should receive prophylaxis with a cephalosporin, such as cefazolin, cefamandole, or cefonicid, for no longer than 24 hours. This regimen should be seen as an adjuvant to thorough and careful wound debridement; a decision regarding the method and timing of wound closure should be made after consideration of the local conditions in the wound.

Prophylaxis in Amputation

Most lower extremity amputations are carried out for ischemic necrosis; other indications include severe open fractures with irretrievable soft-tissue damage (16) and chronic osteomyelitis (30). In each circumstance, use of antimicrobial prophylaxis is intuitively indicated. In a placebo-controlled, randomized study in amputation for ischemia, use of a broad-spectrum agent, cefoxitin, for 24 hours significantly reduced the infection rate compared with placebo (31). In another randomized study, methicillin was as effective as cephalothin (32). Antibiotic prophylaxis is indicated in lower extremity amputation.

Evaluation and Management of Infected Osteosynthesis

Figure 10-1 illustrates a management algorithm for infected osteosynthesis. The principles on which it is established are based on the cumulative experience of many investigators (4,10,19,21,26,29,33–37) rather than comparative studies. The main principle is retention of fracture fixation. Whether debridement and implant exchange are required depends on the natural history of the individual infection.

When infection becomes apparent, evaluation of the wound using ultrasound will determine the presence or absence of a collection requiring drainage (38). Occasional small fascial collections, which may be seen in cellulitis, are not an indication for surgical drainage, but their aspiration may identify the causative organism. In the absence of a collection or a wound discharge, empiric antibiotic therapy with a broad-spectrum agent should be begun.

If a collection or a wound discharge is present, drainage and debridement should be carried out and empiric antimicrobial therapy begun pending identification of an organism. We believe it is appropriate to delay skin closure for 2 to 3 days, but the decision should be individualized. Antibiotic therapy should be adjusted once sensitivi-

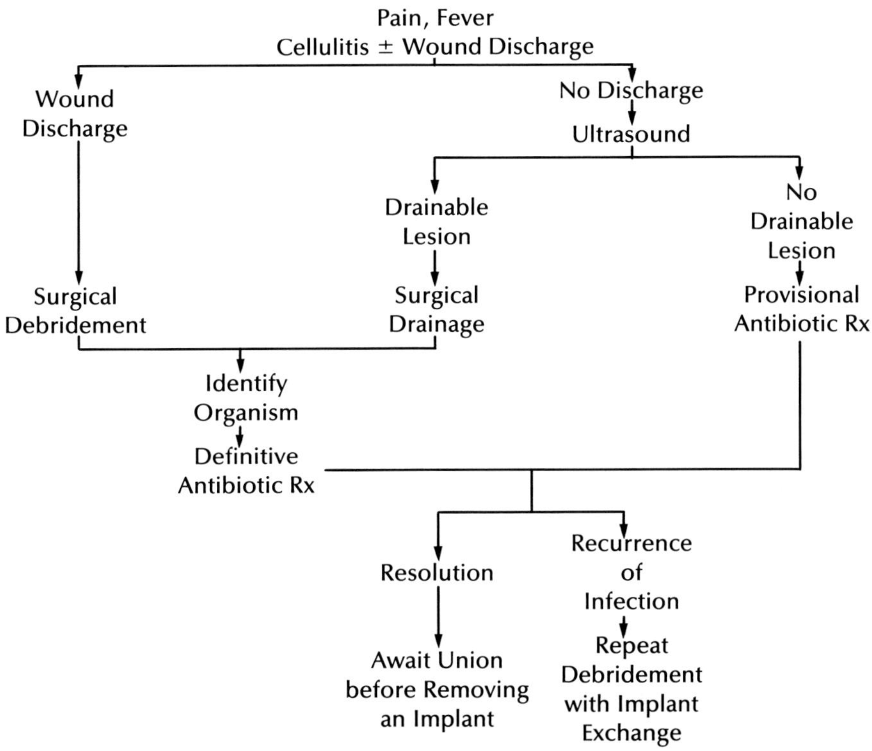

Figure 10-1 *Algorithm for investigation and management of post-traumatic or post-surgical osteomyelitis*

ties are known. Features suggesting the presence of necrotizing soft-tissue infection (see Chapter 20) demand the use of aggressive, multidrug antimicrobial therapy and radical soft-tissue debridement.

If this program of early management results in resolution of the episode of infection, the implant should be retained until either fracture union or nonunion has clearly occurred. No data are available comparing outcome with the length of antimicrobial therapy; we recommend that it be continued for a minimum of 3 weeks.

If discharge persists following initial debridement and antimicrobial therapy, repeat debridement with implant exchange is indicated. This procedure should include removal of all devitalized bone and poor quality soft tissue, with bone grafting and flap coverage to fill the defect. Although use of external fixation has been recommended to restabilize diaphyseal fractures following debridement (35), results of exchanging both plates (33) and intramedullary nails (21) have been satisfactory, provided debridement has been thorough.

Infected Puncture Wounds of the Foot

Puncture wounds of the foot from nails or glass are common, particularly in childhood. If a retained foreign body is suspected, ultrasound examination may be used to seek it (39). In the absence of foreign material, clean punctures without evidence of infection need not be surgically enlarged; however, the decision should be individualized (40).

Osteomyelitis develops in approximately 2% of puncture wounds of the foot (41). Bone may have been penetrated directly, or infection may spread from soft tissues to affect one or more contiguous bones. If secondary osteomyelitis does occur, there is typically a period of 2 to 3 days when the initial pain settles, only to worsen thereafter. Symptoms and signs are local and are rarely systemic (42,43). The calcaneum is frequently involved (42,44). Radiological features are usually present, including soft-tissue swelling, osteopenia, and localized bone destruction. *Pseudomonas aeruginosa* is the most common isolate in this presentation and is thought to survive commonly in the inner soles of footwear (45). If osteomyelitis develops, surgical debridement followed by 14 to 21 days of antibiotic therapy is usually effective treatment (46,47).

Osteomyelitis in Decubitus Ulcers

Osteomyelitis may be confirmed by biopsy from the base of a significant percentage of decubitus ulcers; recent estimates range from 28% to 70% (48,49). The most useful diagnostic test is needle bone biopsy (50). The majority of patients with biopsy-proven osteomyelitis also have radiological changes (48,50,51), although it may be difficult to distinguish between healed and active osteomyelitis. In one study, any positive result from serial testing of erythrocyte sedimentation rate, white cell count, and pelvic radiograph was the best noninvasive predictor of osteomyelitis (50).

Although not recommended for management of uncomplicated pressure sores (52), antibiotics are indicated in the management of contiguous osteomyelitis. The choice should be based on the organism or organisms grown from the bone biopsy. Almost all pressure ulcers will contain large numbers of infected bacteria in the base (53). Surgical resection of the infected bone may permit local skin closure (54) but careful planning is necessary because significant bone resection may unbalance pressure patterns, particularly in the pelvis in paraplegic patients, giving rise to recurrence locally and to the development of contralateral ulcers (55). Myocutaneous flaps are superior to skin flaps in achieving secure cover of debrided areas (50).

In prophylaxis against contiguous osteomyelitis, prevention of pressure sores is both desirable and, to a considerable extent, achievable. A number of risk scales have been described, of which the Braden Scale appears to be the best predictor (58). It uses six subscales: sensory perception, skin moisture, activity, mobility, friction and shear, and nutritional status. Identification of high-risk individuals assists deployment of preventive measures; the key elements are high nursing standards, which ensure minimization of pressure and shear, and management programs that reduce immobility, promote activity, and preserve nutritional status.

Osteitis Pubis

A syndrome of pubic pain, radiating to the adductor region of one or both thighs; exacerbated by walking, coughing, micturition and defecation; with radiological signs of perisymphyseal bone resorption (Figure 10-2) has been described following suprapubic surgery (57). It seems clear that this syndrome is an example of osteomyelitis arising from a

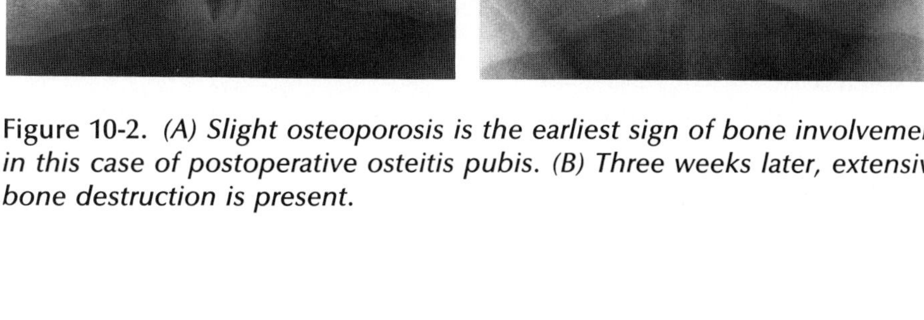

Figure 10-2. *(A) Slight osteoporosis is the earliest sign of bone involvement in this case of postoperative osteitis pubis. (B) Three weeks later, extensive bone destruction is present.*

contiguous low grade soft-tissue infection (58). Hematogenous infection of the pubis also occurs (59). Both presentations are uncommon.

Confusion over the use of the term *osteitis pubis* has arisen, because similar clinical and radiological findings have since been described in situations where infection is improbable (e.g., after pregnancy, in polyarthritis, after trauma [60], and in athletes [61] [see Chapter 16]).

If the context of the presentation suggests infection, aspiration of the symphysis or needle biopsy of the pubis is indicated. Any collection present should be drained, and antibiotic therapy should be administered. The optimum duration is unknown. We suggest that the recommendations for vertebral infection should be followed. Persisting symptoms may require debridement and symphyseal fusion.

Conclusions

Despite the power of contemporary antimicrobial agents and despite clear evidence of the value of wound debridement and, if necessary, early flap coverage, infection after injury or surgery remains a complication associated with significant morbidity. Prior risk assessment and reduction is possible in discretionary surgery (see Chapters 15 and 17) but not in the management of open or penetrating injury. In these circumstances, decreasing the burden of morbidity will require above all changes in social behavior, which can only be addressed at a political level. There are also, however, technical issues. How wide is the gap between outcomes achieved by different centers? Are antimicrobial agents used cost-effectively according to established principles? What are the most effective techniques of managing early postsurgical infections? There are few comparative studies. Finally, because the nature of soft-tissue wounds appears to be the main determinant of outcome in both infection and fracture healing, do health care systems afford the proper priority to the care of the injured to allow rapid skilled wound management to be instituted?

References

1. Waldvogel FA, Medoff G, Swartz MN. Oseomyelitis: a review of clinical features, therapeutic considerations and unusual aspects. N Engl J Med 1970;282:198–206.

2. Platt R. Methodologic aspects of clinical studies of perioperative antibiotic prophylaxis. Rev Infect Dis 1991;13(suppl 10):S810–S814.
3. Braun R, Enzler MA, Rittmann WW. A double-blind clinical trial of prophylactic cloxacillin in open fractures. J Orthop Trauma 1987;1:12–17.
4. O'Brien PJ, Meek RN, Powell JN, Blachut PA. Primary intramedullary nailing of open femoral shaft fractures. J Trauma 1991;31:113–116.
5. Marshall PD, Saleh M, Douglas DL. Risk of deep infection with intramedullary nailing following the use of external fixators. J R Coll Surg Edinb 1991;36:268–271.
6. Dellinger EP, Miller SD, Wertz MJ, Grypma M, Droppert B, Anderson PA. Risk of infection after open fracture of the arm or leg. Arch Surg 1988;123:1320–1327.
7. Haley RW, Hootin TM, Culver DH. Nosocomial infections in US hospitals 1975–76. Estimated frequency by selected characteristics of patients. Am J Med 1981;70:947–959.
8. McQueen MM, Littlejohn MA, Miles RS, Hughes SPF. Antibiotic prophylaxis in proximal femoral fracture. Injury 1990;21:104–106.
9. Bodoky A, Neff U, Heberer M, Harder F. Antibiotic prophylaxis with two doses of cephalosporin in patients managed with internal fixation for a fracture of the hip. J Bone Joint Surg [Am] 1993;75:61–65.
10. Gustilo RB, Merkow RL, Templeman D. The management of open fractures. J Bone Joint Surg [Am] 1990;72:299–304.
11. Boyd RJ, Burke JF, Colton T. A double-blind clinical trial of prophylactic antibiotics in hip fractures. J Bone Joint Surg [Am] 1973;55:1251–1258.
12. Burnett JW, Gustilo RB, Wiliams DN, Kind AC. Prophylactic antibiotics in hip fractures. J Bone Joint Surg [Am] 1980;62:457–462.
13. Tengve B, Kjellander J. Antibiotic prophylaxis in operations on trochanteric femoral fractures. J Bone Joint Surg [Am] 1978;60:97–99.
14. Gatell JM, Riba J, Lozano L, Mana J, Ramon R, San Miguel J. Prophylactic cephamandole in orthopaedic surgery. J Bone Joint Surg [Am] 1984;66:1219–1222.
15. Hughes SP, Miles RS, Littlejohn M, Brown E. Is antibiotic prophylaxis necessary for internal fixation of low-energy fractures? Injury 1991;22:111–113.
16. Helfet DL, Howey T, Sanders R, Johansen K. Limb salvage versus amputation. Preliminary results of the mangled extremity severity score. Clin Orthop 1990;256:80–86.
17. Dellinger EP, Caplan ES, Weaver LD, et al. Duration of preventive antibiotic administration for open extremity fractures. Arch Surg 1988;123:333–338.
18. Trueta J "Closed" treatment of war fractures. Lancet 1939;1:1452–1455.
19. Byrd HS, Cierney G, Tebbetts JB. The management of open tibial fractures with associated soft tissue loss. External pin fixation with early flap coverage. Plast Reconstr Surg 1981;68:73–82.
20. Merritt K. Factors increasing the risk of infection in patients with open fractures. J Trauma 1988;28:823–827.
21. Court Brown CM, Keating JF, McQueen MM. Infection after intramedullary

nailing of the tibia. Incidence and protocol for management. J Bone Joint Surg [Br] 1992;74:770–774.
22. Benson DR, Riggins RS, Lawrence RM, Hoeprich PD, Huston AC, Harrison JA. Treatment of open fractures: a prospective study. J Trauma 1983;23:25–30.
23. Miles AA, Miles EM, Burke J. The value and duration of defence reactions of the skin to the primary lodgment of bacteria. Br J Exp Pathol 1957;38: 79–96.
24. Burke JF. The effective period of preventive antibiotic action in experimental incisions and dermal lesions. Surgery 1961;50:161–168.
25. Edlich RF, Smith QT, Edgerton MT. Resistance of the surgical wound to antimicrobial prophylaxis and its mechanisms of development. Am J Surg 1973;126:583–591.
26. Patzakis MJ, Harvey P, Ivler D. The role of antibiotics in the management of open fractures. J Bone Joint Surg [Am] 1974;56:532–541.
27. Dellinger EP, Wertz MJ, Lennard ES, Oreskovich MR. Efficacy of short course antibiotic prophylaxis after penetrating intestinal injury: a prospective randomized trial. Arch Surg 1986;121:23–30.
28. Pollard JP, Hughes SPF, Scott JE, Evans MJ, Benson MKD. Antibiotic prophylaxis in total hip replacement, Br Med J 1979;1:707–709.
29. Johnson KD, Bone LB, Scheinberg R. Severe open tibial fractures; a study protocol. J Orthop Trauma 1988;2:175–180.
30. Lerner RK, Esterhai JL, Polomono RC, Cheatle MC, Heppenstall RB, Brighton CT. Psychosocial, functional and quality of life assessment of patients with post-traumatic fracture nonunion, chronic refractory osteomyelitis, and lower extremity amputation. Arch Phys Med Rehabil 1991;72:122–126.
31. Sonne-Holm S, Menck H, Boeckstyns M, et al. Prophylactic antibiotics in amputation of the lower extremity for ischaemia. A placebo-controlled, randomized trial of cefoxitin. J Bone Joint Surg [Am] 1985;67:800–803.
32. Thomsen S, Jakobsen BW, Wethelund JO, Dalsgaard J, Gregersen HN, Lucht U. Antibiotic prophylaxis in lower-extremity amputations due to ischaemia. A prospective, randomized trial of cephalothin versus methicillin. Arch Orthop Trauma Surg 1990;109:72–74.
33. Rittmann WW, Schibli M, Matter P, Allgower M. Open fractures. Long term results in 200 consecutive cases. Clin Orthop 1979;138:132–140.
34. Cierny G, Byrd HS, Jones RE. Primary versus delayed soft tissue coverage for severe open tibial fractures. A comparison of the results. Clin Orthop 1983;178:54–63.
35. Johnson K. Management of open fractures and infections. In: D'Ambrosia RD, Marier RL, eds. Orthopaedic Infections. Thorofare, NJ: Slack, 1989: 517–528.
36. Caudle RJ, Stern PJ. Severe open fractures of the tibia. J Bone Joint Surg [Am] 1987;69:801–807.
37. Patzakis MJ, Wilkins J. Factors influencing infection rates in open fracture wounds. Clin Orthop 1989;243:36–40.

38. Abiri MM, Kirkepar M, Ablow RC. Osteomyelitis; detection with ultrasound. Radiology 1989;172:509–511.
39. Groleau S, Chem RK, Younge D, Basora J. Ultrasonography of foreign body tenosynovitis. Can Assoc Radiol J 1992;43:454–456.
40. Inaba AS, Zukin DD, Perro M. An update on the evaluation and management of plantar puncture wounds and Pseudomonas osteomyelitis. Pediatr Emerg Care 1992;8:38–44.
41. Fitzgerald RH, Cowan JDE. Puncture wounds of the foot. Orthop Clin North Am 1975;6:965–972.
42. Green NE, Bruno J. Pseudomonas infections of the foot after puncture wounds. South Med J 1980;73:146–149.
43. Crosby LA, Powell DA. The potential value of sedimentation rate in monitoring treatment outcome in puncture-wound related Pseudomonas osteomyelitis. Clin Orthop 1984;188:168–172.
44. Gale DW, Scott R. Puncture wound of the foot? Persistent pain? Think of Pseudomonas aeruginosa osteomyelitis. Injury 1991;22:427–428.
45. Fisher MC, Goldsmith JF, Gilligan PH. Sneakers as a source of Pseudomonas aeruginosa in children with osteomyelitis following puncture wounds. J Pediatr 1985;106:607–609.
46. Jacobs RF, Adelman L, Sack CM, Wilson CB. Management of Pseudomonas osteochondritis complicating puncture wounds of the foot. Pediatrics 1982;69:432–435.
47. Brand RA, Black H. Pseudomonas osteomyelitis following puncture wounds in children. J Bone Joint Surg [Am] 1974;56:1637–1642.
48. Bruck JC, Buttemeyer R, Grabosch A, Gruhl L. More arguments in favour of myocutaneous flaps for the treatment of pelvic pressure sores. Ann Plast Surg 1991;26:85–88.
49. Bohm E, Kuhlmann I, Botel U. Decubitus ulcer in paraplegic patients—a comparative clinico-pathological study. Unfallchirurgie 1988;14:335–342.
50. Lewis VL, Bailey MH, Pulawski G, Kind G, Bashioum RW, Hendrix RW. The diagnosis of osteomyelitis in patients with pressure sores. Plast Reconstr Surg 1988;81:229–232.
51. Borgstrom PS, Ekberg O, Lasson A. Radiography of pressure ulcers. Acta Radiol 1988;29:581–584.
52. Melcher RE, Longe RL, Gelbart AO. Pressure sores in the elderly. A systematic approach to management. Postgrad Med 1988;83:299–308.
53. Alterescu V, Alterescu KB. Pressure ulcers: assessment and treatment. Orthop Nurs 1992;11:37–49.
54. Dimant J, Tanael L. Decubitus ulcers: when to suspect osteomyelitis. Geriatrics 1987;42:74,79,83.
55. Berlemont M, Keromest R. Dangers of ischiectomy in ulcers in the paraplegic patient. Review of 236 records. Rev Chir Orthop 1987;73: 656–664.
56. Bergstrom N, Demuth PJ, Braden BJ. A clinical trial of the Braden scale for predicting pressure sore risk. Nurs Clin North Am 1987;22:417–428.

57. Beer E. Periostitis of symphysis and descending rami of pubes following suprapubic operations. Int J Med Surg 1924;37:224–225.
58. Bouza E, Winston DW, Hewitt WL. Infectious osteitis pubis. Urology 1978;12:663–669.
59. Rutherford A. Osteomyelitis of the symphysis pubis. NZ Med J 1983;96:332–333.
60. Coventry MB, Mitchell WO. Osteitis pubis. JAMA 1961;178:898–905.
61. Harris NH, Murray RO. Lesions of the symphysis in athletes. Br Med J 1974;4:211–214.

CHAPTER 11

Infections of Bone in Patients with Diabetes

Predisposing Factors in Groups at Risk

The epidemiology and importance of foot infections in diabetic patients are well described (1). Infection of the foot is the complication of diabetes that most frequently leads to hospitalization. Foot problems will develop in approximately one fourth of diabetic patients, and approximately 6% will undergo amputation of a limb during their lifetime. The average duration of hospitalization for diagnosis and treatment of foot infections in diabetic patients ranges from 22 to 36 days (2). Finally, diabetic patients have an increased risk of lower extremity amputation of 5- to 15-fold (3), and one half the non-traumatic amputations performed each year in the United States are in patients with diabetes (4,5).

Pathophysiology

Although alterations in cellular and humoral responses to bacterial infection have been associated with diabetes, local factors in the foot are probably most important in understanding the pathogenesis of this type of osteomyelitis, which is almost always secondary to a contiguous focus of infection. The major pathological condition that enhances infection in the diabetic patient is the loss of the normally protective skin barrier caused by ulceration of the foot; however, an obvious ulcer is not always seen.

Once a cutaneous portal is available, bacteria initially cause a soft-tissue infection, which may move rapidly but usually persists as an indolent local infection. A local infection may spread contiguously to involve deep structures, including bone. Even with appropriate therapy, opportunities for recurrent infection exist until healing and re-epithelialization of the ulcer is complete.

Three major factors responsible for foot ulcers and their sequelae in diabetic patients are neuropathy, ischemia, and infection (6,7). Neuropathy predisposes to foot injuries from minor trauma; lack of protective sensation often causes foot ulcers to be neglected. In addition to sensory neuropathy, neuropathy affecting motor nerves can cause changes in gait, alterations in pressure distribution, and deformity of the foot. Autonomic neuropathy, when it occurs, produces alterations in blood flow and abnormalities in skin hydration.

Limb ischemia in diabetics is frequently caused by arteriosclerosis obliterans. Peripheral vascular disease develops after 10 and 20 years' duration of diabetes in 15% and 45%, respectively (8). Atherosclerosis in diabetics usually involves distal as well as proximal vessels (9). Alterations of small cutaneous vessels, leading to abnormalities in cutaneous capillary flow, is well documented in diabetes. These alterations may occur with arteriovenous shunting caused by autonomic neuropathy (10), but may also be secondary to tissue edema (11).

Clinical and Laboratory Findings

The most common clinical presentation of infection in the diabetic foot is in association with an ulcer (Figure 11-1). "Complicated" infections are those associated with involvement of deep spaces (e.g., fascia, bone), the presence of tissue gas, or gangrene. The presence of a foul odor suggests infection with anaerobes, but the presence of gangrene due to ischemia may also cause a fetid odor (12). The presence of crepitus suggests gas in the deeper tissues and should produce suspicion of either aerobic gram-negative infection or anaerobic infection. Large amounts of pus may be clinically undetectable in the fascial planes and spaces; probing of the ulcer by blunt dissection with a hemostat may reveal unexpected purulent material. Infections in the diabetic foot infrequently present with severe systemic symptoms unless the process is rapidly spreading or is associated with massive tissue destruction. Some sign of inflammation such as unexplained painless swelling of one or more toes usually indicates the presence of infection. Laboratory tests are nonspecific; the white blood cell count

A B C D

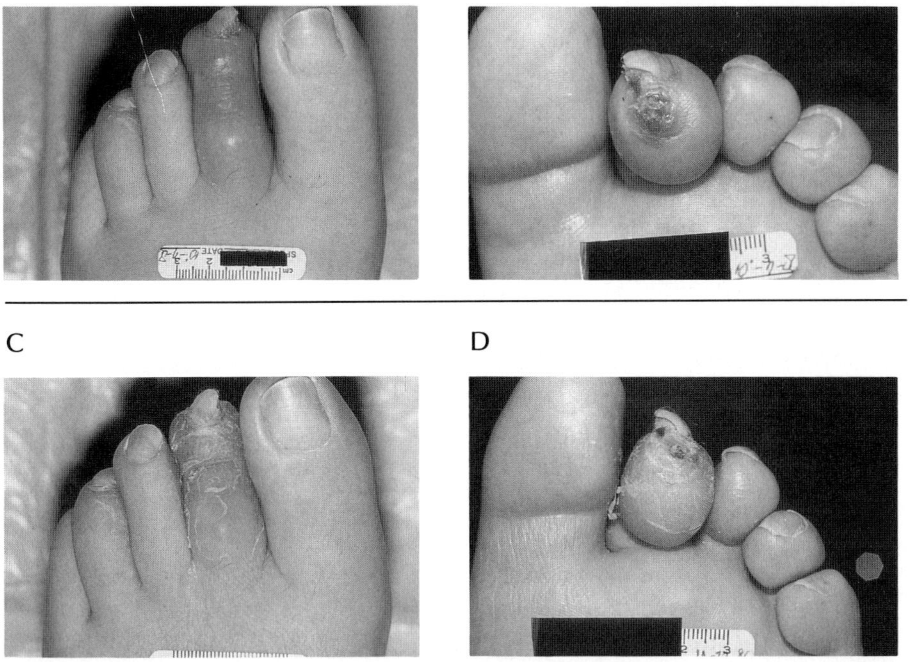

Figure 11-1. *(A,B) A 50-year-old man presented with a 3-day history of pain and swelling in his second toe. Cultures (curettage and aspiration) yielded* Staphylococcus aureus. *(C,D) After 2 weeks of antibiotic treatment, the infection was clinically and microbiologically cured.* (Reproduced by permission from Lipsky BA, Pecoraro RE, Larson SA, Hanley ME, Ahroni JH. Outpatient management of uncomplicated lower extremity infections in diabetic patients. Arch Intern Med 1990;150:790–797.)

may be elevated. Blood cultures are frequently negative unless there is evidence of disseminated infection.

Microbiology

The usefulness of cultures in diabetic patients with a foot infection is related to the quality and type of specimen collected. The easiest to obtain are swabs taken from the ulcer, but these specimens are often misleading. Even if purulent, the specimen is difficult to interpret because it samples the surface of the wound, which may contain both pathogens and colonizing organisms. "Nonpathogens," such as normal skin flora (coagulase-negative staphylococci and *Corynebacteria*), may be potential pathogens in diabetic hosts. Two studies (13,14) compared culture specimens that could not be collected without contact with an open lesion ("unreliable") with simultaneously obtained deep specimens ("reliable"); there was an extremely poor correlation, with identical results in only 27% and 17% for the two studies. Curettage specimens, which more often yield anaerobic organisms and fewer superficial colonizers, may be useful (1,12). Such specimens are obtained after cleansing the surface of the open wound and then scraping tissue from the base and edge of the ulcer with a dental curette or a scalpel blade. Needle aspiration is also useful in providing cultures but may be less sensitive than curettage, particularly if the ulcer is dry. All culture specimens, regardless of how they are obtained, should be transported promptly to the microbiology laboratory and processed for both aerobic and anaerobic organisms.

Many bacterial species, either alone or in combination, are associated with foot infections in diabetic patients. Staphylococci (both coagulase-positive and coagulase-negative) and streptococci are major pathogens. If only a single organism is present, it is generally *Staphylococcus aureus*. Aerobic gram-negative bacteria are usually recovered as part of a mixed infection. *Proteus* is the most frequent isolate, followed by *Escherichia coli, Klebsiella,* and *Pseudomonas.* Anaerobic organisms are also frequently found in mixed infections and often exhibit denser growth than aerobes.

Table 11-1 categorizes the types of bacteria isolated in selected

Table 11-1. Categorization of bacteria isolated in selected series of diabetic foot infections

CATEGORY OF BACTERIA (%)	REF. 15	REF. 16	REF. 17	REF. 12	REF. 13	REF. 2
Anaerobic only	5	0	8	3	0	0
Aerobic only	5	43	17	19	61	87
Aerobic and anaerobic	90	57	75	78	39	13

Reproduced by permission from Lipsky BA, Pecoraro RE, Wheat LJ. The diabetic foot. Soft tissue and bone infection. Infect Dis Clin North Am 1990;4:409–432.

series of diabetic foot infections. In most (but not all), mixed aerobic and anaerobic organisms predominate; infection with anaerobes alone was uncommon. Most series are comprised of hospitalized patients, usually with serious soft-tissue infections; some patients received antimicrobial agents before the culture was taken.

Diagnosis

Diagnosis of osteomyelitis in diabetic patients with foot infections is difficult. The clinical features are not reliable indicators of deep-tissue infection underlying an indolent ulcer. In our opinion, biopsy and culture of bone remains the gold standard for diagnosis, but a variety of noninvasive techniques are available and should be reviewed critically against this "gold standard."

Diabetic patients with osteopathy have several and varied radiographic abnormalities (Figures 11-2, 11-3). The earliest changes include soft-tissue swelling and joint effusion, which are often followed by subluxation and small fractures (18). With progression of the disease, more significant subluxation may occur and bony destruction becomes more severe. Progression of the process includes periosteal new bone formation, primarily in the metatarsal bones and phalanges, and ultimately there is destruction of the articular surface. This process may occur within several weeks, but usually requires much longer periods.

Osteomyelitis, in contrast, shows radiological changes of patchy bone destruction, often with periosteal reaction and usually with loss

A B

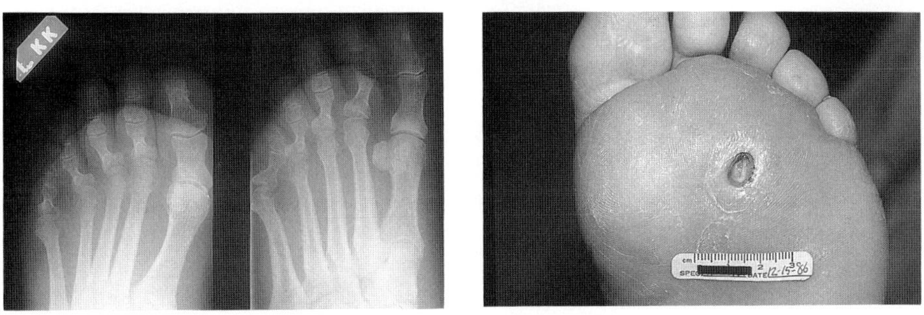

Figure 11-2. *(A) An elderly man with a plantar ulcer of long duration. Bone biopsy culture was sterile. (B) Overlying ulcer healed; patient continued to walk and bony destruction progressed, ultimately leading to amputation. Destruction of underlying bone is due to neuropathic bone changes.* (Provided by Dr. Benjamin Lipsky.)

A B

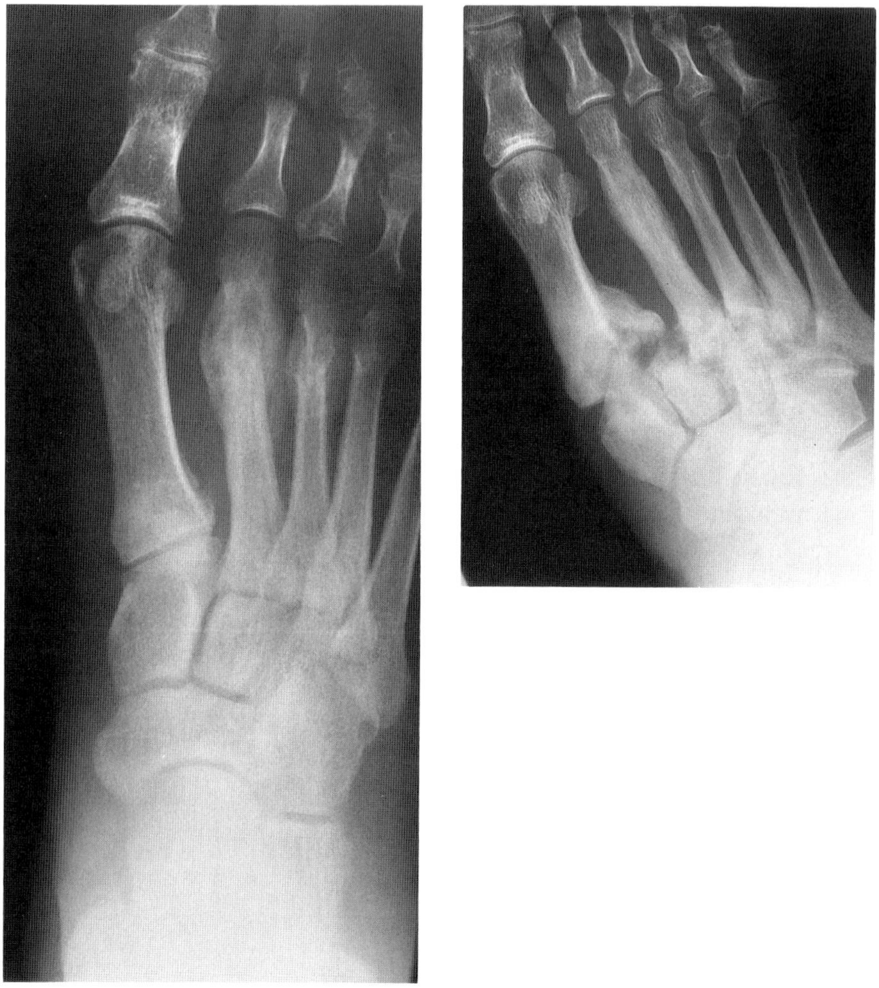

Figure 11-3. *Neuropathic bone changes. (A) Exuberant bone growth; joint spaces are preserved. (B) Six months later, Charcot joints are present, with loss of normal bony architecture.* (Provided by Dr. Alex Norman.)

of definition of the margins of bone (Figure 11-4). It is difficult to confidently differentiate between osteopathy and osteomyelitis (1,18). The sensitivity of plain radiography in the diagnosis of osteomyelitis of the foot in diabetic patients ranges from 62% to 100%, but specificity was no better than 69% (1). Therefore, alternative procedures

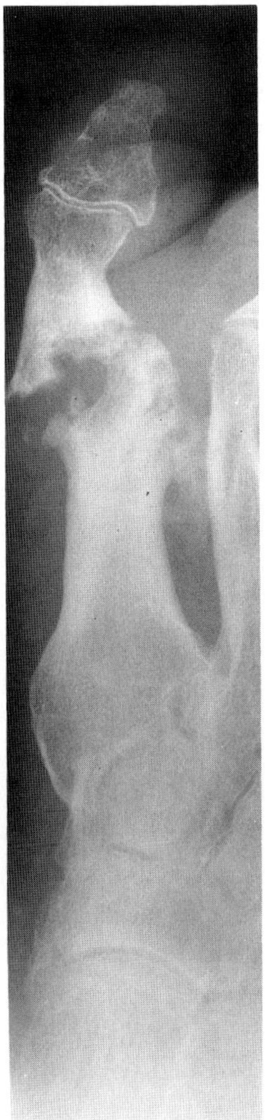

Figure 11-4. *Patient with severe osteomyelitis and destruction of great toe.* (Provided by Dr. Alex Norman.)

have been evaluated. However, many of the available studies are limited: they were retrospective, unblinded, had too small sample size, and, most importantly, did not clearly define the standards by which osteomyelitis was diagnosed.

Bone scanning, using technetium (^{99}Tc-MDP) with three phases, is considered positive when increased uptake localizes to bone in the late phase. This technique is quite sensitive—it identifies 70% to 100% of cases of osteomyelitis—but its limitation is the frequent occurrence of false-positive results in the presence of osteopathy or in the healing phase after treatment of osteomyelitis. Specificity was 43% or less in several studies (1). In a review of technetium bone scanning by meta-analysis (19), the technique was shown to have low specificity with a false-positive rate that was at best 20% occurring at sensitivities of 70% to 80%. As sensitivity increased, the false-positive rate increased such that small increases in sensitivity led to larger decreases in specificity. Thus, the high false-positive rate suggests that if osteomyelitis is suspected, a positive bone scan will not be helpful. Perhaps more value may be found in a negative scan if it indicates that osteomyelitis is unlikely.

^{67}Gallium scanning has not gained great favor in diagnosing osteomyelitis in the diabetic foot. Theoretically, scanning agents such as technetium and gallium should localize to sites of inflammation of any cause, whereas ^{111}indium-labeled leukocytes should aggregate only in areas of active infection. However, white blood cells will aggregate not only when there is infection in bone, but also in overlying soft tissue. To remedy this defect in white blood cell scans and to provide better anatomical localization of infection, many workers now recommend performing both a technetium three-phase bone scan and then an ^{111}indium white blood cell scan. A sensitivity of 100% using these two techniques and a specificity of 83% was reported (20). When considering only patients with a positive indium leukocyte study, the combined bone scan and leukocyte study correctly localized infection to the soft tissues or bone in 89%. Other studies differed in that they found no additional value in adding the three-phase bone scan to the leukocyte scan and therefore argued that white blood cell scanning alone is adequate for evaluation of suspected osteomyelitis (21). In another series, osteomyelitis was present in bone in 68% of patients with diabetic foot ulcers (this high prevalence may be due to selection of patients for this series). A clinical diagnosis of osteomyelitis was only made in 30% of those patients. Leukocyte scans with indium demonstrated a sensitivity of 89% and a specificity of 69% in patients with bone biopsy–confirmed diagnosis of osteomyelitis (22). In another series of biopsy-positive patients (23), a sensitivity of 73%, a specificity of 91%, and a positive predictive value of 89% was found for positive leukocyte scans (Figure 11-5). Limitations of leukocyte scanning are that the technique is not yet widely available, the test is time-consuming because of the need to radiolabel the patient's white

A B

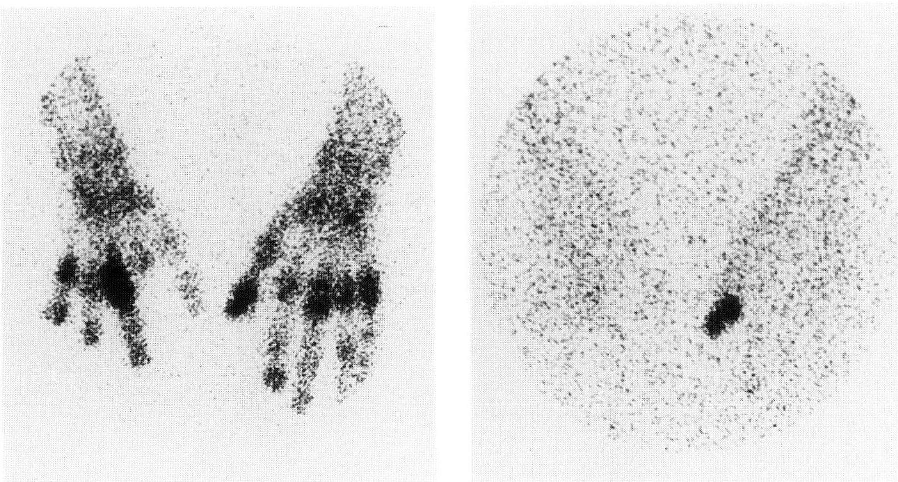

Figure 11-5. *Twenty-four hour bone (A) and leukocyte (B) scintigrams of hands of a 50-year-old diabetic patient with draining ulcer at top of right thumb show intense uptake in distal first phalanx. Biopsy grew* Staphylococcus aureus. *Bone image shows increased uptake in multiple neuropathic joints, which do not show increased accumulation of leukocytes.* (Reproduced by permission from Jacobson AF, Harley J, Lipsky B, Pecoraro R. Diagnosis of osteomyelitis in the presence of soft tissue infection and radiologic evidence of osseous abnormalities. AJR 1991;157:807–812.)

blood cells, and it is expensive. We believe that no definitive recommendation can be made regarding the best single test or combination of radioisotope scanning techniques and that these tests form only part of the approach to the diabetic foot outlined in the algorithm (Figure 11-6).

Magnetic resonance imaging (MRI) has been compared with three-phase bone scans and plain radiographs (24). MRI was not associated with false-positive or false-negative results in patients with a tissue-proven diagnosis of osteomyelitis; there were two false-positive results in 19 patients without osteomyelitis. These results and others (25) are extremely promising; however, although MRI provides a great deal of information about anatomical abnormalities involving the bone and soft tissue, it does not clearly distinguish infection from other causes of bone disease (Figure 11-7; see Chapter 6).

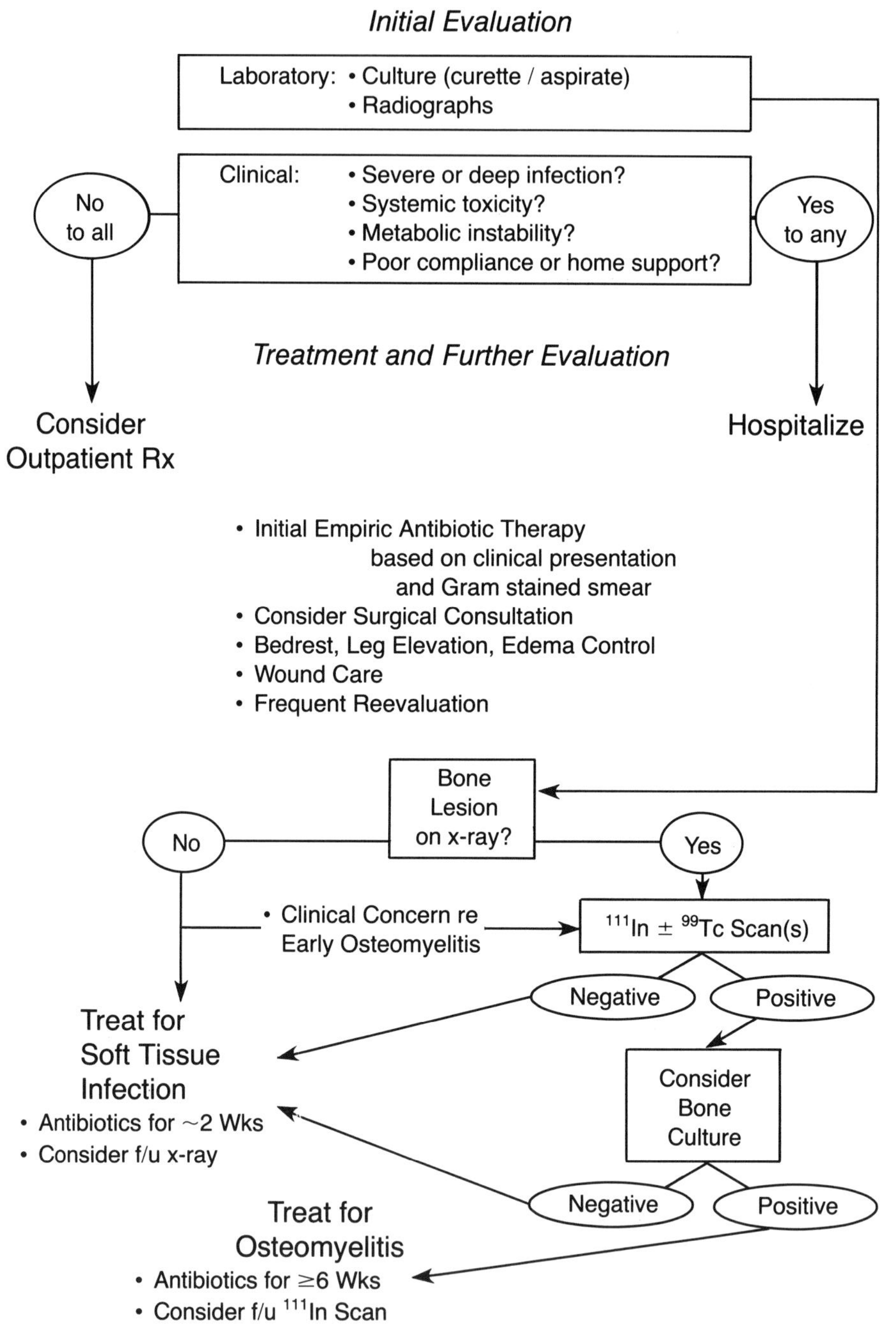

Figure 11-6. *Suggested algorithmic approach to diagnosis and treatment of foot infection in diabetic patients.* (Reproduced with permission from Lipsky BA, Pecoraro RE, Wheat LJ. The diabetic foot. Soft tissue and infection. Infect Dis Clin North Am 1990;4:409–432.)

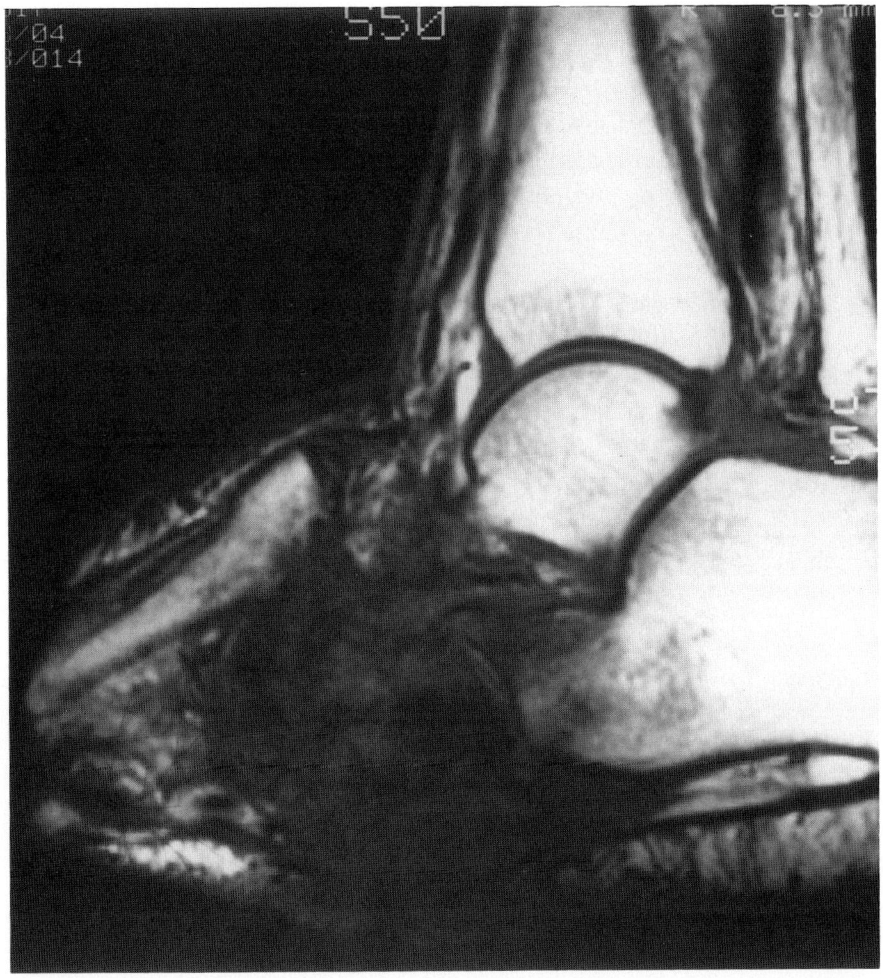

Figure 11-7. *T1-weighted image reveals forefoot amputation and normal signal in distal tibia, talus, and posterior calcaneus. The interior portion of calcaneus has edema. The remainder of the tarsal bones are destroyed and replaced by a dark heterogeneous inflammatory mass.* (Provided by Dr. Denise Leslie.)

Culture of the infected bone remains the most precise test for diagnosing osteomyelitis. Either percutaneous needle biopsy or material obtained at surgery is adequate for study. In a retrospective series (26) of 13 patients, 71% of bones biopsied had a positive culture, and the bone culture results usually differed from that obtained from overlying ulcers. Biopsy, avoiding soft-tissue infections and ulcers, was safe and the diagnosis of osteomyelitis appeared to be well founded. Only eight patients (40%) had a positive bone culture; the others appeared to have osteopathy. Many diabetic patients with bone lesions that appear to be osteomyelitis may not have osteomyelitis (1). The limitations of percutaneous biopsy include sampling error because of the small piece of tissue that is obtained and the imprecise localization of the biopsy; possible false-negative cultures if the patient receives antibiotics; possible contamination by soft-tissue organisms; and a potential risk of damage to the bone as a result of the biopsy.

A sensible approach to the diagnosis of osteomyelitis in the diabetic foot uses an algorithm (see Figure 11-6). The approach is systematic and moves from clinical grounds to conventional radiographs to surgical probing. From there it includes other radiographic and scintigraphic examinations. Because no radiographic or scan features are totally specific for osteomyelitis, surgical debridement or percutaneous biopsy with a specimen of bone submitted for histology and culture is recommended if diagnosis is not clear.

Therapy

The approach to treatment of foot infections in diabetic patients is conceptually simpler if they are divided into uncomplicated and complicated. Complicated infections have deep soft-tissue involvement, osteomyelitis, or gangrene. Uncomplicated infections include patients lacking signs of systemic toxicity, extensive cellulitis, fasciitis, osteomyelitis, or gangrene. Outpatient management has been reviewed (2); necessary requirements to treat such patients outside the hospital include availability of an appropriate oral antimicrobial agent, absence of severe metabolic abnormalities, and presence of a home environment in which the patient can be in a nonweight-bearing state. Failure to respond to out-patient treatment is an indication for hospitalization. Clindamycin, cephalexin, dicloxacillin, or erythromycin appeared adequate in a few studies (2,6,27). If clinical or laboratory findings indicate infection with gram-negative aerobic bacilli, agents such as trimethoprim-sulfamethoxazole, amoxicillin-clavulanic acid, or quinolones (i.e., ofloxacin or ciprofloxacin) may be used. If enterococci are present, ampicillin may be used; in the presence of a foul odor, anaerobes should be suspected and metronidazole may be used. There is no clear evidence as to whether all organisms isolated must be covered by the antimicrobial agents. For example, it is unclear whether treatment for Enterococci, which are found in approximately one third of reported diabetic foot infections, is critical. Treatment for Enterococci in infections of the foot in diabetic patients is usually not necessary except in complicated infections (1,28). The optimal duration of treatment with antimicrobial agents is unclear; we recommend 1 to 2 weeks for uncomplicated infections.

Appropriate local surgical treatment is always indicated. Any pus in the foot must be drained. Patients need to stay off their feet and to elevate the infected extremity. Any necrotic debris overlying the wound should be removed, if necessary, by surgical debridement. Draining wounds can be treated with wet to damp dressings using saline-moistened gauze. Hyperbaric oxygen has not been shown to be beneficial (29).

In complicated infections of the lower extremity in diabetic patients, choice of initial antimicrobial therapy is often empiric. The agents chosen should be effective against organisms commonly isolated; as discussed earlier, these usually include Staphylococci (coagulase-positive and coagulase-negative) Streptococci, gram-negative aerobic bacilli, and anaerobic organisms. Once specific and reliable cultures (as defined earlier) have been obtained, antimicrobial therapy may be adjusted. There are many choices for empiric initial therapy, including a broad-spectrum cephalosporin plus an agent active against anaerobes (e.g., metronidazole or clindamycin); combination of a penicillin and a beta-lactamase inhibitor; or a carbapenem as the sole agent. This broad-spectrum approach to therapy should be modified once the results of cultures are available. There are no reliable data concerning the optimal duration of therapy or for how long agents should be given parenterally before switching to oral agents. In one study (28), use of appropriate antimicrobial therapy (active against the isolated pathogens) for at least 4 weeks intravenously, or a combination of parenteral and oral therapy for at least 10 weeks, was associated with a favorable outcome.

Surgical debridement of infected tissue has two purposes. First, when there is necrotic material present, it may hasten eradication of infection; second, it may provide specimens for culture. In some patients, amputation may significantly shorten the period of hospitalization without compromising functional activity and rehabilitation, particularly for removal of a toe. We recommend this approach in preference to prolonged antimicrobial therapy, especially if hospitalization is required (30). Amputations should generally be reserved for patients for whom (a) there is no acceptable antimicrobial agent (i.e., none to which the organism is susceptible in vitro and the patient is not allergic); (b) there is no response to antimicrobial therapy; and (c) the infection has already destroyed the integrity of the foot.

Prognosis and Complications

In uncomplicated lower extremity infections, an excellent outcome using the therapeutic approach described has been reported (2). Of 56 patients in one series, randomized to outpatient treatment with either cephalexin or clindamycin for 2 weeks, 42 were clinically cured after 2 weeks and nine showed significant improvement (2). Of these nine, seven showed ultimate resolution and in two, new soft-tissue infection developed. Five patients were considered clinical failures. Results did not differ between the two antibiotic regimens. In long-term follow-up among the 42 patients whose infections were classified as cured, new infection developed at the same site in only three. Six of the nine patients whose infections were classified as improved became reinfected; of these, all but one reinfection occurred in patients who still had open wounds after 2 weeks of therapy. Culture specimens yielded an average of only two organisms per patient, and the majority of infections were caused by gram-positive cocci, particularly Staphylococci, which would respond to either of the antimicrobial agents selected. Enterococci were isolated from five patients, of whom four had polymicrobial infections. Although neither cephalexin nor clindamycin is active against *Enterococcus,* all infections were cured, supporting the argument that antimicrobial therapy for uncomplicated infections need not have specific activity for enterococci.

The prognosis for diabetic patients with complicated infections of the lower extremity is less sanguine. One of the studies most frequently quoted reporting an unhappy outcome is from the Massachusetts General Hospital in 1970 (31). Of 31 patients with vascular insufficiency and osteomyelitis of the feet, 25 were diabetic, five had severe atherosclerosis, and one had vasculitis secondary to rheumatoid arthritis. Eventually, 28 of the 31 patients underwent amputation, most within 6 months of diagnosis. The majority of cultures reported included gram-positive and gram-negative aerobic organisms, but not anaerobic organisms. Although antimicrobial therapy is not detailed, treatment for anaerobic organisms was presumably not given. The authors' feelings are clearly stated: "Because of the progressive nature of this illness, we have included successful amputation as cure of the disease since it halted its continuing advance" (31).

Seventeen years later, a series of 51 episodes of osteomyelitis in the lower extremities of 42 patients with diabetes was reported (28); some patients did not have bone biopsy to confirm the diagnosis. More than half (27 episodes) had a favorable outcome with a follow-up time of approximately 1.5 years. The majority of the episodes with a successful outcome did not require major surgical procedures. Two prognostic factors were noted: In the poor outcome group, there was a more frequent presence of necrosis, and in the good outcome group, there was swelling. Also associated with a favorable outcome was the use of specific antimicrobial therapy for at least 4 weeks intravenously or therapy with intravenous and oral antimicrobial agents for 10 weeks. Unlike previous studies (30,31), the majority of patients (without evidence on examination of necrosis or gangrene who received high doses of appropriate systemic antibiotics early in their hospitalization) had a favorable response to therapy without a need for surgical ablation (28). Earlier reports of poor results may have been associated with the fact that antimicrobial therapy use was more limited and often not active against anaerobic organisms.

In an era of decreasing reimbursement for hospitalization costs, treatment with oral agents from the onset of therapy would offer significant economic advantages. In one series (32), 48 patients with peripheral vascular disease were treated with oral ciprofloxacin for lower extremity infections; 31 had osteomyelitis. Sixty-one percent of the patients with osteomyelitis had a good clinical response after long-term follow-up (32). The authors recognized the variable anaerobic coverage of ciprofloxacin, but believed that drainage and debridement might partially explain favorable results even when anaerobic organisms were present. It was noted that the initial presence of gangrene was associated with early amputation, that a prolonged course of therapy correlated with a successful outcome, and that failure of the wound to close augured poorly for one-year successful outcome.

Unresolved Problems

It would appear from the literature reviewed herein, that there has been an improvement in the outcome of diabetic foot infections since 1970 (31). Some of the factors that may have contributed to improvement include increased antibiotic potency and spectrum; improvement in diagnosis, including new scanning techniques; improvements in surgical procedures and revascularization techniques; improvements in general medical and surgical care, as well as critical care, for diabetic patients with severe metabolic derangements; an increased awareness of diabetic foot problems, which has resulted in specialty clinics and advanced and specific care; and availability of outpatient antimicrobial therapy, both parenteral and oral, which has increased the length of time antibiotics can be administered successfully.

Despite these optimistic observations, certain problems and unanswered questions remain. What is the cause of osteopathy (noninfected bone lesions)? In polymicrobial infections, is therapy for *Enterococcus, Corynebacteria,* and other "dubious" pathogens necessary? Does an initial period of parenteral antibiotic therapy improve long-term outcome or could oral therapy with appropriately active agents be utilized from the inception of therapy? What can be done to enhance wound closure or ulcer healing because failure to do so is associated with reinfection? How does one extend the advances being made in a few centers with a keen interest in infection of the diabetic foot to the large majority of patients who are not being treated in such facilities?

References

1. Lipsky BA, Pecoraro RE, Wheat LJ. The diabetic foot. Soft tissue and bone infection. Infect Dis Clin North Am 1990;4:409–432.
2. Lipsky BA, Pecoraro RE, Larson SA, Hanley ME, Ahroni JH. Outpatient management of uncomplicated lower-extremity infections in diabetic patients. Arch Intern Med 1990;150:790–797.
3. Most RS, Sinnock P. The epidemiology of lower extremity amputations in diabetic individuals. Diabetes Care 1983;6:87–91.
4. National Diabetes Advisory Board. The National Long-range Plan to Combat Diabetes. Washington, DC: US Government Printing Office, DHEW Publ. No. NIH87-1587, 1987:ix.

5. Rutkow IM. Orthopaedic operations in the United States, 1979 through 1983. J Bone Joint Surg [Am] 1986;68:716–719.
6. Boulton AJM. The diabetic foot. Med Clin North Am 1988;72:1513–1530.
7. Edmonds ME. The diabetic foot: pathophysiology and treatment. Clin Endocrinol Metab 1986;15:889–916.
8. Palumbo PJ, Melton LJ. Peripheral vascular disease in diabetes. In: Harris MI, Hamman RF, eds. Diabetes in America. Washington, DC: US Government Printing Office, NIH Publ. No 85-1468, 1985:16–21.
9. Faris I, Duncan H. Vascular disease and vascular function in the lower limb in diabetes. Diabetes Res 1984;1:171–177.
10. Edmonds ME, Roberts VC, Watkins PJ. Blood flow in the diabetic neuropathic foot. Diabetologia 1982;22:9–15.
11. Pecoraro RE, Reiber GE, Labbe RF. Nutrition, wound failure, and diabetic amputation (abstract POS-003-082). From the 13th congress of the International Diabetes Federation, Sydney, Australia, Nov 20–25, 1988. Amsterdam: Elsevier Science Publishers, S398.
12. Sapico FL, Witte JL, Canawati HN, Montgomerie JZ, Bessman AN. The infected foot of the diabetic patient. Quantitative microbiology and analysis of clinical features. Rev Infect Dis 1984;6(suppl 1):S171–176.
13. Wheat LJ, Allen SD, Henry M, et al. Diabetic foot infections. Bacteriologic analysis. Arch Intern Med 1986;146:1935–1940.
14. Sharp CS, Bessman AN, Wagner FW Jr, Garland D. Microbiology of superficial and deep tissues in infected diabetic gangrene. Surg Gynecol Obstet 1979;149:217–219.
15. Louie TJ, Bartlett JG, Tally FP, Gorbach SL. Aerobic and anaerobic bacteria in diabetic foot ulcers. Ann Intern Med 1976;85:461–463.
16. Fierer J, Daniel D, Davis C. The fetid foot: lower-extremity infection in patients with diabetes mellitus. Rev Infect Dis 1979;1:210–217.
17. LeFrock JL, Blais F, Schell RF, et al. Cefoxitin in the treatment of diabetic patients with lower extremity infections. Infect Surg 1983;2:361–374.
18. Zlatkin MB, Pathria M, Sartoris DJ, Resnick D. The diabetic foot. Radiol Clin North Am 1987;25:1095–1105.
19. Littenberg B, Mushlin A. Technetium bone scanning in the diagnosis of osteomyelitis: a meta-analysis of test performance. J Gen Intern Med 1992;7:158–163.
20. Schauwecker DS, Park HM, Burt RW, Mock BH, Wellman HN. Combined bone scintigraphy and indium-111 leukocyte scans in neuropathic foot disease. J Nucl Med 1988;29:1651–1655.
21. Keenan AM, Tindel NL, Alavi A. Diagnosis of pedal osteomyelitis in diabetic patients using current scintigraphic techniques. Arch Intern Med 1989;149:2262–2266.
22. Neuman L, Waller J, Palestro CJ, et al. Unsuspected osteomyelitis in diabetic foot ulcers. JAMA 1991;266:1246–1251.
23. Jacobson A, Harley J, Lipsky B, Pecoraro R. Diagnosis of osteomyelitis in the presence of soft tissue infection and radiologic evidence of

osseous abnormalities: value of leukocyte scintigraphy. AJR 1991;157: 807–812.
24. Yuh WTC, Corson JD, Baranlewski HM, et al. Osteomyelitis of the foot in diabetic patients: evaluation with plain film, ^{99}Tc-MDP bone scintigraphy, and MR Imaging. AJR 1989;152:795–800.
25. Weinstein D, Wang A, Chambers R, Stewart C, Motz H. Evaluation of magnetic resonance imaging in the diagnosis of osteomyelitis in diabetic foot infections. Foot Ankle 1993;14:18–22.
26. Caprioli R, Testa J, Cournoyer R Jr, Esposito FJ. Prompt diagnosis of suspected osteomyelitis by utilizing percutaneous bone culture. J Foot Surg 1986;25:263–269.
27. Edmonds ME, Blundell MP, Morris MC. Improved survival of the diabetic foot. The role of the specialized foot clinic. Q J Med 1986;60:763–771.
28. Bamberger DM, Daws GP, Gerding DN. Osteomyelitis in the feet of diabetic patients. Long-term results, prognostic factors, and the role of antimicrobial and surgical therapy. Am J Med 1987;83:653–660.
29. Mizel MS. Diabetic foot infections. Orthop Rev 1989;18:572–577.
30. Benton GS, Kerstein MD. Cost effectiveness of early digit amputation in the patient with diabetes. Surg Gynecol Obstet 1985;161:523–524.
31. Waldvogel FA, Medoff G, Swartz MN. Osteomyelitis: a review of clinical features, therapeutic considerations and unusual aspects. N Engl J Med 1970;282:198–322.
32. Peterson LR, Lissack LM, Canter K, Fasching CE, Clabots C, Gerding DN. Therapy of lower extremity infections with ciprofloxacin in patients with diabetes mellitus, peripheral vascular disease, or both. Am J Med 1989;86: 801–808.

CHAPTER 12

Osteomyelitis Associated with Special Risk Groups

Certain groups of patients appear to be at increased risk for development of osteomyelitis. Although the reasons for this association are not always clear, there does appear to be an increased incidence of osteomyelitis in patients with hemoglobinopathies, in patients undergoing hemodialysis, and in patients who are intravenous drug abusers. In patients who are immunocompromised (particularly due to the human immunodeficiency virus [HIV] infection), it is less clear whether the incidence of osteomyelitis is really greater. In this chapter, the clinical presentations, infecting organisms, management, and outcome of osteomyelitis in these patients are reviewed.

Osteomyelitis in Patients with Hemoglobinopathies

There is an increased risk of significant bacterial infections in individuals with hemoglobinopathies, particularly sickle-cell disease (1). The most common infection is overwhelming sepsis, and *Streptococcus pneumoniae* is the primary infecting organism. In one series following 70 patients with complete major sickling disorders for a 10-year period, 20 had at least one hospitalization for treatment of osteomyelitis (2). The frequency of osteomyelitis or suppurative arthritis is low, but the fact that an organism not frequently associated with bone and joint infections (*Salmonella*) is often reported has brought attention to these entities. Among 166 patients with sickle-cell anemia over an 11-year period, nine were hospitalized for osteomyelitis; in another series of 315 patients with either SS or SC disease, only eight of 315 had osteoarticular infection (3).

The mechanism for increased susceptibility to bone infection, particularly with *Salmonella,* is not clear. One mechanism postulated is the impaired function of macrophages; it has been suggested that in patients with hemoglobinopathies, phagocytosis of red cell breakdown products so satiates the macrophages that they are incapable of ingesting and killing *Salmonella* (4). Some support for this hypothesis was obtained in experimental studies (5). A second predisposing factor is that following ingestion, *Salmonella* characteristically invades intestinal lympathics, regional lymph nodes, and the reticuloendothelial system, which includes the bone marrow. In normal hosts, *Salmonella* is presumably cleared from the bone marrow because osteomyelitis due to this organism is quite infrequent. In contrast, in patients with sickle-cell disease, bone marrow thrombosis and infarction, which are usually present, may allow the organism to produce infection.

Salmonella and other gram-negative organisms are the major agents that cause osteomyelitis in patients with hemoglobinopathies (2,3). In patients without sickle-cell disease, *Salmonella* was the etiological agent of osteomyelitis in less than 1% (2,3). The distribution of etiological agents for septic arthritis was also quite different between patients with and without hemoglobinopathies. Five of six patients with sickle-cell disease and septic arthritis had infections due to *S. pneumoniae,* and one was due to *Hemophilus influenzae* type B. In patients without sickle-cell disease, *S. pneumoniae* was the etiological agent in only 2.5% with suppurative arthritis, and *H. influenzae* was responsible for one fourth of infections in children without hemoglobinopathy (3).

Diagnosis of osteomyelitis in a child with sickle-cell disease can be extremely difficult. Osteomyelitis may have a subacute or insidious onset and be difficult to distinguish from sickle-cell crisis. Symptoms of mild fever and bone tenderness at multiple sites, which could persist for one to 2 weeks before clinical and radiographic signs of bone infection become apparent, has been noted (2). The early signs and symptoms of osteomyelitis can be identical to those of thrombotic marrow crises. High fever is less common in patients with bone infarction than in those with osteomyelitis, but it can occur in either (3). Local physical findings, such as swelling, may be more prominent in osteomyelitis, but can occur in patients with both entities. One series suggests that involvement of multiple sites makes the diagnosis of bone infarction more likely than osteomyelitis (3), but in another, seven of ten children with osteomyelitis had multiple sites of bone infection (2). Leukocytosis is generally present in both conditions, although a finding of an absolute band neutrophil count greater than 500 may be useful in suggesting osteomyelitis (3). Positive cultures are clearly the most important factor in distinguishing these entities. Positive blood cultures strongly favor the diagnosis of osteomyelitis. Stool cultures that yield *Salmonella* increase the suspicion for osteomyelitis. Radiographic findings are usually not present until 10 to 14 days after onset of illness; these findings include periosteal reaction and destruction of bone, features that occur in both osteomyelitis and bone infarction (Figure 12-1).

Newer radionuclide bone imaging studies may have some use in differentiation of osteomyelitis from infarction in sickle-cell disease. ^{99}Technetium-MDP bone imaging and ^{67}gallium imaging (6–9) appear

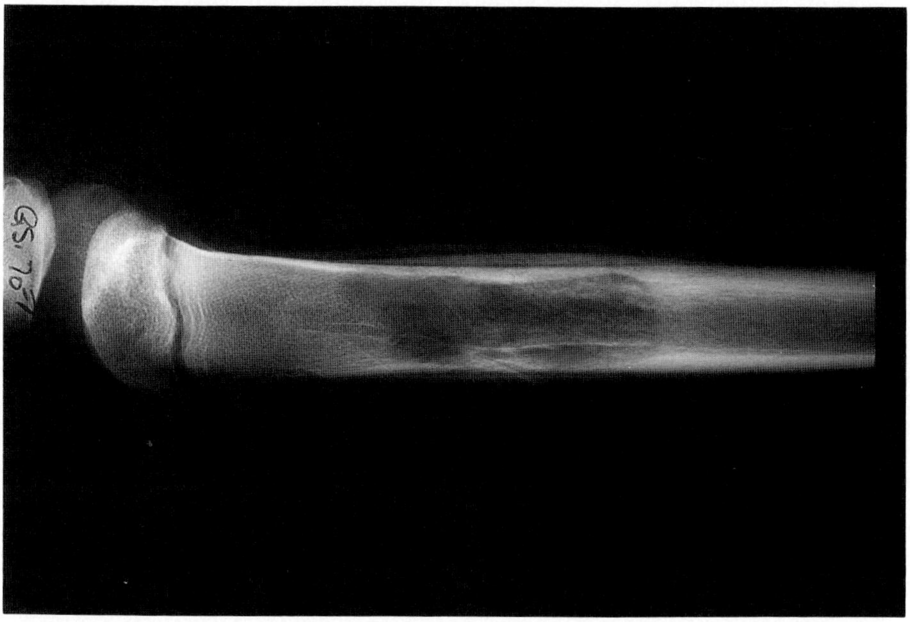

Figure 12-1. *Radiograph of the femur showing a lesion of the shaft in a child with sickle-cell disease. The initial appearance raised concerns about a Ewing's sarcoma, but* Streptococcus pneumoniae *was isolated from culture.*

to lack the necessary specificity to make a definitive diagnosis. Bone marrow imaging, although very sensitive, did not appear to distinguish osteomyelitis from infarction (8).

In an attempt to define further the usefulness of bone marrow scans and bone scans, one study (10) examined the two techniques in relation to the time after onset of symptoms and argued that both tests should be performed within 72 hours of the onset of pain. If the bone marrow scan revealed large abnormalities, with normal or decreased uptake on bone scan, infarction was likely. Increased uptake of the bone scan during the same period was more indicative of infection of bone or joints, particularly if the bone marrow scan was normal or minimally abnormal. Studies done 7 or more days after onset of pain were generally not valuable in differentiating infarction from osteomyelitis. Bone marrow scan may not be sensitive enough to detect small infarcts.

Another study (11) reported on the use of combined bone marrow and gallium imaging and indicated that in osteomyelitis, gallium uptake at the site of infection was incongruently increased relative to bone marrow activity, whereas in bone infarction, there was congruent activity with both isotopes. This promising study needs confirmation and a larger series to determine whether the technique will have significant clinical usefulness.

The role of ^{111}indium labeled white blood cell scans was examined in patients with sickle-cell disease. Acute osteomyelitis in a patient with sickle-cell disease in which the ^{99}Tc-MDP bone images and conventional radiographs were not diagnostic of osteomyelitis, has been reported; ^{111}indium white blood cell imaging was positive and pointed to a site for biopsy (12). ^{111}Indium scanning, if positive, may be a valuable tool in establishing the diagnosis of osteomyelitis in patients with sickle-cell disease, prior bone infarcts, and abnormal ^{99}Tc-MDP bone images. The import of a negative examination is not yet clear. Use of this scanning technique, as well as the others previously described, should be reserved for those patients in whom the diagnosis of osteomyelitis is strongly suspected but is difficult to prove by conventional methods.

Identification of a subperiosteal abscess by ultrasound or computerized tomography suggests infection, which can then be confirmed by aspiration (13). Conversely, absence of such a collection supports a provisional diagnosis of bone infarct. How should a patient with sickle-cell disease who presents with bone pain be approached? Factors favoring a painful bone crisis include relatively normal temperature, multiple sites of pain, relative absence of physical findings, a low absolute band neutrophil count, and a normal sedimentation rate. Most children with sickle-cell disease present in this manner. We suggest obtaining blood and stool cultures and observing the child; if remission of symptoms occurs in a few days without antibiotics, the diagnosis of bone infarction is supported. In contrast, one should strongly suspect osteomyelitis if high fever, toxic appearance, local findings with point tenderness, high band neutrophil count, and elevated sedimentation rate are present. In such patients (before culture results are available), therapy should be selected that includes antimicrobial agents with a spectrum broad enough to cover gram-positive and gram-negative organisms, including *Salmonella.* Local antimicrobial sensitivity patterns for *Salmonella* need to be considered; therapy with a third-generation cephalosporin or a carbapenem may be appropriate. Surgical drainage and debridement may be required.

Suppurative arthritis is easier to diagnose because joint aspiration provides a gold standard. A positive culture is confirmatory of the diagnosis of suppurative arthritis. If joint tap chemistries and cytology are suspicious for infection, broad-spectrum antimicrobial therapy that encompasses *S. pneumoniae, Salmonella, H. influenzae,* and *Staphylococcus aureus* should be instituted. As noted, local antimicrobial sensitivity patterns for *Salmonella* need to be considered; treatment with a third-generation cephalosporin or a carbapenem may be appropriate as initial empiric therapy. Effective arthrolavage, repeated if necessary, must be considered; for infection of the hip joint, open surgical drainage is usually necessary (see Chapter 18).

Osteomyelitis in Patients Undergoing Hemodialysis

One of the risks of hemodialysis is the development of osteomyelitis (Figure 12-2). One series (14) described five patients undergoing regular hemodialysis in whom osteomyelitis developed. It was speculated that the diagnosis was frequently not considered in the absence of bone pain or fracture, that the clinical and radiographic signs and symptoms of osteomyelitis could mimic those of renal osteodystrophy, and that fracture sites were infrequently biopsied and examined for osteomyelitis. All five patients had preceding bacteremia, and the organism infecting bone and blood was usually the same.

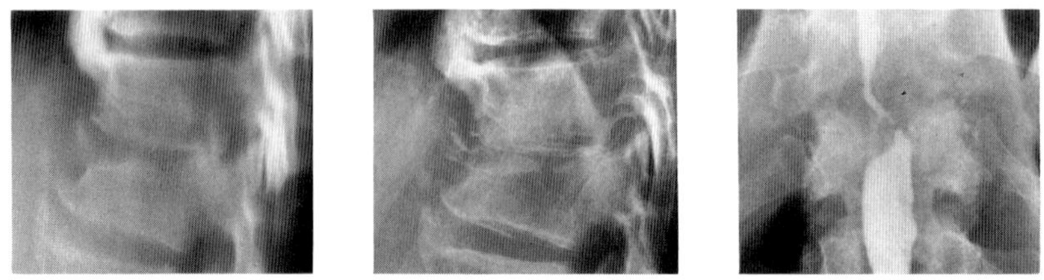

Figure 12-2. *Patient with chronic renal failure maintained on intermittent hemodialysis in whom bacteremia developed due to* Staphylococcus aureus *and subsequent vertebral osteomyelitis. (A) Lateral tomogram of thoracic spine 50 days after onset of bacteremia, showing decrease in vertical height of T11, narrowing of vertebral interspace, and loss of normal architecture of vertebral end plates of T11 and T12. (B) Lateral radiograph taken 63 days after onset of bacteremia shows further progression of disease, with obliteration of interspace between T11 and T12. (C) Thoracic myelogram performed 83 days after onset of bacteremia showing marked extradural constriction behind T11 to T12 disk space. Patient was found to have an epidural abscess causing compression of the spinal cord.* Staphylococcus aureus *was isolated from the abscess 74 days after onset of bacteremia.* (Provided by Dr. Martin McHenry.)

Staphylococci (either *S. aureus* or *S. epidermidis*) were found in four of the five patients, and *Pseudomonas aeruginosa* was found in the fifth. Patients had been on dialysis for an average of 30 months (range, 12–72 mo) when the diagnosis of osteomyelitis was made. The ribs and the thoracic spine were the most common sites of involvement. All patients were treated with antimicrobial agents; three of the five were considered cured, although recurrence of osteomyelitis subsequently developed in one in the same area and responded favorably to retreatment.

Two cases of cervical osteomyelitis due to *S. epidermidis* were reported in long-term hemodialysis patients (15). The initial complaint in both was neck pain; both responded well to antibiotic therapy without surgical drainage. It is postulated that the osteomyelitis presumably results from seeding due to bacteremia (bacteremia that develops secondary to infection of indwelling cannulae).

There must be a high index of suspicion of bone infections in hemodialysis patients who present with bony pain (14,15). The diagnosis may be difficult to make, and patients may present without fever, elevated white blood cell count, or radiographic abnormalities. We recommend biopsy at the involved area whenever feasible for both histological examination and microbiology. The danger of empiric antimicrobial therapy is failure to detect an unusual organism or a nonbacterial pathogen (i.e., fungi) and therefore treatment with an inappropriate agent. *S. epidermidis,* often discarded as a contaminant, must be regarded as a potential pathogen in these patients, particularly if it is recovered frequently.

Bone and Joint Infections in Intravenous Drug Abusers

The frequency of bone and joint infections in intravenous drug abusers is well documented (16). In one study over a one-year period, approximately 1,600 intravenous drug abusers were admitted to the hospital; 45 met the well-defined inclusion criteria as having osteomyelitis or septic arthritis. Septic arthritis was noted in 33, osteomyelitis in seven, and both in five. Two thirds of the patients were men. The majority of patients were heroin addicts, most of whom injected into the groin. The left groin was the site of injection twice as often as the right groin (presumably related to the handedness of the patients), and the left knee was the most commonly involved joint (one third of patients with septic arthritis). For those patients with osteomyelitis alone, sites of involvement were the vertebral column (3), the femur (2), and the fingers (2).

Pain and tenderness were the most constant features in all patients. Pyrexia was present in three fourths of the patients with septic arthritis, but in only two of seven patients with osteomyelitis. In those patients with osteomyelitis, with or without septic arthritis, admission radiographs were useful and revealed abnormalities (Figure 12-3). Among those patients with septic arthritis, radiographs were valuable only in patients with sacroiliac joint involvement. Technetium bone scans were of diagnostic value when radiographs were normal and when the sternal-clavicular joint, the sacroiliac joint, or the pubic symphysis were involved.

The infecting agent in patients with septic arthritis was diagnosed by either synovial fluid cultures (76% positive) or blood cultures. In patients with osteomyelitis, the etiological agent was recovered from cultures of pus overlying the bony lesion by bone biopsy and by blood

A B

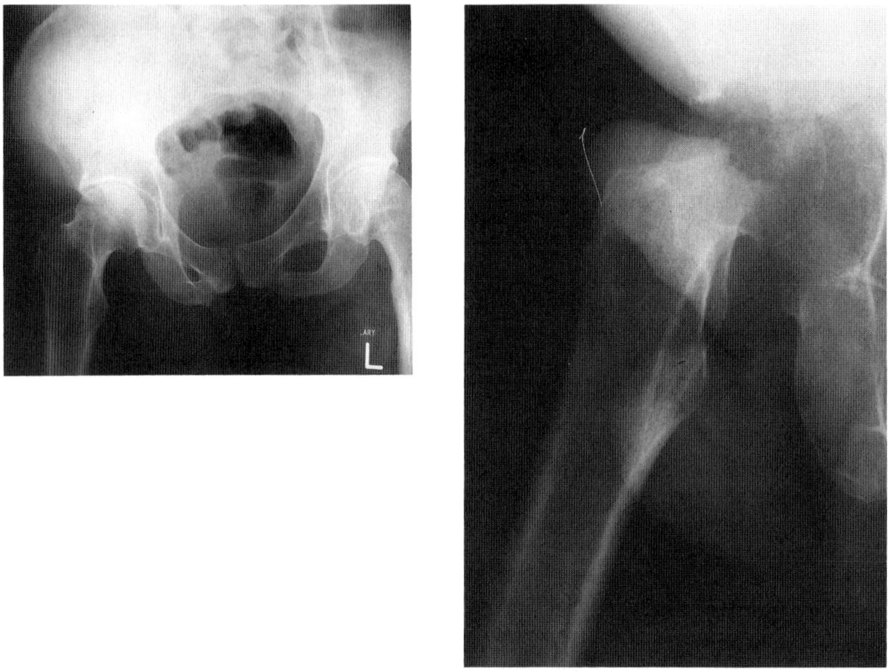

Figure 12-3. *Patient was an intravenous drug abuser with* Staphylococcus aureus *septicemia treated for one week before signing out against advice. (A) Radiograph of hip at time of discharge is essentially normal. (B) Four months later, patient returned with hip pain and radiograph showed destruction of acetabulum.* (Provided by Dr. Alex Norman.)

cultures. Staphylococci and streptococci were recovered from 82% of patients; *P. aeruginosa* was found in 11% of patients.

The majority of patients appeared to recover with antimicrobial therapy and with arthrocentesis for those with septic arthritis. Patients with osteomyelitis appeared to respond well to intravenous antibiotics and surgical treatment when necessary; however, long-term follow-up was difficult to obtain. Nonetheless, the immediate prognosis of bone and joint disease in intravenous drug abusers appeared to be excellent.

Prior studies have reported a high prevalence of gram-negative infections of bones or joints in intravenous drug abusers; *P. aeruginosa* is the major pathogen (16). In one study there was a shift in etiological agents from gram-negative pathogens to staphylococci and streptococci (16). A concurrent study at the same medical center found that bacteremia due to *P. aeruginosa* was seen in only 9% of intravenous drug abusers with bacteremia. Thus, the frequency of bone and joint involvement in intravenous drug abusers with gram-positive organisms appears to parallel the experience with bacteremia in the same population.

One presentation of osteomyelitis in intravenous drug abusers is infection of the pubis. In the general population, osteomyelitis of the pubis accounts for less than 1% of all cases of hematogenous osteomyelitis. In many of the cases reported in the literature, the disease developed as a complication of pelvic surgery; however, two studies published in 1982 (17,18) indicate that infection of the pubic symphysis may be seen in intravenous drug abusers. Patients were identified because they had tenderness over the pubic symphysis, radiological evidence of osteomyelitis, or an abnormal bone scan and positive cultures from either blood or bone biopsy.

In the usual presentation of pubic osteomyelitis in drug addicts, the mean duration of symptoms was three weeks. Radiographs on admission were frequently normal; abnormal findings included irregularity of the margins of the pubic bones and widening of the pubic symphysis with bone destruction. Radioisotope bone scans were often helpful and demonstrated activity at the site. In the majority of patients, *P. aeruginosa* was the responsible pathogen. In both series, patients responded to antibiotic treatment and debridement satisfactorily. The optimal duration of therapy for pubic osteomyelitis is not clear.

The pubic symphysis is a fibrocartilaginous joint. Infections of such joints are relatively uncommon in the general population, but infection of the sternoclavicular and sternochondral articulations (19) have also been reported in heroin users. As with osteomyelitis of the pubis, *P. aeruginosa* appears to be the most common infecting organism of the sternoclavicular and sternochondral joints.

The reasons for the frequency of bone and joint infections in somewhat unusual sites of presentation among drug addicts are not clear. There appears to be a relationship between the site of injection in the left groin and the site of disease (16). Organisms may enter the arterial circulation in the groin by arteriovenous channels produced by multiple needle punctures and then travel to produce disease in weight-bearing, frequently traumatized joints, such as the knee. Involvement of fibrocartilaginous joints, such as the pubis and the sternoclavicular joints, is difficult to explain. Degenerative changes of these joints, with damaged cartilage, have been noted in humans by the third decade (20) and might serve as a focus for infection, but there are no studies to suggest that such changes occur more frequently or more prominently in drug abusers. Thirty-eight heroin addicts were studied in 1974, and a high incidence of abnormalities, including hypergammaglobulinemia and impaired in vitro responsiveness in lymphocyte culture studies to at least one of three mitogens, were found (21). However, it was somewhat difficult to exclude the effects of liver disease in accounting for the defects seen in the humoral immune system in this series. Currently, the reasons for increased infection among intravenous drug abusers, other than direct injection of contaminated material and subsequent vascular damage by foreign materials and altered immune status (i.e., HIV), are not known.

Bone and Joint Infections in Patients with HIV Infection

In a large series of 1,400 patients with the acquired immunodeficiency syndrome (AIDS), only six had manifestations of bone disease; only one of the six had osteomyelitis; the others had lymphoma or reflex sympathetic dystrophy (22). In another series (23), ten infections involving bone, joint, or muscle occurred in an HIV-positive population of approximately 3,000 individuals. Septic arthritis occurred in seven patients (with accompanying osteomyelitis in two), and osteomyelitis, myositis, and bursitis occurred in three others. Although *S. aureus* was the most common organism isolated, the organisms recovered include *Sporothrix, Cryptococcus, S. pneumoniae, Histoplasma capsulatum,* and *Mycobacterium avium* complex. In all infections occurring in patients with AIDS, the CD4 lymphocyte count was markedly reduced. One case report (24) described a patient with indolent osteomyelitis of the tibia from which a biopsy grew *Mycobacterium kansasii,* and simultaneous blood cultures grew *Salmonella* species, indicating that organisms associated with HIV infection may cause infection of bone. Another case report (25) of osteomyelitis due to *S. aureus* in a patient with AIDS illustrates the rapidity of severe bony destructive changes over an 8-day period and calls attention to the fact that the immunocompromised state may allow a more fulminant presentation and progression of disease.

References

1. Barrett-Connor E. Bacterial infection and sickle cell anemia: an analysis of 250 infections in 166 patients and a review of the literature. Medicine 1971;50:97–112.
2. Engh CA, Hughes JL, Abrams RC, Bowerman JW. Osteomyelitis in the patient with sickle-cell disease. J Bone Joint Surg [Am] 1971;53:1–15.
3. Syrogiannopoulos GA, McCracken GH, Nelson JD. Osteoarticular infections in children with sickle cell disease. Pediatrics 1986;78:1090–1096.
4. Hook EW, Kay D, Gill FA. Factors influencing host resistance to Salmonella infection: the effects of hemolysis and erythrophagocytosis. Trans Am Clin Climatol Assoc 1967;78:230–241.
5. Kaye D, Hook EW. The influence of hemolysis or blood loss on susceptibility to infection. J Immunol 1963;91:65–75.
6. Majd M, Frankel RS. Radionuclide imaging in skeletal inflammatory and ischemic disease in children. Am J Roentgenol 1976;126:832–841.
7. Sain A, Sham R, Silver L. Bone scan in sickle cell crisis. Clin Nucl Med 1978;3:85.
8. Lutzker LG, Alavi A. Bone and marrow imaging in sickle cell disease: diagnosis of infarction. Semin Nucl Med 1976;6:83–93.
9. Greenwald L, Fajman W. Utility of gallium scans in differentiating osteomyelitis from infarction in sickle cell patients (abstract). Clin Nucl Med 1982;10:71.
10. Kim HC, Alavi A, Russell MO, Schwartz E. Differentiation of bone and bone marrow infarcts from osteomyelitis in sickle cell disorders. Clin Nucl Med 1989;14:249–254.
11. Kahn CE, Ryan JW, Malcolm KH, Martin WB. Combined bone marrow and gallium imaging. Differentiation of osteomyelitis and infarction in sickle hemoglobinopathy. Clin Nucl Med 1988;13:443–449.
12. Fernandex-Ulloa M, Vasavada PJ, Black RR. Detection of acute osteomyelitis with ^{111}indium labeled white blood cells in a patient with sickle cell disease. Clin Nucl Med 1989;14:97–100.
13. Howard C, Einhorn M, Dagan R, Nygha M. Ultrasound in diagnosis and management of acute haematogenous osteomyelitis in children. J Bone Joint Surg [Br] 1993;75:79–82.
14. Leonard A, Comty CM, Shapiro FL, Raij L. Osteomyelitis in hemodialysis patients. Ann Intern Med 1973;78:651–658.
15. Parker MA, Tuazon CU. Cervical osteomyelitis. Infection due to Staphylococcus epidermidis in hemodialysis patients. JAMA 1978;240:50–51.
16. Chandrasekar PH, Narula AP. Bone and joint infections in intravenous drug abusers. Rev Infect Dis 1986;8:904–911.
17. del Busto R, Quinn EL, Fisher EJ, Madhavan T. Osteomyelitis of the pubis. Report of seven cases. JAMA 1982;248:1498–1500.

18. Sequeira W, Jones E, Siegel ME, Lorenz M, Kallick C. Pyogenic infections of the pubic symphysis. Ann Intern Med 1982;96:604–606.
19. Goldin RH, Chow AW, Edwards JE Jr, Louie JS, Guze LB. Sternoarticular septic arthritis in heroin users. N Engl J Med 1973;289:616–618.
20. Silberg M, Frank EL, Jarrett SR, et al. Aging and osteoarthritis of the human sternoclavicular joint. Am J Pathol 1959;35:851–863.
21. Brown SM, Stimmel B, Taub RN, Kochwa S, Rosenfield RE. Immunologic dysfunction in heroin addicts. Arch Intern Med 1974;134:1001–1006.
22. Sabbagh M, Meyer O, De Bandt M, et al. Bone manifestations associated with acquired immunodeficiency syndrome (AIDS). Ann Intern Med 1992; 148:50–56.
23. Hughes R, Rowe I, Shanson D, Keat A. Septic bone, joint and muscle lesions associated with human immunodeficiency virus infection. Br J Rheumatol 1992;31:381–388.
24. Crawfurd EJP, Baird PRE. An orthopaedic presentation of AIDS: brief report. J Bone Joint Surg [Br] 1987;69:672–673.
25. Goh BT, Jawad ASM, Chapman D, Winceslaus SJ, Forster GE, Perry JD. Osteomyelitis presenting as a swollen elbow in a patient with the acquired immune deficiency syndrome. Ann Rheum Dis 1988;47:695–696.

CHAPTER 13

Mycobacterial Infections of the Musculoskeletal System

Prior to the introduction of chemotherapy in the middle 1940s, skeletal tuberculosis was a significant cause of morbidity in most communities (1). In the developing world, it is still a major problem, but in the developed world, the incidence has decreased dramatically (2,3). In the last decade, however, that trend has slowed (4) and may be reversing in keeping with the recrudescence of tuberculosis in a number of developed communities. Mycobacterial bone and joint infections associated with human immunodeficiency virus (HIV) infection have been increasingly reported (5,6). Many are caused by atypical mycobacteria. Most skeletal tuberculosis, however, still occurs in the developing world, from which much of the recent literature has come (7–9).

Epidemiology

Bone or joint infections have accounted for 2% to 5% of notified tuberculosis cases (10–14). By the 1980s, the incidence in developed societies had decreased to less than 1 per 100,000 per year (2,3,11,15). In the developing world, however, and in immigrants and some ethnic minorities in developed societies, it remains much higher (14,15).

Until recognition of the frequency of mycobacterial infections in immunocompromised hosts, the percentage of cases of osteoarticular tuberculosis with concurrent active disease elsewhere appeared to have decreased steadily since the introduction of chemotherapy (11,16–19). Multiple sites, however, are present in 25% to 70% of patients with HIV infection and tuberculosis. Up to 6% of patients with HIV are on the tuberculosis registers in the United States and in Great Britain (5,6). Between 5% and 10% of notifications of nontuberculous mycobacterial (NTM) infections have skeletal involvement (20).

Notifications of nonrespiratory tuberculosis show no seasonal trends. Annual notification rates and hospital morbidity data confirm the dramatic decrease in incidence of osteoarticular tuberculosis in the developed world since 1948 (2,3). Where BCG vaccination is carried out, BCG osteitis is endemic, and occasional epidemics have been reported (21).

In the developing world (8,22), as in Europe and North America prior to the introduction of chemotherapy (1,16), the highest incidence rates of osteoarticular tuberculosis have been recorded in those less than 45 years of age. In contrast, in developed countries, the highest incidence currently occurs in those more than 65 years of age (3,4,11,14,23). In individuals with a normal immune response, there may be a long latent period between a primary tuberculous focus and the onset of an episode of bone and joint disease. Indeed, no primary focus may have been recorded. In a recent study, only 30% of patients gave a history of previous tuberculosis (4).

Case Characteristics

Reviews of osteoarticular tuberculosis suggest that approximately half the affected individuals have spinal infection; 10% to 20% have tuberculous osteomyelitis, or extra-articular synovial or bursal disease. The remainder have tuberculous arthritis; the hip and knee are particularly affected (3,8,11,16,22). BCG osteomyelitis rarely involves the spine (24).

In addition to immunocompromised individuals, other groups at risk include those with known primary infections more than 10 years previously; health staff; migrant groups from areas of high incidence; and patients with diabetes, asbestosis, chronic renal failure, malabsorption, steroid therapy, or alcoholism (15,25–28). Current or recent corticosteroid therapy is strongly associated with NTM infections (29).

Microbiology and Pathology

The organisms causing human skeletal mycobacterial infections are listed in Table 13-1. Human acquisition is by airborne droplet nu-

Table 13-1. Mycobacteria known to cause musculoskeletal infection in humans

Tuberculosis
Mycobacterium tuberculosis
M. bovis
M. ulcerans
Nontuberculous mycobacteria
Group I
M. kansasii
M. marinum
M. simiae
M. asiaticum
Group II
M. scrofulaceum complex
Group III
M. avium-intracellulare complex
M. terrae complex
Group IV
M. fortuitum complex
Leprosy
M. leprae

clei, by the gastrointestinal tract, or occasionally from direct inoculation (30). BCG osteomyelitis is exclusively the result of inoculation. The majority of musculoskeletal infections arise from hematogenous spread from lesions elsewhere, but direct spread from adjacent infected lymph nodes may also occur (31).

The characteristic granulomatous lesion of tuberculosis is seen on histological examination in the majority of infection by the *M. tuberculosis/bovis* group (32). NTM infections, however, may show only a diffuse nonspecific chronic inflammatory infiltrate surrounding areas of bone death and necrosis (33). Typical histological changes of tuberculosis may be found in bone in apparently cured disease 10 or more years later (34).

Diagnostic and Laboratory Investigations

Hematological investigation is nonspecific and may be misleading. The erythrocyte sedimentation rate is usually increased but may be normal (19). The white cell count is increased in less than 10% of patients (35).

In osteoarticular tuberculosis in immunocompetent individuals, the tuberculin (Mantoux) test is almost always positive (36,37). However, false-negative results may occur early in the course of the disease, in individuals who have become anergic in response to extensive disease, in those immunocompromised by disease or medication, and in individuals with active viral infections, such as measles. Where the prevalence of active tuberculosis is low, as it currently is in the developed world, the positive predictive value of the Mantoux test is low (38). Furthermore, in patients with tuberculosis and acquired immunodeficiency syndrome (AIDS), one third to one half will have a positive tuberculin test result, although up to 80% of those who are HIV-positive but without AIDS may do so (5,6). Currently, enzyme-linked immunosorbent assay antibody studies and DNA probes remain research tools: They are not yet sufficiently specific to allow serological diagnosis of active osteoarticular tuberculosis on a routine basis (39–41).

Demonstration of mycobacteria from pus or tissue is still the most efficient route to a proven diagnosis. Unfortunately, in osteoarticular tuberculosis, the bacterial population may be very small (42). Thus, although Ziehl-Neelsen staining of suitable material can give quick identification, this direct examination is seldom positive. The yield of positive cultures can be improved by provision of adequate material for examination (43). At least 1 mL and preferably 10 mL pus or caseous material, as well as specimens of the abscess wall, if available, should be sent to the microbiology laboratory. Abscess wall specimens should also be sent for histological examination. Use of guinea pig inoculation is no longer recommended (44). A number of different solid and liquid media are now available (45), and culture processing may take up to 10 weeks.

Histological examination of suitable specimens is characteristic of mycobacterial infection in most patients. In immunocompromised and anergic individuals, however, only nonspecific inflammatory changes may be seen (32). It has been suggested that histological examination is more reliable than culture (46). In experienced hands, interpretation of material from fine-needle aspiration may also be diagnostic (47).

Imaging

The characteristic radiological appearance of skeletal mycobacterial infection is a destructive lesion involving a joint with marked regional osteoporosis, little surrounding sclerosis, and associated soft-tissue swelling (Figure 13-1); however, other patterns are recognized, including cystic tuberculosis (Figure 13-2) and lesions with marked reactive sclerosis or periostitis (Figure 13-3). Sequestra and pathological fractures may occur. Dystrophic calcification in the walls of tuberculous abscesses (Figure 13-4) is a suggestive radiological sign, but may also occur in brucellosis and in staphylococcal infections. A four-stage radiological classification has been described (8).

Other imaging techniques are available and may be useful but rarely contribute significantly to confirming diagnosis. Tomography and computerized axial tomography (48) elegantly demonstrate localization and extent of bone and soft-tissue lesions, particularly in

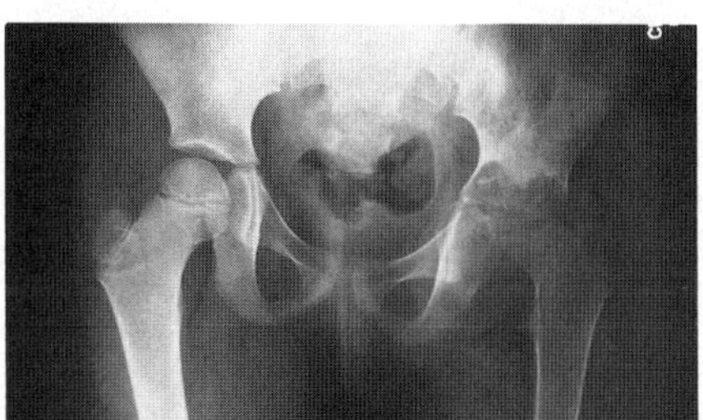

Figure 13-1. *Tuberculosis of the left hip, with regional osteoporosis and destruction of the left hip.*

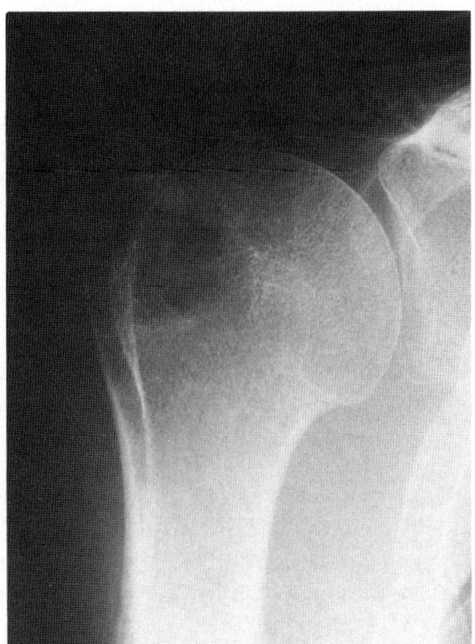

Figure 13-2. *Cystic tuberculosis. Tuberculous osteomyelitis of the greater tuberosity of the humerus.*

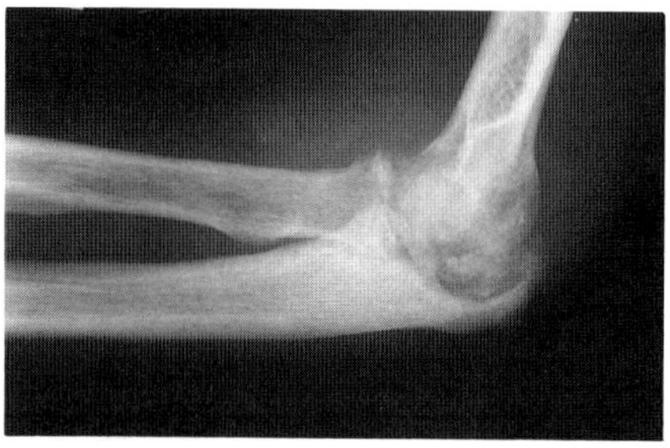

Figure 13-3. *Tuberculous arthritis of the left elbow. Some reactive new bone is present in the medial aspect of the proximal ulna. The radiocapitellar articulation is narrowed and sclerotic, but destruction of the olecranon suggests an infective lesion.*

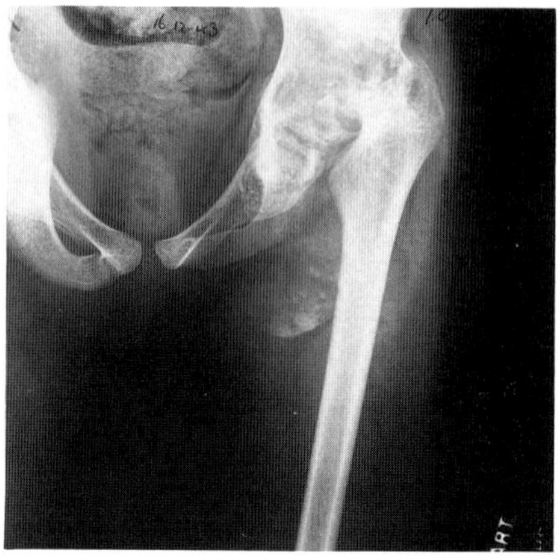

Figure 13-4. *Dystrophic calcification in the wall of a tuberculous abscess associated with destruction of the hip joint.*

spinal disease (Figure 13-5), thus aiding biopsy and surgical planning (49).

It was recognized early that ^{99m}Tc scintigraphy showed increased uptake at sites of tuberculous infection. In miliary tuberculosis, and in the presence of skip lesions in the spine, the appearances may be misinterpreted as metastatic disease (50). A potential radio tracer for tuberculosis, I^{124}-2-iodoisonicotinic acid hydrazide, has been synthesized (51), but its use in clinical practice has yet to be evaluated.

Soft-tissue abscesses, including psoas abscesses, are well demonstrated by ultrasound (52). Magnetic resonance imaging is comparable to computed tomography in the evaluation of both bone and articular destruction, as well as of soft-tissue abscesses (53).

Antibiotic Management

Before the introduction of chemotherapy, up to one third of those who contracted tuberculosis achieved control of their disease assisted by general conservative measures, including rest and improved

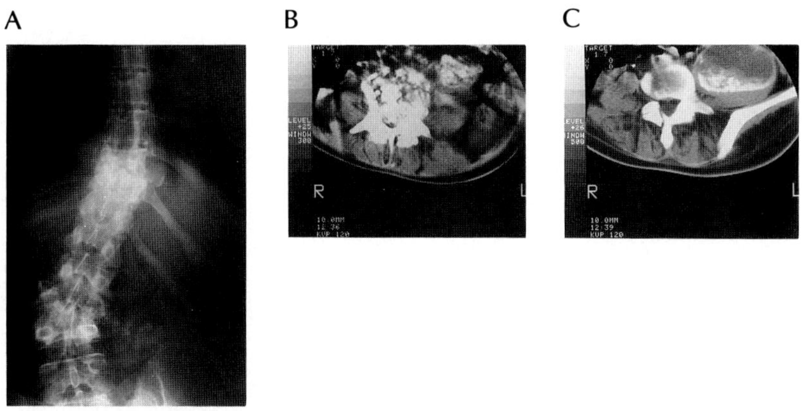

Figure 13-5. *(A) Tuberculous spondylitis at three levels: T10/11, L2/3, and L3/4. (B) Computerized tomography through L3 showing extensive destruction of the vertebral body with canal compromise. (C) A large left psoas abscess is well demonstrated in a section at the level of L5.*

nutrition (54). In skeletal tuberculosis, this figure was probably higher. In 1935, Seddon (55) reported a 70% recovery in patients with tuberculous spondylitis complicated by paraplegia. Contemporary results should be viewed against this background, which attests to the resilience of the host; however, without treatment, the potential for relapse is obviously higher.

Drug treatment alone is extremely effective, particularly in tuberculous spondylitis. Until recently, most studies reported protracted periods of 12 to 24 months of drug treatment. Short-course chemotherapeutic regimens have been evaluated; their results are comparable to those of 2-year programs (7,56).

While awaiting precise identification of the organism and its sensitivities, provisional treatment with one of the standard antibiotic regimens should be begun. The great majority of osteoarticular infections with the *M. tuberculosis/bovis* group remain sensitive. However, within certain geographical areas (such as New York City and Los Angeles) and particularly among immunocompromised hosts, the epidemiology has shifted to include an increasing frequency of multiple drug-resistant strains (57). For such patients (presumed or proven), therapy should be instituted with 5-, 6-, or 7-drug regimens until antimicrobial sensitivities are known. Of the atypical mycobacteria, some, particularly *M. kansasii,* generally respond well to standard antituberculous regimens. Complex strains of *M. avium,* however, are frequently drug-resistant in vitro (58). Other aminoglycosides and quinolones (59) may be effective in vitro. Clinical outcomes in NTM infection in HIV-positive patients are generally poor (60).

Surgical Treatment

The role of surgery in osteoarticular infection include acquisition of tissue or pus for diagnosis, drainage of large abscesses, and reconstructive procedures designed to restore function or stability. In accessible sites, needle biopsy may provide a diagnosis, although in paucibacterial disease, larger quantities of material may be required.

Spinal Tuberculosis

In countries where tuberculosis has a high prevalence, most infections occur in patients less than 45 years of age (1,22). In developed societies, the majority of cases occur in older patients. Dorsolumbar and lumbar disease are most common. Skip lesions, relatively uncommon in pyogenic vertebral osteomyelitis, occur in up to one third of patients with tuberculous spondylitis (1).

The characteristic lesion involves vertebral bodies with destruction of the intervening disk or disks (49; Figure 13-6). However, foci confined to vertebral bodies (61) or to the neural arch are also seen (62). Significant soft-tissue abscesses occur in approximately 20% of patients (8). These abscesses may be paravertebral, extradural, or in the buttock or thigh. Kyphosis results in approximately two thirds of typical cases.

The clinical features are spinal pain, stiffness, and deformity. Girdle pain occurs in thoracic and upper lumbar disease and may be misleading. Biopsy is essential for a proven diagnosis. In developed societies, where the incidence of pyogenic vertebral infections currently exceeds that of tuberculosis and where the predictive value of a positive Mantoux test result may be low, a needle biopsy should be attempted. If the diagnosis remains in doubt, open biopsy is required. If tuberculosis is confirmed, other tuberculous foci should be sought by chest radiography, sputum smear, and examination of the urinary tract.

A controlled study of large treatment groups showed that in the

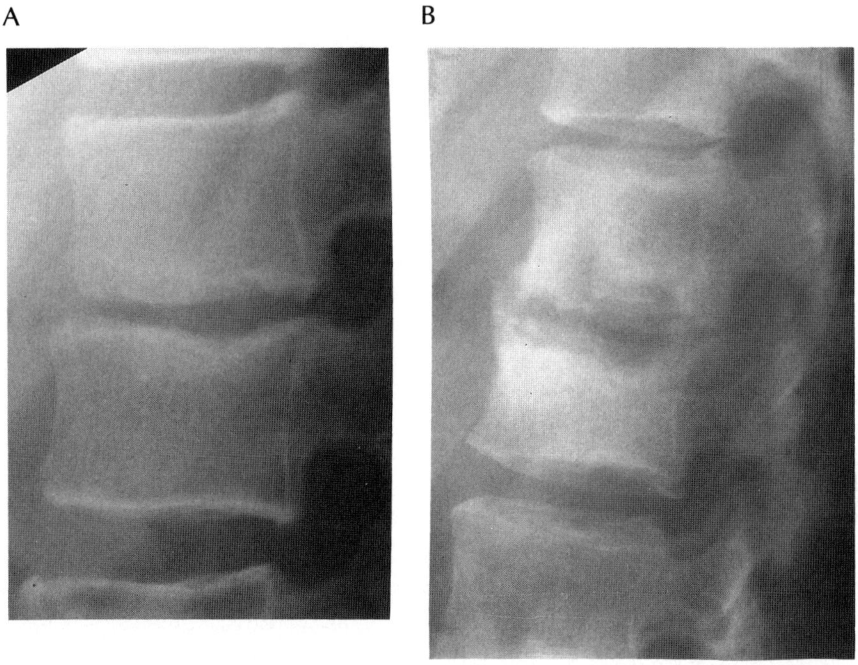

Figure 13-6. *(A) Appearance of L1/2 in an adult with tuberculous spondylitis at presentation. There is disk space narrowing and loss of end-plate definition anteriorly and in the posterior third. (B) After 4 months of antituberculous chemotherapy, intervertebral bridging is occurring. Typically, the appearances of bone destruction persist for some time; radiological resolution lags behind clinical response to therapy. Bone destruction is greater than at presentation. Provided there is evidence of systemic improvement and stabilization by intervertebral bridging, these appearances should not be considered evidence of failure of antimicrobial therapy.*

absence of significant neurological involvement, control of infection achieved by ambulant chemotherapy alone is comparable to that achieved by the addition of bed rest, plaster immobilization, or surgical debridement with or without grafting (63). However, the design of the study leaves unanswered questions about comparability of the treatment groups and a number of relative indications for surgery.

Laminectomy for surgical debridement of typical lesions is strongly contraindicated. Radical anterior debridement with grafting has been considered to result in more rapid bony fusion, less kyphosis, and quicker resolution of abscesses (18,64,65), but kyphosis may progress if the graft spans more than two disk spaces (9). Significant deformity in the presence of active tuberculosis has been considered an indication for decompression, correction, and stabilization by the anterior route (65). Severe kyphosis may require both anterior and posterior stabilization with instrumentation (66).

Surgical treatment requires experience and sophisticated resources. Other groups have achieved encouraging results with predominantly conservative management (8).

Tuberculosis Paraplegia (Pott's Disease)

In 1924, Sorel and Sorel-Dejerine (67) classified tuberculous paraplegia as early (< 2 years) or late onset. Currently, the preferred division is "paraplegia with active disease" and "paraplegia with healed disease" (68). Most cases of paraplegia with active disease are caused by an extradural abscess arising from a typical vertebral lesion, in which debris from the lesion is pushed back as kyphosis develops. Other rarer causes include collapse of an isolated vertebral body lesion (69), tuberculosis of the neural arch (62), and extradural extraosseus tuberculosis (64,67).

Management of paraplegia with typical active disease is somewhat controversial. As noted earlier, the outcome of protracted bed rest without chemotherapy or surgical debridement, reported by Seddon in 1935, was 70% recovery. Hodgson and colleagues from Hong Kong (64) reported 75% complete recovery with anterior decompression, grafting, and chemotherapy. Others have supported this approach (18,70). In a study from North Africa, however, bed rest and chemotherapy (71) gave superior results.

A "middle path" regimen beginning with 3 to 4 weeks of recumbent chemotherapy has been described and reviewed (72,73). If recovery began during the period of recumbency, surgical decompression was not performed. If there was no change, or if deterioration occurred, decompression was performed. The 78% success rate of this regimen is similar to the published results from surgical or conservative policies.

In the presence of severe kyphosis, there is a risk of late recurrence of paraplegia, which may arise either from reactivation of disease or from hard ridges of bone with healed disease (74). Decompression of healed disease is technically difficult and results are relatively poor.

The presence of a significant kyphus in active disease is therefore a strong relative indication for decompression, grafting, and possibly posterior fusion to restore trunk balance and to reduce the risk of late paraplegia.

The cervical spine may be the site of very extensive diffuse disease, particularly in childhood, and the value of ambulant chemotherapy has not been clearly established. Anterior surgical debridement and stabilization are recommended, using the transoral route for the upper cervical spine (75,76).

Tuberculous Arthritis

The objectives of current management are diagnosis; antibiotic control of disease; and restoration of a painless, stable, and preferably mobile joint. The choice of reconstructive procedure and the outcome are predominantly influenced by the stage of the disease (8,77) and by cultural and technical considerations.

In tuberculosis of the hip, although chemotherapy has significantly improved the outcome, the incidence of stiff, painful hips requiring reconstructive surgery is still high. Prior to the introduction of chemotherapy, arthrodesis was the treatment of choice (1), but it is culturally unacceptable in many societies. Excision arthroplasty can give good relief of pain with preservation of an acceptable range of movement. Provided that adequate chemotherapy is given both before and after the operation, cemented or cementless total hip arthroplasty gives good results in hips destroyed by tuberculosis, although there may be little or no improvement in the range of movement (78–80). Tuberculosis may be reactivated by total hip replacement (81), which is not an insuperable problem, and stability of the prosthesis may be regained by chemotherapy. In summary, total joint arthroplasty is recommended, if available, in older patients. In children and young adults, arthrodesis, or if arthrodesis is culturally unacceptable, excision arthroplasty, should be considered.

In the knee, monoarticular arthritis may be identified at an early stage, while disease is confined to the synovium (82). Radiological appearances are nonspecific. Synovitis presents as a severe regional osteopenia. Bony changes are predominantly destructive, but occasionally marked reactive sclerosis simulates osteoarthritis. In more typical appearances, arthroscopic inspection and biopsy should allow diagnosis. If there is extensive synovitis and debris, operative debridement may be indicated (22). Early mobilization is recommended in early disease in young patients (83), because debridement and prolonged immobilization lead to stiffness. Surgical reconstruction should be reserved for instability, deformity, and extensive joint destruction. Despite apparent good response to chemotherapy, histological examination of material from knees subjected to reconstructive surgery has sometimes demonstrated synovial tuberculous granulomata (84). Arthrodesis of the knee is an alternative to replacement arthroplasty in young patients and in those in whom replacement arthroplasty fails.

In the last decade, management of tuberculosis of the ankle (85), elbow (86), and sacroiliac joint (87) has been reviewed. For these joints, as for the others, chemotherapy is the keystone of management; surgery should be reserved for drainage of large abscesses and for instability or deformity.

Tuberculosis in the Wrist and Hand

Tuberculosis in the wrist and hand accounts for approximately 5% of skeletal tuberculosis (88). Synovitis, arthritis, and osteomyelitis (dactylitis) occur as isolated lesions or in combination. Dactylitis is more common in childhood; it may occur as one site in multiple disease (89). Three patterns of bony radiological change occur (90) (Figure 13-7).

A B C

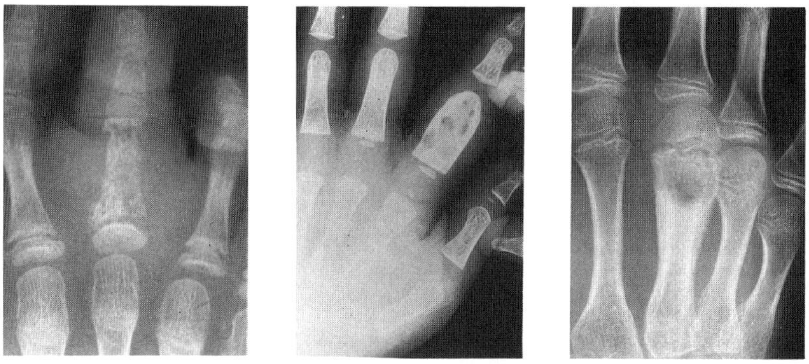

Figure 13-7. *(A) Honeycomb pattern of tuberculous dactylitis. (B) Longstanding spina ventosa with cystic cavities in a phalanx symmetrically enlarged by periosteal bone accretion. (C) Cystic tuberculosis in the third metacarpal.*

"Spina ventosa" is an expanding destructive lesion of both cortical and cancellous bone with periostitis; "honeycombing" is a diffuse uniform infiltration with small cavities and relatively little osteoporosis; and single cystic lesions also occur. Dactylitis may extend to involve joints or palmar tenosynovium (91). Most tuberculosis of the wrist occurs in older adults (92,93).

Any part of the tenosynovium of the hand may be involved in mycobacterial infections. The natural history was described in detail in 1923 by Kanavel (94). Stiffness, with swelling following the anatomical outline of the sheath involved, is an early sign. Initially, synovitis alone is present, but granulation, rice bodies, and eventually extensive necrosis occur. In the classic compound palmar ganglion, synovial hyperplasia may be sufficiently severe to produce compression of the median nerve. The local lesion closely resembles rheumatoid arthritis (95). Many synovial lesions recently reported have been associated with NTM infections (96,97).

Bacteriological diagnosis and chemotherapy are the fundamentals of treatment, but drainage of septic arthritis or occasionally debridement of a bony lesion may be required. Some have advocated synovectomy in tenosynovitis (91), but if the synovitis is not extensive, chemotherapy and immobilization alone may suffice (96,98). Flexor synovectomy is technically demanding and should be used only when skilled surgeons and rehabilitation are available.

Tuberculosis Osteomyelitis

Historically, the small bones of the hand and foot accounted for 30% to 50% of cases of tuberculosis involving bone alone (15). Other common sites include rib, sternum, and the metaphyses of long bones, particularly in children. However, any site, including skull and facial bones, may be affected. Because radiological appearances are not diagnostic, biopsy is essential. Surgical debridement has been the traditional treatment, but chemotherapy alone may suffice for a primary lesion (99).

Bursitis

Any bursa may be affected by tuberculosis (100). Radiological changes may be subtle, with soft-tissue swelling, minor calcification, and under-

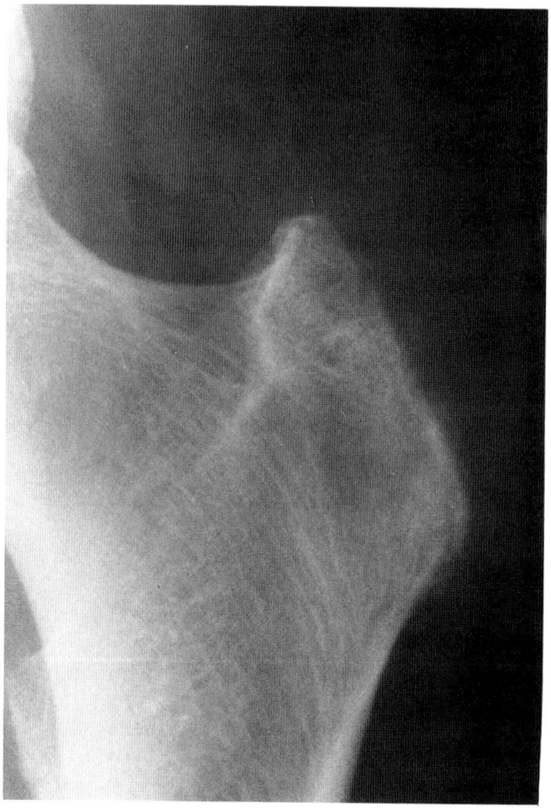

Figure 13-8. *Tuberculous bursitis over the greater trochanter produced irregularity and reaction of the underlying femoral cortex.*

lying bone erosion (Figure 13-8). Chemotherapy has been supplemented by block excision in some circumstances (101).

Management of Sinuses

More than 80% of tuberculous sinuses heal with drug treatment (102); however, secondary bacterial infection may occur (83), leading to persistence of the sinus and risking misdiagnosis.

Leprosy (Hansen's Disease)

Two types of infective bone lesions occur in leprosy (*Mycobacterium leprae*). In primary or specific leprous osteitis, which is extremely rare, multiple poorly marginated lytic lesions may be seen. Occasionally, significant cysts form, from which bacteria may be isolated

(103,104). Periostitis may also be seen (105). However, secondary or nonspecific leprous osteitis, the result of neuropathy, is common and important. Extensive secondary infections occur, usually with pyogenic organisms.

Poncet's Disease

Poncet (106) described polyarthritis occurring in patients with tuberculosis. The status of this condition has been controversial (107); however, polyarthralgia and polyarthritis associated with localized tuberculosis, usually extra-articular, continue to be described (108,109). Occasionally, one symptomatic joint may be culture-positive (110). The reactive arthritis usually responds rapidly to antituberculous and anti-inflammatory drugs.

References

1. Girdlestone GR. Tuberculosis of bone and joint. London: Oxford University Press, 1940.
2. Paus B. The changed pattern of bone, joint tuberculosis in Norway. Acta Orthop Scand 1977;48:277–279.
3. Gillespie WJ, Mayo KM, Johnstone V. Skeletal tuberculosis in New Zealand since the introduction of chemotherapy. Aust NZ J Surg 1987;57:727–732.
4. Autzen B, Elberg JJ. Bone and joint tuberculosis in Denmark. Acta Orthop Scand 1988;59:50–52.
5. Watson JN, Gill ON. HIV infection and tuberculosis. Br Med J 1990;300: 63–65.
6. Chaisson RE, Slutkin G. Tuberculosis and human immunodeficiency virus. J Infect Dis 1989;159:96–100.
7. Hannachi MR. Comparison of three chemotherapeutic regimens of short duration (6 months) in osteo-articular tuberculosis—results after 5 years. Working group on osteo-articular tuberculosis in Algeria. Bull Int Union Tuberc Lung Dis 1988;63:14–15.
8. Martini M, Ouahes M. Bone and joint tuberculosis: a review of 652 cases. Orthopedics 1988;11:861–866.
9. Rajasekaran S, Soundarapandian S. Progression of kyphosis in tuberculosis of the spine treated by anterior arthrodesis. J Bone Joint Surg [Am] 1989;71:1314–1323.
10. United Kingdom medical research council tuberculosis and chest disease unit. National survey of tuberculosis notification in England, Wales in 1983. Tubercle 1987;68:19–32.

11. Enarson DA, Fujii M, Nakielna EM, Grzybowski S. Bone and joint tuberculosis: a continuing problem. Can Med Assoc J 1979;120:139–145.
12. Hamblett EP. Tuberculosis in the Gilbert and Ellice islands colony (1964–1968). South Pacific Commission, Technical Paper No. 161, 1969.
13. De Hamel FA. Tuberculosis in Canterbury. New Zealand: Department of Health, Special Report No. 7. Wellington, 1962.
14. Rieder HL, Snider DE, Cauthen GM. Extrapulmonary tuberculosis in the United States. Am Rev Respir Dis 1990;141:347–351.
15. Davies PD, Humphries MJ, Byfield SP, et al. Bone and joint tuberculosis. A survey of notifications in England and Wales. J Bone Joint Surg [Br] 1984;66:326–330.
16. Nathanson L, Cohen W. A statistical and roentgen analysis of two hundred cases of bone and joint tuberculosis. Radiology 1941;36:550–567.
17. Berney S, Goldstein M, Bishko F. Clinical and diagnostic features of tuberculous arthritis. Am J Med 1972;53:36–42.
18. Chahal AS, Jyoti SP. The radical treatment of tuberculosis of the spine. Int Orthop 1980;4:93–99.
19. Halsey JP, Reeback JS, Barnes CG. A decade of skeletal tuberculosis. Ann Rheum Dis 1982;41:7–10.
20. Tuberculous notifications in New South Wales 1989. State Health Publication 89-086. Department of Health, New South Wales, Australia.
21. Bottiger M. Romanus V, de Verdier C, Boman G. Osteitis and other complications caused by generalized BCG-itis. Experiences in Sweden. Acta Paediatr Scand 1982;71:471–478.
22. Silva JF. A review of patients with skeletal tuberculosis treated at the University Hospital, Kuala Lumpur. Int Orthop 1980;4:79–81.
23. Garrido G, Gomez-Reino JJ, Fernandez-Dapica P, Palenque E. A review of peripheral tuberculous arthritis. Semin Arthritis Rheum 1988;18:142–149.
24. Bergdahl S, Fellander M, Robertson B. BCG osteomyelitis. J Bone Joint Surg [Br] 1976;58:212–216.
25. WHO Expert Committee on Tuberculosis Ninth Report. WHO Tech Rep Series 1974;552.
26. Papavasiliou VA, Petropoulous AV. Bone and joint tuberculosis in childhood. Acta Orthop Scand 1981;52:1–4.
27. Sasaki S, Akiba T, Suenaga M, Tomura S, Yoshiyama N, Nakagawa S. Ten years survey of dialysis associated tuberculosis. Nephron 1979;24:141–145.
28. Feng PH, Tan TH. Tuberculosis in patients with systemic lupus erythematosus. Ann Rheum Dis 1982;41:11–14.
29. Wallace RJJ, Brown BA, Onyi GO. Skin, soft tissue and bone infections due to Mycobacterium chelonae: importance of prior corticosteroid therapy, frequency of disseminated infections, and resistance to oral antimicrobials other than clarithromycin. J Infect Dis 1992;166:405–412.
30. Shea JM. Bilateral tuberculous osteomyelitis of medial humeral condyles. Infection secondary to cutaneous inoculation. JAMA 1982;247:821–822.
31. Kaufmann R. Quinze observations d'attaque ganglionnaire dan le mal de

Pott et autres localisations de la tuberculose. Mem Acad Chir 1948;74: 238–256.
32. Collins DH. Pathology of bone. London: Butterworths, 1966.
33. Klah EC, Jensen DF, Meyer PR. Pathology of Mycobacterium avium-intracellulare infection in acquired immunodeficiency syndrome. Hum Pathol 1987;18:709–714.
34. Kim YY, Ko CU, Lee SW, Kwak BM. Replacement arthroplasty using the Charnley prosthesis in old tuberculosis of the hip. Int Orthop 1979;3:81–88.
35. Hutchins, PM. Skeletal tuberculosis in the Lothian region of Scotland. A ten year survey. J Coll Surg Edinb 1984;29:167–171.
36. Jones WC, Miller WE. Skeletal tuberculosis 1963. South Med J 1964; 57:964–971.
37. Newton P, Sharp J, Barnes KL. Bone and joint tuberculosis in greater Manchester. Ann Rheum Dis 1982;41:1–6.
38. Snider DE. The tuberculin skin test. Am Rev Respir Dis 1982;125:108–118.
39. Lau JHK, Leong JCY, Stroebel AB. A longitudinal study of antibody titres to antigen 6 in patients with bone and joint tuberculosis. Int Orthrop 1983; 7:205–208.
40. Daniel TM, Debanne SM. The serodiagnosis of tuberculosis and other mycobacterial diseases by enzyme-linked immunoabsorbent assay. Am Rev Respir Dis 1987;135:1137–1151.
41. Grange JM. The rapid diagnosis of paucibacillary tuberculosis. Tubercle 1989;70:1–4.
42. Debaumont A. Bacteriologie de la tuberculose osteo-articulaire sous chemotherapie. Adv Tuberc Res 1966;15:125–128.
43. Allen BW, Mitchison DA, Darbyshire J, Chew WW, Gabriel M. Examination of operation specimens from patients with spinal tuberculosis for tubercle bacilli. J Clin Pathol 1983;36:662–666.
44. Pallen ML. The inoculation of tissue specimens into guinea pigs in suspected cases of mycobacterial infection: does it aid diagnosis and treatment? Tubercle 1987;68:51–57.
45. Martin T, Cheke D, Natyshak I. Broth culture: the modern "guinea pig" for isolation of mycobacteria. Tubercle 1989;70:53–56.
46. Reisis N, Dendrinos G, Fragiadakis E, Trouli H, Hartofylakides G. Value of tissue biopsy in bone and joint tuberculosis. Acta Orthop Belg 1989;55: 12–16.
47. Masood S. Diagnosis of tuberculosis of bone and soft tissue by fine needle aspiration biopsy. Diagn Cytopathol 1992;8:451–455.
48. Whelan MA, Naidich DP, Post JD. Computed tomography of spinal tuberculosis. J Comput Assist Tomogr 1983;7:25–30.
49. Sankaran-Kutty M, Chowdhary UM, Corea JR, Al-Majid MH. The role of computerised tomography in the management of spinal tuberculosis. Int Orthop 1991;15:319–321.
50. Rust RTJ, Park HM, Robb JA. Skeletal scintigraphy in miliary tuberculosis: photopenia after treatment. Am J Roentgenol 1981;137:877–879.

51. Somanardhana CW, Lambrecht RH. Iodine^{124}-2-iodoisonicotinic acid hydrazide—a potential radiotracer for tuberculosis. J Nucl Med 1989; 30:1756.
52. Rubaltelli L, de Gerone E, Caterino G. Echographic evaluation of tubercular abscesses in lumbar spondylitis. J Ultrasound Med 1990;9:67–70.
53. de Roos A, van Meerten EL, Bloem JL, Bluemm RG. MRI of tuberculous spondylitis. Am J Roentgenol 1986;146:79–82.
54. Fox W. Whither short course chemotherapy. Br J Dis Chest 1981;65: 331–357.
55. Seddon HJ. Potts paraplegia: prognosis and treatment. Br J Surg 1935; 22:769–799.
56. United Kingdom Medical Research Council. A ten year assessment of a controlled trial comparing debridement and anterior spinal fusion in the management of tuberculosis of the spine in patients on standard chemotherapy in Hong Kong. Eighth report of the Medical Research Council Working Party on tuberculosis of the spine. J Bone Joint Surg [Br] 1982;64:393–398.
57. Frieden TR, Sterling T, Pascal-Mendez A, et al. The emergence of drug resistant tuberculosis in New York City. N Engl J Med 1993;328:521–526.
58. Chapman JS. The atypical mycobacteria. Am Rev Respir Dis 1982;125: 119–124.
59. Leysen DC, Hamers A, Pattyn SR. Mycobacteria and the new quinolones. Antimicrob Agents Chemother 1989;33:1–5.
60. Young LS. Mycobacterium avium complex infection. J Infect Dis 1988; 157:863–867.
61. Abdelwahab IF, Norman A, Hermann G, Santini L, Klein MJ. Atypical radiographic appearances of tuberculous granulomas of bone. Can Assoc Radiol J 1990;41:72–75.
62. Arthornthurasook A, Chongpieboonpatna A. Spinal tuberculosis with posterior element involvement. Spine 1990;15:191–194.
63. Rand C, Smith MA. Anterior spinal tuberculosis: paraplegia following laminectomy. Ann R Coll Surg Engl 1989;71:105–109.
64. Hodgson AR, Stock FE. Anterior spinal fusion for the treatment of tuberculosis of the spine. J Bone Joint Surg [Am] 1960;42:295–310.
65. Pun WK, Cwow SP, Luk KD, Cheng CL, Hsu LC, Leong JC. Tuberculosis of the lumbo-sacral junction. J Bone Joint Surg [Br] 1990;72:675–678.
66. Hillinger J, Kehr P, Lang G. Stabilization of the spinal column in spondylitis using Harrington instrumentation. Zentralb Chir 1982:107:879–885.
67. Sorrel E, Sorrel-Dejerine Y. Recherches sur la transit due lipiodal par voie sousarachnoidienne dan les differentes formes de paraplegie pottique. Rev Neurol (Paris) 1924;2:88–96.
68. Griffiths DL. The treatment of tuberculosis of bone and joint. Trans R Soc Trop Med Hyg 1978;72:559–563.
69. Girdlestone GR. The operative treatment of Pott's paraplegia. Br J Surg 1931;19:121–141.
70. Govender S, Charles RW, Naidoo KS, Goga IE. Results of surgical decompression in chronic tuberculous paraplegia. S Afr Med J 1988;74:59–69.

71. Moula T, Fowles JV, Kassab MT. Pott's paraplegia: a clinical review of operative and conservative treatment in 63 adults and children. Int Orthop 1981;5:23–29.
72. Tuli SM. Treatment of neurological complications in tuberculosis of the spine. J Bone Joint Surg [Am] 1969;51:680–692.
73. Tuli SM. Results of treatment of spinal tuberculosis by "middle path" regime. J Bone Joint Surg [Br] 1975;52:13–23.
74. Hsu LC, Cheng CL, Leong JC. Pott's paraplegia of late onset. The cause of compression and results after anterior decompression. J Bone Joint Surg [Br] 1988;70:534–538.
75. Fang D, Leong JCY, Fang HSY. Tuberculosis of the upper cervical spine. J Bone Joint Surg [Br] 1983;65:47–50.
76. Hsu LC, Leong JCY. Tuberculosis of the lower cervical spine (C2–C7). A report of 40 cases. J Bone Joint Surg [Br] 1984;66:1–5.
77. Marmor L, Chan KP, Ho KC, Justin M. Surgical treatment of tuberculosis of the hip in children. Clin Orthop 1969;67:133–142.
78. Kim YY, Ko CU, Ahn JY, Yoon YS, Kwak BM. Charnley low friction arthroplasty in tuberculosis of the hip. An eight to thirteen year follow up. J Bone Joint Surg [Br] 1988;70:756–760.
79. Santavirta S, Eskola A, Konntinen YT, Tallroth K, Lindholm ST. Total hip replacement in old tuberculosis. Acta Orthop Scand 1988;59:391–395.
80. Eskola A, Santavirta S, Kontinnen YT, Tallroth K, Hoikka V, Lindholm ST. Cementless total hip replacement for old tuberculosis of the hip. J Bone Joint Surg [Br] 1988;70:603–606.
81. Hecht RH, Meyers MM, Thornhill-Joynes M, Montgomerie JZ. Reactivation of tuberculous infection following total joint replacement. J Bone Joint Surg [Am] 1983;65:1015–1016.
82. Girdlestone GR. The pathology and treatment of tuberculosis of the knee joint. Br J Surg 1932;19:488–507.
83. Chow SP, Yau A. Tuberculosis of the knee—a long term follow up. Int Orthop 1980;4:87–92.
84. Kim YY. Total knee arthroplasty for tuberculous arthritis. J Bone Joint Surg [Am] 1988;70;1322–1330.
85. Martini M, Adjrad A, Daoud A. Les osteoarthrites tuberculeuses du pied et de la cheville. Int Orthop 1984;8:203–209.
86. Parkinson RW, Hodgson SP, Noble J. Tuberculosis of the elbow. J Bone Joint Surg [Br] 1990;72:523–524.
87. Goldberg J, Jovarsky J. Tuberculous sacroiliitis. South Med J 1983;76:1175–1176.
88. Benkeddache Y, Gottesman H. Skeletal tuberculosis of the wrist and hand—a study of 27 cases. J Hand Surg 1982;7:593–600.
89. Umansky AL, Schlesinger PT, Greenberg BB. Tuberculous dactylitis in adults. Arch Surg 1947;54:67–78.
90. Feldman F, Auerbach R, Johnston A. Tuberculous dactylitis in the adult. Am J Roentgenol 1971;112:460–479.

91. Leung PC. Tuberculosis of the hand. Hand 1978;10:285–291.
92. Robins RHC. Tuberculosis of wrist and hand. Br J Surg 1967;54:211–218.
93. Hodgson AR, Smith TK. Tuberculosis of the wrist. Clin Orthop 1972; 83:73–83.
94. Kanavel AB. Tuberculous tenosynovitis of the hand. Surg Gynaecol Obstet 1923;37:635–647.
95. Bush DC, Schneider LH. Tuberculosis of the hand and wrist. J Hand Surg [Am] 1984;9:391–398.
96. Jones MW, Wahid IA. Mycobacterium marinum infections of the hand and wrist. Results of conservative treatment in 24 cases. J Bone Joint Surg [Am] 1988;70:631–632.
97. Deenstra W. Synovial hand infection from Mycobacterium terrae. J Hand Surg [Br] 1988;13:335–336.
98. Brashear HR, Winfield HG. Tuberculosis of the wrist: a report of ten cases. South Med J 1975;68:1345–1349.
99. Versfeld GA, Solomon A. A diagnostic approach to tuberculosis of bones and joints. J Bone Joint Surg [Br] 1982;64:446–449.
100. Rehm-Graves S, Weinstein AJ, Calabrese LH, Cook SA, Boumphrey FR. Tuberculosis of the greater trochanteric bursa. Arthritis Rheum 1983; 26:77–81.
101. Sharma SV, Varma BP, Khanna S. Dystrophic calcification in tubercular lesions of bursae. Acta Orthop Scand 1978;49:445–447.
102. Bosworth DM, Della Pietra A, Farrell RF. Streptomycin in tuberculous bone, joint lesions with mixed infections and sinuses. J Bone Joint Surg [Am] 1950;32:103–108.
103. Lechat MF. Bone lesions in leprosy. In: Doull JA, ed. Transactions of the Symposium on Research in Leprosy. Baltimore: Johns Hopkins University, 1961:14–24.
104. Lechat MF, Chardome J. Alterations radiologiques des os de la face chez le lepreux congolais. Ann Soc Belg Med Trop 1955;35:603–611.
105. Oberdoeffer MJ, Collier MD. Roentgenological observations in leprosy. Am J Roentgenol 1940;44:386–395.
106. Poncet A. De la polyarthrite tuberculeuse deformante ou pseudo-rhumatisme chronique tuberculeux. Assoc Franc Chir 1897;11:732–739.
107. Summers GD, Jayson MIV. Does Poncet's disease exist? Rheum Rehabil 1980;19:149–150.
108. Allen SC. A case in favour of Poncet's disease. Br Med J 1981;283:952.
109. Southwood TF, Hancock EJ, Petty RF. Tuberculous rheumatism (Poncet's disease) in a child. Arthritis Rheum 1988;31:1311–1313.
110. Wilkinson AG, Roy S. Two cases of Poncet's disease. Tubercle 1984; 65:301–303.

CHAPTER 14

Vertebral Osteomyelitis and Disk Space Infection

The spinal column is the most common site of osteomyelitis in adults; the reasons for this incidence are not known. The clinical presentation is sometimes obscured and diagnosis may be delayed, perhaps because the characteristic radiological changes take days or weeks to develop and because episodic back pain is an almost universal human experience.

The main risk factors for vertebral osteomyelitis include infection and instrumentation of the urinary tract (1), diabetes mellitus (2), and intravenous drug abuse (2). Other risk factors for disk space infection and vertebral osteomyelitis include prior laminectomy; direct inoculation of the disk space, as in shootings, stabbings, or penetration by objects; and iatrogenic introduction of organisms, as during lumbar punctures, myelograms, and translumbar aortagrams (3). Chemonucleolysis has also been reported to be associated with the complication of disk space infection.

There is confusion in the literature about the entity called "diskitis," regarding whether it is distinct from vertebral osteomyelitis. The term is usually used to describe a relatively benign disorder in children that causes primary intervertebral disk inflammation (4). This disease has no sex or racial predilection and most often occurs in individuals age 3 to 6 years (with a much wider range). The role of trauma, in both diskitis and vertebral osteomyelitis, is plausible; the idea that the trauma creates a "locus minoris resistantiae" is attractive. However, it is difficult to establish an association and it has been said that trauma "is often noted as preceding various disorders of childhood and infancy and may only mirror the fact that infants and children live dangerously" (4).

Pathophysiology

There is general agreement that vertebral osteomyelitis is a process involving bacterial seeding; there is less agreement as to whether the route is arterial or venous. In animals and in human cadavers, it has been shown that abdominal pressure caused dye injected into the pelvic venous system to reflux into the paravertebral venous plexus (5). This effect was used to explain the association of urinary tract infection with vertebral osteomyelitis. Others demonstrated similar phenomena but questioned whether the amount of abdominal pressure needed was nonphysiological. A voluminous vertebral arterial network has been demonstrated and used to support the argument that arterial seeding leads to vertebral osteomyelitis (6). The frequency with which *Staphylococcus* is found as a pathogen in vertebrae would certainly support the arterial supply as important in the pathogenesis of these infections. It has also been argued that the association of urinary tract infection with vertebral osteomyelitis may simply reflect high-grade bacteremia and arterial seeding rather than reflux through the venous plexus. It seems that the two routes of seeding are not mutually exclusive and that it is not possible to determine which is more important.

In diskitis that occurs after surgery or needling, histopathological findings are chronic inflammation with invasion and replacement of disk by granulation tissue (7). Because in clinical practice prophylactic antibiotics reduce the incidence of diskitis, it is plausible to propose that this process is initiated by bacteria (8). Experimental studies (7–10) have confirmed that implantation of small numbers of bacteria into sheep intervertebral disks is associated initially with the development of localized zones of inflammation on the vertebral side of the contiguous end plates, usually in a central situation. By approximately 3 weeks, the end plates are breached by the inflammation and the disk herniates into the vertebral body, allowing access of the host defenses to the bacteria. The bacteria are then usually eradicated. By 6 weeks, extensive granulation has grown into the disk. In a few patients, osteomyelitis supervenes in the vertebrae.

In iatrogenic diskitis, infection clearly begins in the disk. In childhood diskitis—which, if infective (which it sometimes may not be), is hematogenous (11)—the initial site of the infection must be on the vertebral side of the end plate. The vascular anatomy of the juvenile vertebral end plate may allow localization of infection more readily than in adults (12), thus plausibly explaining the characteristic course of juvenile diskitis.

In adults, primary diskitis has been reported in which the disk space was completely replaced by granulation without significant damage to the growth plate (13). However, the typical vertebral osteomyelitis, although characteristically showing disk destruction, also demonstrates major involvement of the adjacent vertebrae. We hypothesize that the same sequence of events may account for both vertebral osteomyelitis and diskitis; therefore, they represent different points in the balance between infecting organisms and host defenses.

Clinical and Laboratory Findings

Depending on the part of the spine involved, pain with accompanying stiffness is the most common presentation of vertebral osteomyelitis or diskitis. Localization of pain and tenderness usually predicts the site of infection.

The most typical presentation involves back pain, which is a prominent symptom in adults. Children, if not able to verbalize the back pain, will manifest it by reluctance to walk, sit, or stand. Pain is accentuated by motion and relieved by rest. Pain often seems out of proportion to the examination; some physical findings that may be present include decreased range of motion of the spine, loss of lumbar lordosis, and local tenderness. A positive straight leg raising test may be present, and paravertebral muscle spasm may be seen.

A second presentation includes hip joint pain, particularly in children. The explanation for this is that the nerve supply to the hip joint comes from the L2-S1 distribution.

A presentation that often confuses the diagnosis is abdominal pain. Abdominal pain may occur because the segmental nerves of the spinal cord (thoracic and lumbar) supply the abdominal wall. An alternative explanation is that disk space infection leads to inflammation in the retroperitoneum, with resultant abdominal pain.

Meningeal signs have been seen in disk space infection, although the spinal fluid obtained on lumbar puncture will be normal. Involvement of the cervical or thoracic spine may lead to presentation with neck stiffness, dysphagia, sore throat, or chest pain.

In one series from New Zealand (1), two clear patterns of presentation in terms of chronology emerged. In approximately 10% of patients, symptoms were present for less than one week, and the illness appeared more severe and hectic with fever, night sweats, elevated white blood cell count, and other systemic signs of infection, such as hypotension. In this presentation, blood cultures were positive in six of seven patients. The remaining 90% had a subacute presentation with symptoms of back pain present for periods of 2 weeks to 2 years prior to diagnosis. The white blood cell count was elevated in only one third of the patients, and fever was present in only 8%.

Vertebral osteomyelitis cannot be ruled out because of the absence of fever. Different series vary in the frequency with which fever is reported, but generally, no more than half the patients seen will be febrile on initial evaluation (14). The erythrocyte sedimentation rate (ESR) is the most consistent laboratory abnormality in vertebral osteomyelitis or disk space infection. Although extremely sensitive, the test is also nonspecific; however, a normal ESR makes the diagnosis of vertebral osteomyelitis or disk space infection open to question; the test should be repeated if persistent symptoms continue to be clinically suspicious.

One other presentation of vertebral osteomyelitis that may be difficult to diagnose is spinal compression fracture in patients with underlying osteoporosis. In patients with osteoporosis and vertebral compression fractures, infection should be considered when there is severe constant back pain, persistent unexplained fever, unexplained elevation of the ESR, or bacteremia without an obvious focus of infection (15). In osteoporotic patients, pre-existing vertebral collapse is common. Destruction of the end plate is likely to be the first sign of infection, but it may not become apparent for 2 to 3 weeks. Diagnosis is best made by biopsy and culture of the collapsed vertebral body. In one series of 45 patients with vertebral osteomyelitis during a 5-year period, 6 presented with the picture of radiological collapse of a single vertebra (Figure 14-1).

If postoperative diskitis occurs, it is important to distinguish between septic and avascular etiologies. One approach is percutaneous disk biopsy because treatment is different depending on the etiology of the lesion. Either etiology produces a distinctive clinical or radiological picture, although bone cysts are more common and larger in

A B C

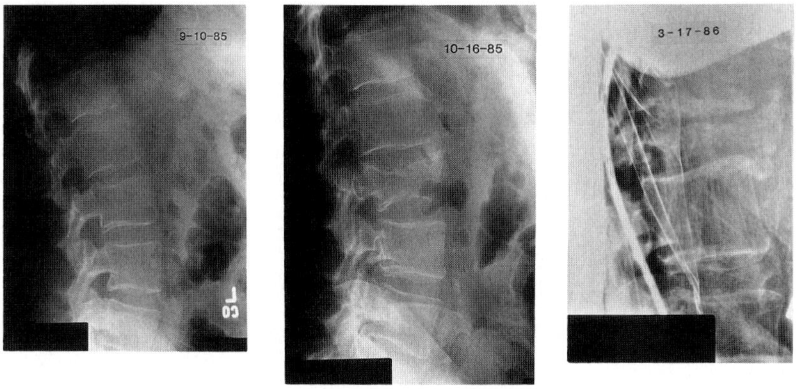

Figure 14-1. *(A) Radiograph of spine showed no evidence of compression fracture. (B) Obvious compression of L-3 vertebra 5 weeks later, with apparently intact end plates. (C) Further destruction of L-3 vertebra 5 months later, with areas of rarefaction, sclerosis, and anterior displacement of vertebral body.* (Reproduced with permission from McHenry MC, Duchesneau PM, Keys TF, Rehm SJ, Boumphry FRS. Vertebral osteomyelitis presenting as spinal compression fracture. Six patients with underlying osteoporosis. Arch Intern Med 1988;148:417–423.)

the septic group. In general, ESR and C-reactive protein levels were significantly higher in patients with infection. For septic diskitis, antimicrobial therapy is critical; for a vascular etiology, rest and physical therapy should suffice (16).

Microbiology

Staphylococcus aureus is the major etiological agent isolated from patients with vertebral osteomyelitis (2). Gram-negative bacillary infection, usually arising from genitourinary tract foci, is also recognized as a major source of infection of the vertebrae. *Pseudomonas aeruginosa,* a rare cause of vertebral osteomyelitis, has been documented in patients using intravenous drugs (17). Patients on hemodialysis also appear to be at risk for vertebral osteomyelitis, both with gram-positive organisms and occasionally with gram-negative organisms, such as *P. aeruginosa.* In an era of medical progress and increasing use of long-term intravascular devices, bacteremia related to these devices may occur, as well as seeding of other organs. Coagulase-negative staphylococci have been reported in one such patient, with identification of the same organism from the vertebrae and from the Hickman catheter as defined by plasmid analysis (18).

Hemophilus influenzae, a relatively rare cause of infection in adults, has been reported to cause vertebral osteomyelitis (19). Preceding infections associated with vertebral osteomyelitis included infections of the respiratory tract and the genitourinary tract.

Hematogenous vertebral osteomyelitis is usually associated with a single organism as the etiological agent. Polymicrobial infection is often seen when osteomyelitis is secondary to a contiguous focus (2). The most common source for this infection is infected pressure sores (decubitii) (2). These infections are frequently mixed aerobic/anaerobic problems. In one series of 40 patients with osteomyelitis involving anaerobes, four patients had spinal involvement; all four had mixed aerobic/anaerobic infections and none had pure anaerobic isolates (20). In a second series of 75 patients reported in the literature with "pure" anaerobic osteomyelitis, three were reported in the spine. This low incidence may be questioned because approximately 15% of patients with osteomyelitis are reported as culture-negative and raise the issue of whether some of these may have been caused by anaerobes (21,22).

Postoperative intervertebral disk infections are rare (23); they occur after less than 1% of procedures. They usually involve coagulase-positive or coagulase-negative staphylococci (2); however, gram-negative aerobic bacilli may also be seen (24). Endemicity of infection should be considered in the diagnosis of vertebral osteomyelitis (e.g., *Brucella* in areas where there is a high prevalence). In one series, approximately 10% of patients with brucellosis had spondylitis (25). Spondylitis involving the cervical region is associated more frequently with compression of spinal roots than involvement of the thoracic or lumbar regions. Also associated with cervical involvement was a higher incidence of paravertebral and epidural masses, with associated neurological involvement and poorer resolution of disease. Similarly, vertebral osteomyelitis due to fungi such as *Coccidioides* and *Blastomyces* is rare in nonendemic areas and is more frequently diagnosed in their more native regions. Tuberculosis is also a cause of vertebral osteomyelitis. The usual presentation of the osteoarticular form involves two or more vertebral bodies and the disks between them. An unusual presentation is tuberculosis of the vertebral arch. This entity, uncommon in western countries, has been reported from highly endemic areas, such as India or Pakistan. Recently, two infections were described in drug addicts who were seropositive for HIV (26). In this presentation, patients usually have signs of spinal cord compression, and surgery to drain "cold abscesses" is usually required.

Diagnosis

It can be difficult to diagnose vertebral osteomyelitis (27–29). Despite the advent of sophisticated scanning techniques, magnetic resonance imaging, and guided biopsies, diagnosis may still be difficult and delayed.

The frequency with which routine radiographic films are reported as positive in vertebral osteomyelitis is variable. In one series (30), 16 of 20 patients had plain spinal films that failed to demonstrate osteomyelitis, but computerized tomography (CT) scanning revealed changes consistent with osteomyelitis in 94%. Routine tomography, however, identified vertebral osteomyelitis in 80% of the patients studied. In contrast, others report that spine films reveal abnormalities in 95% of patients with pyogenic vertebral osteomyelitis and observe that patients whose initial plain radiographs are normal will generally show abnormalities on plain tomograms (2). Our own experience is that either routine radiographs or plain tomograms will frequently allow diagnosis of infection of the vertebrae to be made (Figures 14-2,14-3).

CT scanning may show early bony changes even before they are detectable on routine radiographs (31). CT imaging also allows visualization of paravertebral collections that might be aspirated. CT scanning is exquisitely sensitive for soft-tissue abnormalities, such as paravertebral abscesses, epidural collections, and spinal cord compression. CT may also help differentiate the relative densities of loculated liquid material, such as edema versus pus.

Magnetic resonance imaging (MRI) has great promise in the diagnosis of vertebral osteomyelitis (32) and may allow diagnosis earlier than other imaging techniques (33). It is extremely sensitive in detecting and delineating infective lesions, regardless of their spinal location. Osteomyelitis is associated with edema of the bone marrow and is therefore seen as bright-intensity imaging on a T2-weighted scan and as low-intensity imaging on T1-weighted scans. Limitations of MRI include the difficulty of performing biopsy under MRI guidance

A B

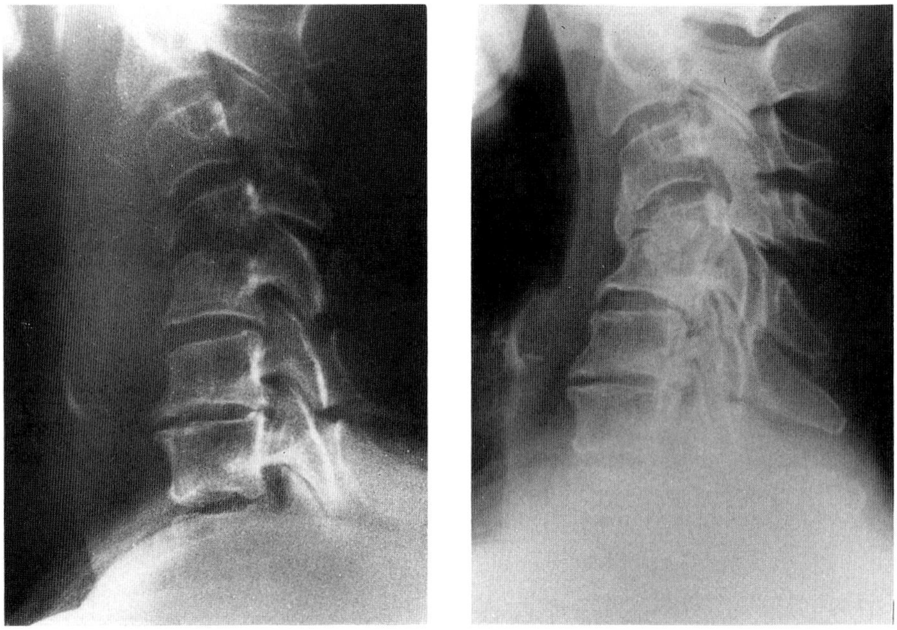

Figure 14-2. *(A) In vertebral infection, two adjacent vertebrae and their intervening disk are characteristically involved. Most destruction has occurred in the upper involved vertebra (C4). A large retropharyngeal abscess is present. (B) Solid fusion between C4 and C5 with inclusion of C3 anteriorly was the outcome of antibiotic treatment and drainage of the abscess.*

and the low specificity for distinguishing granulomatous myelitis or intramedullary infections from neoplasia (34). The procedure is costly, and its advantages need to be convincingly demonstrated before it is used on a routine basis (2).

Scanning techniques are useful in the diagnosis of vertebral osteomyelitis but have definite limitations. The technetium bone scan is extremely sensitive, but relatively nonspecific in that it will show abnormalities in noninfectious processes, such as malignancy or degenerative joint disease. In a review of 15 patients with pyogenic vertebral osteomyelitis, the addition of gallium- or indium-labeled leukocyte scans to technetium scans increased the specificity of the diagnosis of pyogenic vertebral osteomyelitis; however, the number of patients on which this conclusion is based is relatively small (35).

A B

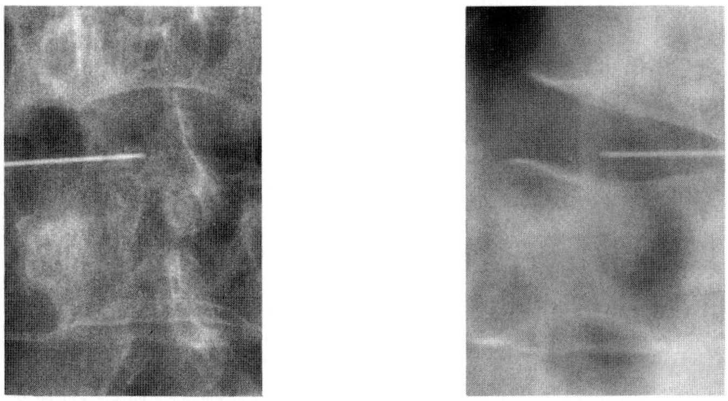

Figure 14-3. *(A) Two months after a translumbar aortogram, this 53-year-old woman presented with back pain, stiffness, malaise, and a raised erythrocyte sedimentation rate. There is localized erosion of the inferior end plate of L3, which is also the site of a previous compression fracture. (B) The disk space between L3 and L4, however, is well preserved.*

It appears that further studies of the positive and negative predictive values of the three scanning techniques currently available (i.e., technetium, gallium, and indium) need to be compared with the "gold standard" of a positive biopsy.

Many organisms may be etiological agents of vertebral osteomyelitis. Therefore, it is imperative to identify the microbial agent causing infection to begin appropriate antimicrobial therapy. Because vertebral osteomyelitis is usually caused by a single agent (with the exception of infections associated with decubitii), it is reasonably safe to assume that an organism isolated from blood cultures also accounts for the bone infection. In the absence of bacteremia, the diagnostic procedure of choice is a bone biopsy, performed with a cutting needle, such as the Craig needle, and guided by fluoroscopy or CT scanning for accurate localization. Specimens should be sent for histological study, including special stains for fungi and acid-fast bacilli. Cultures for aerobic, anaerobic, fungal, and mycobacterial organisms should also be performed. In the literature, as many as 30% of initial bone biopsy cultures were reported as sterile; it is not clear how many were performed under guidance (2). In another series (36), 30 patients with vertebral osteomyelitis underwent percutaneous biopsy. Histology confirmed the diagnosis of osteomyelitis in 90% of patients. Bacteriology, histology, or both, provided a diagnosis of tuberculous osteomyelitis in five of seven patients. The organisms responsible for nontuberculous pyogenic osteomyelitis were identified in 53% of 23 patients. Particularly striking is that the causative organism was isolated in 75% of patients without any previous antimicrobial therapy and in only 27% of those who received antimicrobial agents before the biopsy. Also, the responsible organism was isolated by blood cultures, biopsy, or both, in 18 of 23 patients (36). No complications were reported (36). These good results were obtained performing biopsies with intensifying screen guidance in the radiology room rather than under CT guidance. It is recommended that if the first needle biopsy yields negative results, a repeat biopsy is indicated; if both needle biopsies are sterile, open surgical biopsy should be strongly considered (2). An algorithm is suggested for the diagnostic approach to vertebral osteomyelitis (Figure 14-4).

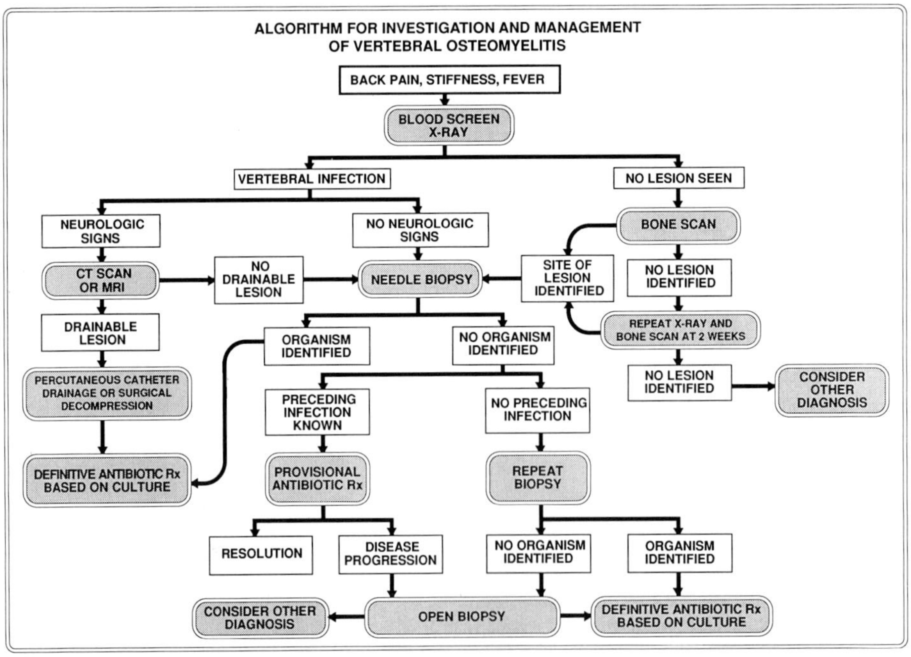

Figure 14-4. *Recommended plan for management of vertebral osteomyelitis.*

Therapy

The objective of therapy in vertebral osteomyelitis is elimination of infection followed by fusion of the involved vertebral bodies. Use of operative techniques to achieve vertebral fusion has diminished greatly in recent years, even in tuberculous infection. In contemporary practice, there are three indications for surgery in vertebral osteomyelitis.

The first is to obtain adequate tissue to confirm the diagnosis and the causative organism when needle biopsy has failed to do so. We recommend that in the absence of other indications, surgical exploration should not be considered until two unsuccessful needle biopsies have been performed.

The presence of an abscess that cannot be adequately drained with a percutaneous catheter (37) is a strong indication. Such abscesses may be in the paravertebral muscles, in iliopsoas muscle, or in other retroperitoneal sites. If within the epidural space, they may be associated with neurological impairment; this finding is a particularly strong indication for exploration. Two points must be made. First, the results of decompression may be disappointing, particularly in long-standing infection, in which the epidural mass may be granulation rather than fluid abscess and the neurological lesion may be the consequence of vascular thrombosis rather than displacement of neural structures (37–39). Second, surgery should be by an anterior or anterolateral route. The posterior approach carries a high risk of destabilizing the spine and precipitating neurological deterioration (40).

The third indication for surgery is the presence of gross bone destruction leading to significant deformity or instability. Such indication may exist at presentation or may develop despite apparently adequate conservative management. Clinical resolution of infection usually precedes radiological healing by many months; thus, support and regular assessment of the spine should be continued until restoration of stability is assured. In the presence of instability or major deformity, excellent results may be obtained from spinal debridement and anterior grafting (40,41).

Apart from surgery, immobilization has been the mainstay of orthopedic management of vertebral osteomyelitis. Previously, prolonged immobilization in a plaster cast extending from chest to knee was recommended. Although there are no controlled studies and the majority of reports indicating that immobilization is not necessary are anecdotal, the consensus is clearly that treatment with antimicrobial agents and bedrest suffices in most uncomplicated cases to achieve satisfactory results. The degree of limitation of activity necessary, in conjunction with antimicrobial therapy, is unknown. We recommend a short period of inactivity dictated by pain, followed by limited activity until the patient is pain free.

Spontaneous fusion is a good indicator of successful therapy, but many patients have been apparently cured without radiographic evidence of fusion. In one study (42), spontaneous fusion was noted in only 37% of the patients studied; relapse did not occur in any. It is postulated that patients who fail to achieve complete fusion achieve a degree of fibrous stabilization (43), which functions as effectively as complete bony fusion.

In general, recommendations for management of patients with vertebral osteomyelitis are bedrest initially plus appropriate antimicrobial agents. Ambulation may be initiated when back pain is minimal and when the spine appears to be stable. In view of the potential for spinal instability, devices to immobilize, such as body or neck braces, may be used. Surgical drainage of significant paravertebral and epidural pyogenic abscesses is indicated. Development of neurological deficits may necessitate surgical intervention and decompression, although this approach may be unrewarding (38,39): the lesion may consist of granulation tissue alone (13,38). The danger of instability following wide laminectomy in the presence of vertebral body destruction should be remembered: it should be reserved for posterior element infections and epidural abscesses only.

Antimicrobial therapy should be chosen according to the isolated infecting organism. Given the number of organisms that can cause vertebral osteomyelitis, the need for diagnostic biopsy to isolate an etiological agent is obvious. Suggested antimicrobial agents and alternative choices are given in Table 14-1. In general, pyogenic vertebral osteomyelitis requires at least 4 weeks of antimicrobial therapy. The ESR is a good tool to monitor the success of therapy, and it should be expected to decrease to at least half to two thirds the pretherapy level (2). Home intravenous antibiotic therapy may be used as part of the 4-week treatment course. Use of oral antimicrobial therapy has not been studied in controlled trials, but with agents that achieve good serum and bone levels and with a compliant patient, it is likely that oral

Table 14-1. Antimicrobial therapy for vertebral osteomyelitis

ORGANISM	PREFERRED IV THERAPY*	PREFERRED ORAL THERAPY*	ALTERNATIVE THERAPY*
Staphylococcus aureus (methicillin-sensitive)	Nafcillin, 2 g every 6 hr	Clindamycin, 300 mg every 6 hr	Clindamycin, 600 mg every 8 hr IV
Staphylococcus aureus (methicillin-resistant)	Vancomycin, 1 g every 12 hr	NA	NA
GpA Streptococci	Penicillin G, 5 million U every 6 hr	Penicillin V-K, 250 mg q.i.d.	Clindamycin, 600 mg every 8 hr IV
GpD Streptococcus (enterococci)	Ampicillin, 2 g every 4 hr	Amoxicillin, 1 g t.i.d.	Vancomycin, 1 g every 12 hr IV
Hemophilus influenzae (beta-lactamase–negative)	Ampicillin, 2 g every 4 hr	Amoxicillin, 1 g t.i.d.	TMP-SMX, 10 mg/kg/day in 4 doses IV
Hemophilus influenzae (beta-lactamase–positive)	Ceftriaxone, 1 g every 12 hr	Amoxicillin/ clavulanate, 500 mg every 6 hr	TMP-SMX, 10 mg/kg/day in 4 doses IV
E. coli	Cefazolin, 1 g every 8 hr	Amoxicillin/ clavulanate, 500 mg every 6 hr	TMP/SMX, 10 mg/kg/day in 4 doses IV
Klebsiella pneumoniae	Ceftriaxone 1 g every 12 hr	Amoxicillin/ clavulanate, 500 mg every 6 hr	Imipenem, 500 mg every 6 hr
Pseudomonas aeruginosa	Ciprofloxacin, 400 mg b.i.d.	Ciprofloxacin, 750 mg every 12 hr	Aztreonam, 1 g every 8 hr IV
Proteus species	Ceftriaxone, 1 g every 12 hr	Amoxicillin/ clavulanate, 500 mg every 6 hr	TMP/SMX, 10 mg/kg/day in 4 doses IV
Bacteroides species	Imipenem-cilastatin, 1 g every 8 hr	Clindamycin, 300 mg every 6 hr	Clindamycin, 600 mg every 8 hr IV

*In all instances, these choices are based on the likelihood that most organisms will be sensitive to the agents listed. Should the isolated organism be resistant to the agents listed, therapy should be switched to an agent to which the organism is sensitive. Also, the doses listed are for adults; for pediatric doses, consult other sources.

agents could be used after an initial 2 weeks of intravenous therapy. Longer courses of therapy are required for certain organisms, such as *Brucella, Actinomyces,* and *M. tuberculosis.*

Prognosis and Complications

The prognosis for pyogenic vertebral osteomyelitis is usually good when it is diagnosed early and managed appropriately. The mortality from this disease in the antibiotic era is less than 5%, and residual neurologic deficits among survivors is approximately 6% (2). In tuberculous osteomyelitis of the spine, the incidence of neurological complications has ranged from 1% to 27% (44); however, the wide range and high incidence of neurological deficits may be due to the variety of locations reporting such statistics and the fact that tuberculosis and its complications are frequently reported from developing countries where the disease is diagnosed late and anatomical abnormalities are already present.

The major complications of vertebral osteomyelitis are neurological symptoms. The usual problem is due to neural compression from intraspinal abscess (epidural abscess), anterior compression of the cord, or spinal deformity.

Spinal epidural abscesses have been reported in 5% to 18% of patients with vertebral osteomyelitis (38,45). Looked at differently, in 38% of patients with epidural abscess, vertebral osteomyelitis appeared to be the precipitating factor (46). Approximately half had acute symptoms with purulent epidural collections and the other half had prolonged courses, with epidural granulation tissue found at operation (46). Gram-positive bacilli, primarily *S. aureus,* accounted for three fourths of infections (46). The classic clinical progression from spinal ache to root pain to weakness followed by paralysis was seen in the majority of patients. In following patients with presumed spinal epidural abscesses, examination of the back and careful neurological examination for a focal deficit are important. Baseline spinal radiographs should be obtained; MRI is then the study of choice for continued evaluation. An MRI can evaluate spinal cord compression, the presence and extent of abscess formation, and determine if a drainable fluid collection exists. An MRI is probably preferable to a CT scan or a myelography (47). Medical therapy can be pursued if neurological progression does not develop, if pain does not become excruciating, and if other parameters, such as white blood cell count and temperature, continue to improve. The need for surgical decompression of the spinal cord would be indicated by increase in neurological deficit, worsening or persistent severe pain, increase in fever, or increase in white blood cell count. If indicated, another approach to the spine is recommended. Clearly, given the devastating consequences of epidural spinal abscess, management must be vigilant and ongoing.

The incidence of kyphosis due to vertebral osteomyelitis has also been reported to range from 2% to 28% (45). In general, kyphosis is not associated with neurological deficits; however, in some patients, anterior compression presents with cord symptoms ranging from mild weakness to paralysis. Anterior cord compression may be due to either localized anterior intraspinal abscess or to deformity. In a series of patients with vertebral osteomyelitis and paralysis, it was postulated that cord compression often arose from structures anterior to the cord, including abscess of the vertebral body and the apex of the kyphosis, if present (39).

Although spinal instability is rare following pyogenic disk or vertebral infection, all patients must be regarded as having the potential for deformity and therefore be maintained with bedrest or braced until the spine appears stable. Stability may occur before actual fusion takes place. It has been argued that spinal instability should be treated definitively in patients whose neurological symptoms could be attributed to their deformity (45) and recommended that either bone fusion or Harrington rod application may be performed safely in the presence of infection; in some patients, anterior decompression without fusion may be sufficient.

Unresolved Problems

One of the major problems with vertebral osteomyelitis is delay in diagnosis. Despite the advent of sophisticated scanning techniques (e.g., MRI), which have very high sensitivity, the disease must first be clinically suspected by physicians before the appropriate tests are ordered. Back pain is a ubiquitous complaint, and vertebral osteomyelitis is an infrequent cause. How to raise the awareness of clinicians who see patients with persistent back pain, with or without low-grade fever, to the possibility of infection of the spine remains an unsolved problem.

A second significant problem is what to do when the bone biopsy returns and is sterile. Craig needle biopsy is unpleasant, and many physicians are reluctant to have patients submit to a second pass. An even more difficult situation arises if a repeat biopsy is also negative. The temptation to institute empiric therapy based on the likely probability of the organism being *S. aureus* is not easy to resist. An open surgical biopsy of the vertebrae requires an anterior approach and in the thoracic or cervical region is a significant surgical procedure with invasion of the chest. The need for precise bacteriological diagnosis is unchallenged; however, the means of obtaining that precise bacteriology are not always simple, and convincing clinicians that it is necessary to repeat procedures or to do open surgical procedures is difficult.

References

1. Silverthorn KG, Gillespie WJ. Pyogenic spinal osteomyelitis: a review of 61 cases. NZ Med J 1986;99:62–65.
2. Sapico FL, Montgomerie JZ. Vertebral osteomyelitis. In: Norden C, ed. Bone and joint infections—new perspectives. Philadelphia: WB Saunders, 1990: 539–550.
3. Schwartz H, Berkow AE, Love L. Vertebral osteomyelitis following translumbar aortography. Angiology 1977;28:555–566.
4. Boscamp JR, Steigbigel NH. Disk space infection. Clinical topics in infectious disease. In: Schlossberg D, ed. Orthopedic infection, New York: Springer-Verlag, 1988:49–68.
5. Batson OV. The function of the vertebral veins and their role in the spread of metastases. Ann Surg 1940;112:138.
6. Wiley AM, Trueta J. The vascular anatomy of the spine and its relationship to pyogenic vertebral osteomyelitis. J Bone Joint Surg [Br] 1959;41: 796–809.
7. Fraser RD, Osti OL, Vernon-Roberts B. Discitis following discography. J Bone Joint Surg [Br] 1986;69:26–35.
8. Fraser RD, Osti OL, Vernon-Roberts B. Iatrogenic discitis: the role of prophylactic antibiotics in prevention and treatment. Spine 1989;14:1025–1032.
9. Fraser RD, Osti OL, Vernon-Roberts B. Discitis following chemonucleolysis: an experimental study. Spine 1986;11:34–43.
10. Osti OL, Fraser RD, Vernon-Roberts B. Discitis after discography: the role of prophylactic antibiotics. J Bone Joint Surg [Br] 1990;72:271–274.
11. Menelaus M. Discitis. J Bone Joint Surg [Br] 1964;46:16–23.
12. Ratcliffe FJ. Anatomic basis for the pathogenesis and radiologic features of vertebral osteomyelitis and its differentiation from childhood discitis. Acta Radiol 1985;26:137–143.

13. Kemp HBS, Jackson JW, Jeremiah JD, et al. Pyogenic infections occurring primarily in intervertebral discs. J Bone Joint Surg [Br] 1973;55:698–714.
14. Sapico FL, Montgomerie JZ. Pyogenic vertebral osteomyelitis: report of nine cases of review of the literature. Rev Infect Dis 1979;1:754–776.
15. McHenry MC, Duchesneau PM, Keys TF, Rehm SJ, Boumphrey FRS. Vertebral osteomyelitis presenting as spinal compression fracture. Six patients with underlying osteoporosis. Arch Intern Med 1988;148:417–423.
16. Fouquet B, Gaupille P, Jattiot F, et al. Discitis after lumbar disc surgery—features of "aseptic" and "septic" forms. Spine 1992;17:356–358.
17. Wiesseman GJ, Wood VE, Kroll LL. Pseudomonas vertebral osteomyelitis in heroin addicts. J Bone Joint Surg [Am] 1973;55:1416–1424.
18. Bryan C, Parisi J, Strike O. Vertebral osteomyelitis due to Staphylococcus worneri attributed to a Hickman catheter. Diagn Microbiol Infect Dis 1987;8:57–59.
19. Beltrani VP, Echols RM, Vedder DK. Verebral osteomyelitis caused by Haemophilus influenzae. J Infect Dis 1987;156:391–394.
20. Hall B, Fitzgerald R, Rosenblatt J. Anaerobic osteomyelitis. J Bone Joint Surg [Am] 1983;65:30–35.
21. Raff M, Melo J. Anaerobic osteomyelitis. Medicine 1978;57:83–103.
22. Singh N, Yu V. Osteomyelitis due to Veillonella parvula. Clin Infect Dis 1992;14:361–363.
23. Lindhamt TS, Pylkkawerr P. Discitis following removal of intervertebral disc. Spine 1982;7:618–622.
24. Thibodeau A. Closed space infection following removal of lumbar intervertebral disc. Clin Neurosurg 1966;14:337–360.
25. Colmenero J, Cisneros J, Orguelo D, et al. Clinical course and progress of brucella spondylitis. Infection 1992;20:38–42.
26. Mallolas J, Gatell JM, Rovera M, Conget JI, Trilla A, Soriano E. Vertebral arch tuberculosis in two human immunodeficiency virus-seropositive heroin addicts. Arch Int Med 1988;148:1125–1127.
27. Musher DM, Thorsteinsson SB, Minuth JN, Luchi RJ. Vertebral osteomyelitis. Still a diagnostic pitfall. Arch Intern Med 1976;136:105–110.
28. Stone DB, Bonfiglio M. Pyogenic vertebral osteomyelitis. Arch Intern Med 1963;112:87–96.
29. Ambrose BG, Alpert M, Neer CS. Vertebral osteomyelitis. A diagnostic problem. JAMA 1966;197:101–104.
30. Abbey DM, Hosea SW. Diagnosis of vertebral osteomyelitis in a community hospital by using computed tomography. Arch Intern Med 1989;149: 2029–2035.
31. Burke DR, Brant-Zazadzki M. CT of pyogenic spine infection. Neuroradiology 1985;27:131–137.
32. Modic MT, Feiglin DH, Piraino DW. Vertebral osteomyelitis: assessment using MR. Radiology 1985;157:157–166.
33. Meyers S, Wiener S. Diagnosis of hematogenous pyogenic vertebral osteomyelitis by magnetic resonance imaging. Arch Intern Med 1991;151:683–687.

34. Sharif H. Role at MR imaging in the management of spinal infections. Am J Radiol 1992;158:1333–1345.
35. Adatepe MH, Parnell OM, Isaacs GH, Nicholas K, Cefola R. Hematogenous pyogenic vertebral osteomyelitis: diagnostic value of radionuclide bone imaging. J Nucl Med 1986;27:1680–1685.
36. Cotty PH, Fouquet B, Pleskof L, et al. Vertebral osteomyelitis: value of percutaneous biopsy. J Neuroradiol 1988;15:13–21.
37. Mueller PF, Ferruci JT, Wittenberg J, Simeone JF, Butch RJ. Iliopsoas abscess. Treatment by CT guided percutaneous catheter drainage. Am J Roentgenol 1984;142:359–362.
38. Kulowski J. Pyogenic osteomyelitis of the spine. An analysis and discussion of 102 cases. J Bone Joint Surg [Am] 1936;18:343–364.
39. Eismont FJ, Bohlman HH, Soni PL, Goldberg VM, Freehafer AA. Pyogenic and fungal osteomyelitis with paralysis. J Bone Joint Surg [Am] 1983;65: 19–29.
40. Ho EKW, Leong JCY. Spinal Osteomyelitis. In: Findlay G, Owen R, eds. Surgery of the spine. Oxford: Blackwell Scientific, 1992:603–619.
41. Kemp HBS, Jackson JW, Jeremiah SD, Cook J. Anterior fusion of the spine for infective lesions in adults. J Bone Joint Surg [Br] 1973;55:715–734.
42. Ambrose BG, Alpert M, Neer CS. Vertebral osteomyelitis: a diagnostic problem. JAMA 1966;197:101–104.
43. Jordan MC, Mirby WMM. Pyogenic vertebral osteomyelitis. Treatment with antimicrobial agents and bed rest. Arch Intern Med 1971;128:405–410.
44. Gorse GJ, Pais MJ, Kusake JA, Cesario TC. Tuberculous spondylitis. Medicine 1983;62:178–193.
45. Abramovitz JN, Batson RA, Yablon JS. Vertebral osteomyelitis. The surgical management of neurologic complications. Spine 1986;11:418–420.
46. Baker AS, Ojemann RG, Swartz MN, Richardson EP Jr. Spinal epidural abscess. N Engl J Med 1975;293:463–468.
47. Baker AS, Ojemann RG, Baker RA. To decompress or not to decompress—spinal epidural abscess. Clin Infect Dis 1992;15:28–29.

CHAPTER 15

Chronic Osteomyelitis

Chronic osteomyelitis is a significant health problem associated with substantial morbidity but a low mortality rate. Whether it arises from hematogenous infection, by spread from a contiguous soft-tissue infection, after trauma, or following a surgical implant, the general principles of management are identical. It is a complex disease, and it is difficult to compare the relative effectiveness of different treatment programs. Although a number of classification systems are available (1–3), the bulk of the extensivc litcrature fails to compare like with like.

Definition and Epidemiology

Chronic osteomyelitis is symptomatic, bacteriologically confirmed osteomyelitis secondary to a known primary infection in which characteristic radiological changes in bone are present. We know of no authentic measures of prevalence, which depend on incidence of new cases, disease activity, and life-expectancy of affected patients. In the developing world, major problems as a sequelae to hematogenous disease still occur (4). In the developed world, less than 5% of cases of acute hematogenous disease become chronic. Accidental injury to bone has become increasingly important; chronic infection occurs in approximately 5% of open fractures and in less than 1% of osteosyntheses for closed fracture. Although infection around a joint replacement is simply a special example of chronic osteomyelitis, it has sufficient distinctive features to merit separate discussion (see Chapter 17).

Microbiology and Pathology

The fundamental problem in chronic bone infection is the prolonged persistence of viable pathogenic organisms. The pathological anatomy reflects the consequences of continuing necrosis (i.e., sequestrum, abscess, and sinus) and repair (i.e., reactive new bone and scar). The balance achieved between these processes determines the outcome; the aim of management is to tip the balance in favor of the host.

Staphylococcus aureus was historically the most common isolate (3,5–7), but other organisms, particularly gram-negative (8) and anaerobic (9–11) organisms, are increasingly reported. Anaerobic infections are seen mainly in association with decubitus or ischemic ulcers. In North America, one third of cases are polymicrobial (3,7,12), the criterion for which is identification of more than one pathogen from adequate deep-tissue specimens. The local pathological anatomy depends on the route of infection, its extent, the frequency of recurrent episodes of exacerbation and extension, and the balance of necrosis and repair in the tissues. Initially, typical hematogenous infection is medullary, extending to involve cortex, subperiosteal space, and soft tissues. Diaphyseal cortical osteomyelitis and post-traumatic osteomyelitis initially involve cortex, although in slightly different ways (13,14).

Frost (15) proposed that the architecture of necrotic bone allowed physical sequestration of bacteria from cellular components of the host defense mechanism and from effective contact with fluid of the interstitial space. This concept fits with clinical experience of remission of infection following discharge or removal of large sequestra. Organisms, however, may be protected from the activity of host defenses and antibiotics in other ways. Bacteria may lodge and survive in sites of allergic inflammation (16). The growth characteristics of organisms adhering either to natural solid surfaces or to prosthetic materials have been extensively studied in the last decade (17). Many bacteria are capable of synthesizing a polysaccharide pseudocapsule, or glycocalyx (18): Individual glycocalyces amalgamate to form protected microcolonies and eventually thick biofilms, which are readily elaborated not only on the surface of implants, but also on the surface of infected bone (17,19) in both experimental osteomyelitis and in human disease. Adherence of *S. aureus* may be promoted by adsorption of fibronectin and other proteins onto surfaces (20,21). Biofilm production protects bacteria from antibodies (22) and phagocytosis (23) and from the majority of cell wall active antimicrobial agents (24).

Surgical implant materials have toxic effects on host defenses that may be of clinical significance (25). Polymethyl methacrylate (PMMA) and some metals (in particular cobalt, nickel, and chromium) inhibit macrophage and monocyte function (26). In foreign body infection, there is poor polymorphonuclear leukocyte function and decreased efficiency of opsonization (27–29). Of greater importance are observations on the effect of lowered oxygen tension (PaO_2) on host defenses (30) and on the process of repair. Intramedullary PaO_2 is reduced in infected experimental fractures (31), for which there may be a number of mechanisms: oxygen consumption by micro-organisms, increased oxygen requirements of the inflammatory cell response, and interference with local perfusion caused by tissue edema. Tissue perfusion in chronic osteomyelitis may be reduced following previous vascular injury, extensive scarring, or small vessel disease. Thus, conditions are suboptimal both for the killing capacity of leukocytes and for the essential elements of repair: accumulation of fibroblasts, proliferation of collagen matrix, and neovascularization (32). Clinical experience confirms the importance of adequate vascularization if management is going to succeed.

Principles of Management

The objectives of management are to reduce the number of bacteria and to improve repair by the host. The principles of management are as follows.

1. Correct and complete microbiological diagnosis.
2. Assessment and modification of host defense mechanisms.
3. Anatomical definition of the extent of local disease, both in bone and in soft tissues.
4. Correct antibiotic therapy.
5. Surgical removal of necrotic and poorly vascularized tissue and of infected granulation.
6. Obliteration of dead space left by debridement.
7. Restoration of functional skeletal stability.
8. Rehabilitation.

These principles apply regardless of the etiology or the anatomy of the infection and are equally applicable to infected total joint replacement.

Microbiological Diagnosis

Superficial sinus tract cultures are poor predictors of the active microbiological flora in chronic osteomyelitis (33) because they may sample symbiotic and contaminant organisms. In general, they overestimate the incidence of polymicrobial infections (12), but active deep organisms may not be identified in the sinus discharge or in needle biopsy. Adequate diagnosis therefore depends on carefully achieved surgical biopsy material.

Assessment and Modification of the Host

The individual is assessed with regard to three categories: (a) social and psychological, (b) systemic disease, and (c) local disease. The significance of the patient's disability in the context of work, home life, and social activities must be evaluated. The patient's social and domestic status should be known, and the opinion of the primary care physician or a community social worker may be valuable. Persistent work loss, frequent hospitalization, foul discharge, and the potential impact of bacteremia at other sites (e.g., rheumatic valvular disease, planned prosthetic implant) argue strongly for intervention. An occasional flare of infection with little or no functional problem, in contrast, does not. The mere presence of chronic osteomyelitis is not an indication for attempts to eradicate it. The cure may be worse than the disease.

Systemic factors that may influence the host's ability to mount an adequate response to infection and surgery should be examined and, when possible, subjected to treatment. Relevant laboratory investigations should be carried out. In uncomplicated chronic osteomyelitis, the erythrocyte sedimentation rate (ESR) may be moderately increased. C-reactive protein is an indicator of disease activity in established bacterial infection, including chronic osteomyelitis (see Chapter 5). When antibiotics have been administered on a long-term basis, blood count, liver function and renal function should be checked.

The extent to which individual factors predict success or failure has not been formally established. Recommended steps include a patient education program, cessation of smoking, adjustment of medication, stabilization of diabetes, appropriate nutritional supplementation, possible use of hyperbaric oxygen (see Chapter 8), and a variety of specific interventions related to organ failure (1).

Patients with chronic osteomyelitis demonstrate impairment of cell-mediated immunity, neutrophil phagocytosis, and microbial killing (34,35). The association may be primary or secondary. Host response may be augmented in a number of different ways: active or passive component transfusion, immunization, administration of colony-stimulating factors (CSFs), and nutritional supplementation.

Prior to the introduction of antibiotics, there was considerable interest in the use of both active and passive immunization to augment the host response to both antitoxic and antibacterial immunity (36). There were probable benefits in the use of *Staphylococcus* antitoxin in patients with acute septicemic osteomyelitis but not in those with chronic osteomyelitis (37). Some European groups have used vaccines, sometimes prepared against organisms from the patient's discharge (38,39). Rigorous evaluation in double-blind trials has not been reported. Recently, as a result of the appreciation of the role of biofilms in chronic infection, there is renewed interest in vaccines against the capsular polysaccharides of *S. aureus* (40). Currently, however, a case for vaccination in the management of chronic osteomyelitis cannot be made. Leukocyte transfusion (41) may be indicated occasionally in the management of severe infections in granulocytopenic patients. There may be a role in the future for CSFs in immunocompromised patients with significant chronic osteomyelitis. In experimental animals, granulocyte-CSF increased resistance to infection (42). Studies of the effect on osteoarticular infections have yet to be published.

Chronic malnutrition is quite common in patients with chronic osteomyelitis (43). Clinical appearances, serum albumin levels, and total lymphocyte count are the most reliable indicators. The safest route of supplementation is oral. Nutritional status may predict wound healing (44), and there is evidence that supplementation is capable of reversing deficient phagocytic responses in patients with chronic infections (45).

Assessment of the Local Disease

For the most part, assessment of skin and soft tissues is clinical. Because eradication of infection and successful reconstruction are unlikely to succeed unless tissue oxygenation is adequate, obliterative arterial disease, venous stasis, chronic lymphedema, and areas of extensive scarring should be assessed and, if significant, should be evaluated for reconstructive surgery. Arteritis and radiation fibrosis justify consideration of hyperbaric oxygen therapy (see Chapter 8). Assessment of the segmental systemic blood pressure with a Doppler probe is predictive of healing in the presence of peripheral vascular disease. In the calf segment, a systolic pressure greater than 70 mm Hg is likely to be associated with healing; systolic pressure less than 40 mm Hg is a poor prognostic sign (46).

Factors evaluated include the history of flares of infection, sinus activity, and the healing and breakdown of scars. Multiple flares of infection are likely to have resolved as scar tissue. A history of recurrent skin breakdown is a clear indication that soft-tissue reconstruction will be required. If present, a sinus should be defined by sinography, preferably in two planes, which may also clarify the activity of radiological cavities in bone. Contractures may indicate scar adherence, which require excision to allow achievement of improved functional range. Extensive soft-tissue loss reduces the potential for repair, and augmentation may be required. If a free flap with microvascular anastomosis is planned to fill a large defect, arteriography to define the vascular anatomy is usually required; it may also be indicated in planning reconstruction in patients with post-traumatic osteomyelitis if previous vascular injury is known or suspected.

In the preoperative assessment of bone involvement, increasingly sophisticated imaging techniques provide useful definition of the pathological anatomy, although the final decision on debridement of an infected area depends on visualization of blood supply. Resnick and Niwayama (47) listed the radiological features that correspond to the different stages and aspects of the disease. Signs of activity in chronic osteomyelitis include change from the previous radiograph, both in bone and soft tissues; ill-defined osteolysis; periostitis, either linear or fluffy; and sequestration (Figures 15-1 to 15-3). When disease has spread from a contiguous soft-tissue infection, cortical lucency and destruction are likely to predominate initially over medullary changes, but the end result may be very similar. Most of these features can be identified on adequate radiographs of the affected limb, but clarification of the extent of the disease and its detailed geography, particularly with respect to sequestra and bone changes,

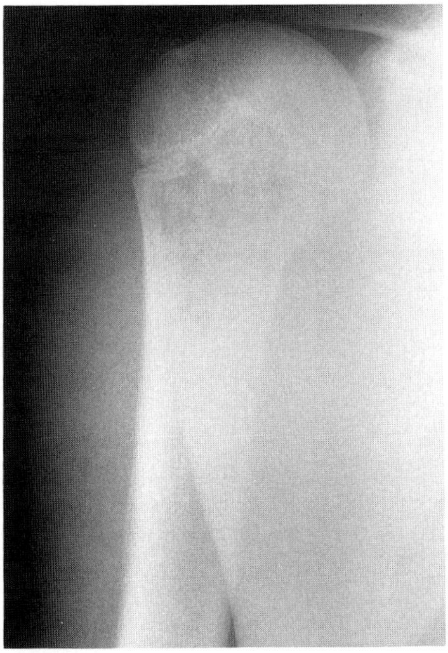

Figure 15-1. *Chronic (hematogenous) osteomyelitis with evidence of active periostitis. This infection subsequently discharged a sequestrum.*

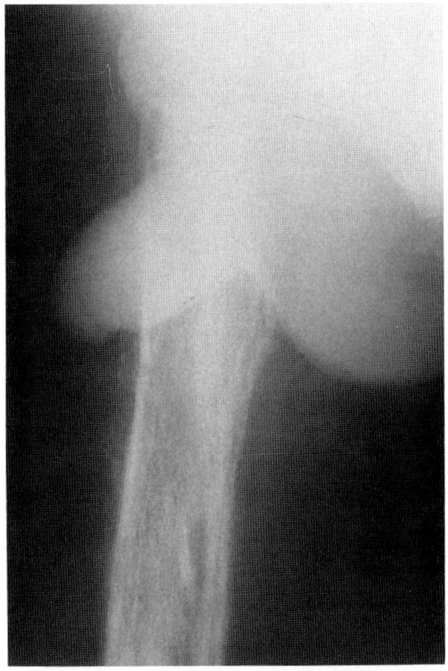

Figure 15-2. *"Fluffy" exuberant periostitis in active chronic osteomyelitis.*

can be obtained by conventional or computerized axial tomography (48) or magnetic resonance imaging (MRI) (see Chapter 6).

MRI is emerging as a powerful tool to define local pathological anatomy. Particularly with gadolinium enhancement, it appears possible to distinguish areas of inflammation and avascular soft tissue (49), which are likely to predict failure if not excised.

The current place of scintigraphy in an ideal management algorithm for chronic osteomyelitis is, in our view, unresolved. In doubtful cases, chronic bone infection can be identified, with quite a high level of accuracy, by contemporary radioisotope imaging techniques. Using ^{99m}Tc-MDP, with 3- or 4-phase studies, high sensitivity for established infection can be achieved (50). Specificity, however, is much less satisfactory. ^{67}Gallium is widely used but may show considerable nonspecific uptake in bone, and a wide range of sensitivities and specificities

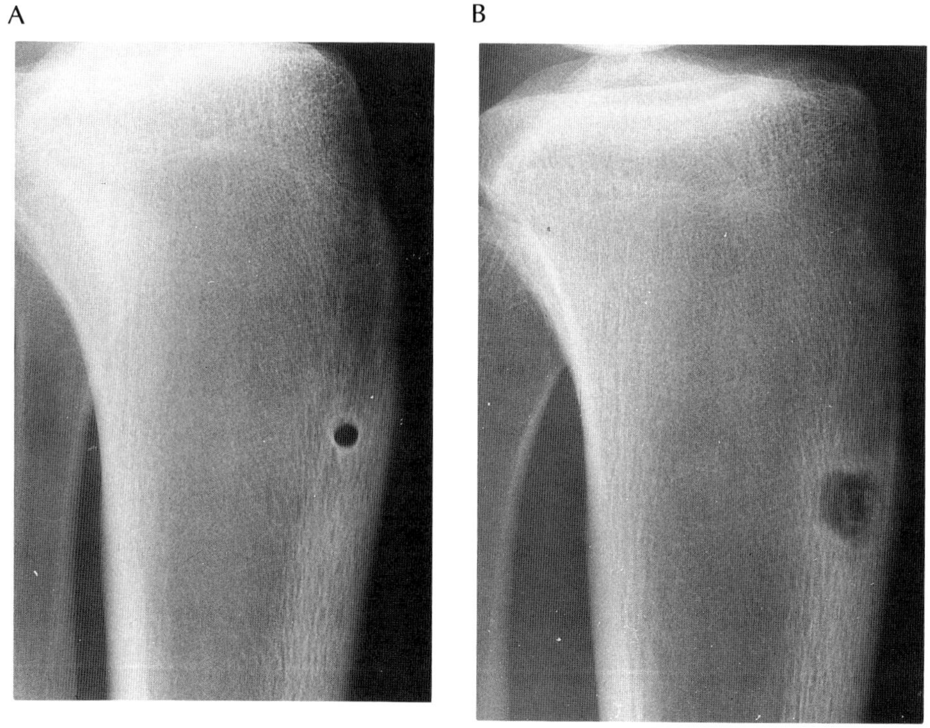

Figure 15-3. *(A) A pin tract with a sclerotic margin, suggesting the possibility of a sequestrum. (B) Two months later, the sequestrum lies within an area of bone resorption with minimal surrounding reaction.*

has been reported (51). For ^{111}Indium-labeled leukocytes, measures of accuracy are more favorable (52). Labeled immunoglobulin techniques are currently under investigation (53).

However, chronic osteomyelitis is often obvious both clinically and with other imaging techniques that define the pathological anatomy more effectively. For example, comparison of ^{111}indium-labeled leukocyte accumulation with ^{99m}Tc-MDP bone scanning can differentiate infected from reactive areas, but MRI is likely to have greater anatomical precision. In surgical management, tissue appearances, assessed visually or by using a laser Doppler flow meter, are at this stage a better guide to the extent of debridement necessary than scintigraphic evaluation. In summary, radioisotope imaging can be justified if it provides the information necessary for planning management more efficiently than other techniques. In practice, it rarely does so. A possible indication would be the provision, by serial examinations, of a minimally invasive objective record of healing. ^{67}Gallium scanning in a rabbit model of osteomyelitis (54) showed that negative scans were associated with negative cultures, but so were nearly 40% of positive scans. In clinical practice, Cierny and Mader (1) used follow-up ^{111}Indium chloride scans every 6 months until they were normal but have not reported their response to an abnormal scan in the absence of clinical disease.

Antibiotic Therapy

Despite some optimistic reports, clinical experience has shown and experimental work has confirmed that antibiotics alone do not produce reliable long-term arrest of chronic osteomyelitis. Nevertheless, antibiotic therapy is a key component of management. Indications for antibiotic therapy in chronic osteomyelitis include the following.

1. Control of systemic and soft-tissue sepsis.
2. Delivery, as an adjunct to surgical debridement and reconstruction, of bactericidal or bacteriostatic levels of antibiotic to vascularized bone.
3. Provision of prophylaxis against flares of infection in individuals with significant disease who are unsuitable candidates for surgery, but who are at special risk (e.g., immunosuppressed patients and those with prosthetic implants or vascular disease).

Empiric antibiotic therapy is indicated only when patients are seriously ill or significantly compromised. It should not be started before aspiration of the site of infection and blood culture.

Choice, Timing, and Route of Antibiotic Agent

Measured levels of antibiotic in bone and the concept of bone penetration may be misleading. Living, perfused bone possesses an interstitial fluid space in equilibrium with the other body spaces (55). Therefore, serum levels of unbound antibiotics should be directly reflected in the interstitial fluid of bone. This correlation has been demonstrated for a number of beta lactam and aminoglycoside agents (56) (see Chapter 8). Diffusion of antibiotics into avascular spaces, such as a fibrin clot, is limited: Effective use of antibiotics therefore depends on the presence of adequate capillary circulation.

The experimental basis for antibiotic choice in the management of chronic osteomyelitis is reviewed in Chapter 3. Briefly, single agents, with the exception of rifampicin and clindamycin, which appear to have degradative effects on protective biofilm, are ineffective in sterilizing bone. Combinations of agents that include rifampicin are particularly effective (57,58). In clinical practice, when appropriate meticulous surgical debridement can be considered, monotherapy directed against known pathogens is widely used.

The route of administration remains controversial and practice has varied. Long periods of intravenous therapy require hospitalization or multiple hospital visits and regular catheter changes to prevent nosocomial infection. Assuming normal absorption, by approximately 60 minutes after administration of the antibiotic by oral, intramuscular, or intravenous routes, the pharmacokinetics are similar and it seems likely that when reliable administration can be assured, oral therapy with beta lactam agents is satisfactory. This technique is certainly safe in children (59), but there has been some reluctance to extend the technique to adults. Use of oral fluoroquinolones has been compared with parenteral therapy, and early results suggest that these agents may prove both safe and effective (8).

Duration of therapy has been determined empirically. Most series report 6 to 12 weeks of therapy. The failure of patients with chronic osteomyelitis to respond reliably to antibiotic therapy alone has encouraged some to use protracted treatment programs (60). Some patients have received antibiotic suppression for more than 20 years (61). We do not recommend this approach. Although intuitively it might be imagined that individuals receiving long-term suppression could experience fewer episodes of recurrent clinical infection, there is no evidence that this effect occurs, and the complications and costs of prolonged administration are difficult to justify. In a patient for whom combined management is inappropriate, occasional flares of infection may be managed effectively by short programs of antibiotic therapy.

Local Administration of Antibiotics

Local administration techniques used have included regional perfusion, external closed-suction irrigation, implantable pump irrigation, and antibiotic-impregnated implants. Temporary control of infection has been reported in the past using perfusion techniques (62,63). Long-term outcomes are not available. Closed-suction irrigation has been examined repeatedly in the last 50 years (64–68). It combines debridement and dead space management with the ability to deliver high local concentrations of antibiotic within the irrigated cavity. Maintaining irrigation without tube blockage is difficult, and the risk of secondary infection increases after 48 hours. Use of implantable pumps has been pioneered by Perry and Pearson (69). In patients with resistant chronic osteomyelitis, with multiple previous procedures, suppression of infection at one year was achieved in 30 of 42 patients. This technique is expensive but provides high levels of antibiotic at the infection site with low systemic titers; it is therefore possible to use powerful but toxic broad-spectrum agents that may not be available by any other route.

High local/serum antibiotic ratios can also be achieved by the use of antibiotic-impregnated implants, of which PMMA has been most widely evaluated. Disadvantages include a slow decline over weeks or months in antibiotic levels and the requirement to remove the PMMA at the end of therapy, leaving a dead space. Nevertheless, this technique has been widely used in staged surgical management of osteomyelitis (70,71), and we consider it a useful option. Biodegradable polymers (72) and impregnated hydroxyapatite implants (73), which would not require removal, are under development.

Surgical Treatment

Ideally, the aim of surgical treatment is cure. If cure is not possible, there are only limited indications for bone surgery. Prerequisites for surgical treatment include the following.

1. Significant disability in the context of the patient's lifestyle and general health.
2. Appropriate patient expectations and commitment to multiple surgeries and prolonged treatment.
3. Prior stabilization of systemic disease.
4. Adequate local conditions in the affected limb.
5. Technical feasibility of any planned reconstruction.

The principles of surgical treatment include the following.

1. Debridement of dead bone, granulation tissue, and poorly vascularized scar.
2. Obliteration of dead space.
3. Restoration of functional stability.

Debridement

Wide debridement was used in the treatment of chronic osteomyelitis in the early twentieth century and was an integral part of the regimen of Orr, which was the mainstay of management of chronic osteomyelitis in the years prior to the introduction of chemotherapy. The introduction of new antimicrobial agents briefly encouraged the expectation that careful excision of all dead and poorly vascularized tissue was no longer necessary (74,75). Experience, however, has confirmed the essential role of removal of such tissue: Penetration of antibiotics into avascular areas is poor and bacterial killing and tissue healing at low PaO_2 are poor. Excision should extend to freely bleeding bone and soft tissue. When viability of bone is in doubt, vital dyes and the laser Doppler flow meter (76) have been used to guide the extent of debridement.

Complex sinus tracks may be outlined by injection of methylene or sulphan blue (77). Adequate debridement may require more than one surgical procedure. In patients with localized diaphyseal medullary disease, debridement may be achieved by intramedullary reaming (78,79).

Obliteration of Dead Space

A number of techniques are available to obliterate the dead space left by debridement. In principle, they fall into four groups, but they may be combined in various ways.

Exteriorization

The cavity is exteriorized and dressed to allow granulation from its base. This approach, formalized in the Orr technique (80), is now more often used as a prelude to cancellous grafting, although skin cover may be occasionally applied directly over the granulation.

Plombage

Inert material is inserted as a temporary space filler to allow granulation around the cavity. In the past, materials used included wax, plaster of Paris, and sand. Current practice combines plombage with local administration of high concentrations of antibiotics using impregnated PMMA (70,71,79).

Cancellous Bone Grafting

Use of cancellous bone grafting to fill defects in chronic osteomyelitis became popular following the introduction of antibiotics. Large series with successful outcomes measured 2 to 5 years following treatment have been published in adults (81) and in children (82). Split skin grafts may be applied successfully to the granulating cancellous bed (83), although coverage may be unstable. Used alone, or in combination with other techniques to correct the defect following debridement, cancellous grafting remains a useful and widely applicable method (84).

Transfer of Living Tissue

Since the introduction of tissue transfer with microvascular anastomosis, its use has become routine, and available transfers have increased rapidly in number and versatility. In patients with chronic osteomyelitis, it is possible to fill large defects created by extensive bone and soft-tissue debridement with well-vascularized tissue, which provides a healing potential and also greatly improves the cosmetic appearance.

Muscle flaps: Local or free muscle flaps provide the opportunity to combine obliteration of the dead space, improved vascularity, and good-quality skin coverage (85–87). Ger (85) popularized use of a number of local muscle flaps around the tibia, utilizing gastrocnemius, soleus, flexor digitorum longus, and abductor hallucis. Local muscle flaps are effective in the upper and middle third of the leg. In the lower third, or in very large proximal defects, free flaps from a range of donor sites are preferred. Five-year results from this approach show probable cure in nearly 90% of patients (88). The muscle flap may be combined with debridement or performed as a second-stage procedure. Split skin cover is applied. Atrophy and reduced vascularity of the flap occur over time.

Composite flaps: McCraw (89) developed composite flaps based on dominant muscular vessels. The gastrocnemius myocutaneous flap (90) is particularly relevant in coverage of the tibia, but a number of other flaps are available for use in both upper and lower limbs.

Versatile and relatively simple fasciocutaneous flaps (91,92) may also be useful in patients in whom only a small cavity requires to be filled. With attention to detail and technique, quite long and narrow flaps may be lifted.

If a substantial bone defect is present, restoration of functional stability may require either incorporation of bone in the transfer (93) or supplementary cancellous grafting, because experience suggests that bone is not induced in cavities obliterated by muscle alone. The incidence of delayed union in transfers incorporating vascularized bone is significant (94), and supplementary grafting may be required.

Restoration of Functional Stability

Long-term functional stability requires restoration of adequate bone structure. There is a risk of fracture after extensive debridement, which should be predictable from preoperative planning or during the procedure itself. Bone grafting or composite transfer including bone do not provide immediate stability. Available options for temporary stabilization include functional bracing, external skeletal fixation, or revision of internal fixation. Currently, there is considerable interest in the use of autogenous local bone transport using the compression-distraction apparatus of Ilizarov and colleagues (95). Using this method, large intercalary deficits created by radical debridement of infected bone may be filled with living autogenous bone by transport of a segment of healthy bone, separated by corticotomy, through the defect to dock with the bone at the other margin of the defect. This technique has many potential local complications, and a considerable learning period is required. However, it appears capable of dealing with problems insoluble by any other means by allowing preservation of functional limbs for which amputation would previously have been advised. Experience in Europe, North America, and other parts of the world is confirming the power of the method (96–100). Special situations, such as patients with large multiloculated cavities in intact bone, may be dealt with by modifications of this technique.

Amputation

Amputation and prosthetic fitting may be preferred if stable reconstruction cannot be obtained by more conservative surgery. Amputation should be as conservative as possible, bearing in mind the prerequisites and principles of surgical treatment. Excision of the calcaneus, for example (101), can result in retention of very useful function in the foot, although its results are better in post-traumatic infection than in contiguous infection with limb ischemia (102). In appropriate patients, relatively early amputation may be associated with less restriction of lifestyle and activity than continuing chronic osteomyelitis (103).

Rehabilitation

Chronic osteomyelitis may produce severe and prolonged disability. It is therefore not surprising that formal studies of outcome using validated functional scales demonstrate that individuals with chronic osteomyelitis have significant psychosocial, functional, and quality of life deficits (103). Careful assessment, informed participation by the patient in decision-making at all stages, and adherence to the principles of management facilitate the outcome.

Special Situations

Pin Track Osteomyelitis

Use of transcutaneous pins to provide skeletal traction or external fixation is frequently associated with infection (104), and residual pin track osteomyelitis occurs in up to 4% of patients. The majority of infections are associated with transfixion pins rather than half-pin assemblies, and with fixation in cortical bone. *S. aureus* is the most common isolate, but in North America, gram-negative aerobes are increasingly common. Nearly all patients demonstrate a ring sequestrum (see Figure 15-3), which may be a heat injury (105) caused by powered insertion of a smooth pointed transfixion pin, but even hand drilling of a screw hole is associated with a small cylindrical sleeve of necrosis around the drill hole (106). The exact temporal relationship of infection and separation of the sequestrum has not been determined, but the small size suggests that if it was not infected, it could readily be assimilated by normal processes of repair and remodeling.

Radiation Necrosis of Bone

Radionecrosis, particularly in the mandible, may lead to refractory chronic osteomyelitis if infection occurs, although the conditions are clearly distinct. The principles of management of infected radiation necrosis of bone are the same as those for managing chronic osteomyelitis; debridement to living tissue may be extensive. Hyperbaric oxygen treatment may be a useful adjunctive treatment (107).

Chronic Osteomyelitis in Children

In the developed world, chronic infection supervenes in less than 5% of patients with treated acute hematogenous osteomyelitis. In the developing world, the situation is very different. Incidence is uncertain; it depends on the availability of early diagnosis and treatment facilities. Extensive established infections, characteristic of the preantibiotic era in Europe and North America, present challenging problems in disease control and reconstruction (108,109).

Some primary presentations with established radiological features of infection have been called primary chronic osteomyelitis, or subacute osteomyelitis. These infections are discussed in Chapter 9.

The possibility of disturbances of skeletal growth is present in childhood chronic osteomyelitis, as it is in severe acute osteomyelitis. A recent review estimates the incidence of shortening or angular deformity at approximately 15% (110).

Complications

Amyloidosis

Secondary amyloidosis, the clinical features of which include fatigue, weight loss, edema, dyspnea, and carpal tunnel syndrome, is a rare complication of chronic osteomyelitis. Wilensky (7) reported four instances in 310 patients with osteomyelitis. Only approximately 10% of amyloid complications are secondary: in this group, rheumatoid arthritis and chronic osteomyelitis account for approximately two thirds (111,112).

Squamous-cell Carcinomas

The occasional occurrence of squamous-cell carcinomas in scar, discharging sinuses, and trophic ulceration has been recognized since the late nineteenth century. Volkmann is reported by Park to have examined 32 patients (113). No carcinomas occurred in the 310 patients with osteomyelitis followed by Wilensky (7). Incidence is estimated at less than 1% of cases of osteomyelitis. Fitzgerald and associates (114) reported 23 patients from the Mayo Clinic. All had had osteomyelitis since childhood (mean, 42 yr); all but one had an active sinus, and the average duration of drainage was 27 years. Clinical features characteristic of malignant change included increased pain, increased drainage, foul odor, and a mass. Regional lymph nodes were usually enlarged. Hemorrhage and pathological fractures were occasionally seen. The ESR was generally greater than 30 mm Hg. The only radiological characteristic was the occasional presence of bone destruction more extensive than that usually seen in patients with uncomplicated osteomyelitis (Figures 15-4,15-5). Although the majority of the tumors are histologically low grade, metastases are discovered in approximately 15% of reported patients (115). Metastasis tends to occur early, and patients surviving 3 years without metastases have a good prognosis.

Amputation is recommended; involvement of all tissues from skin to bone makes any more limited radical resection extremely difficult. The enlarged regional lymph nodes are often inflammatory and should be left alone initially, then watched and biopsied if persistent at 3 months.

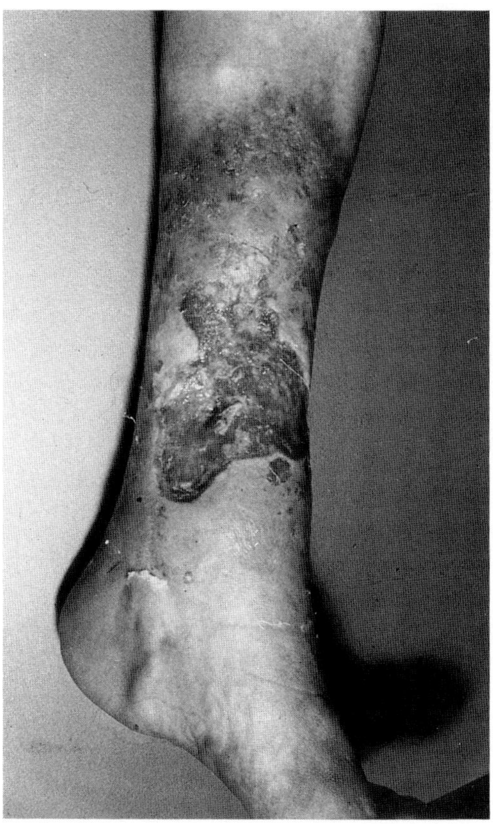

Figure 15-4. *Squamous-cell carcinoma over chronic osteomyelitis of the distal tibia.*

A B

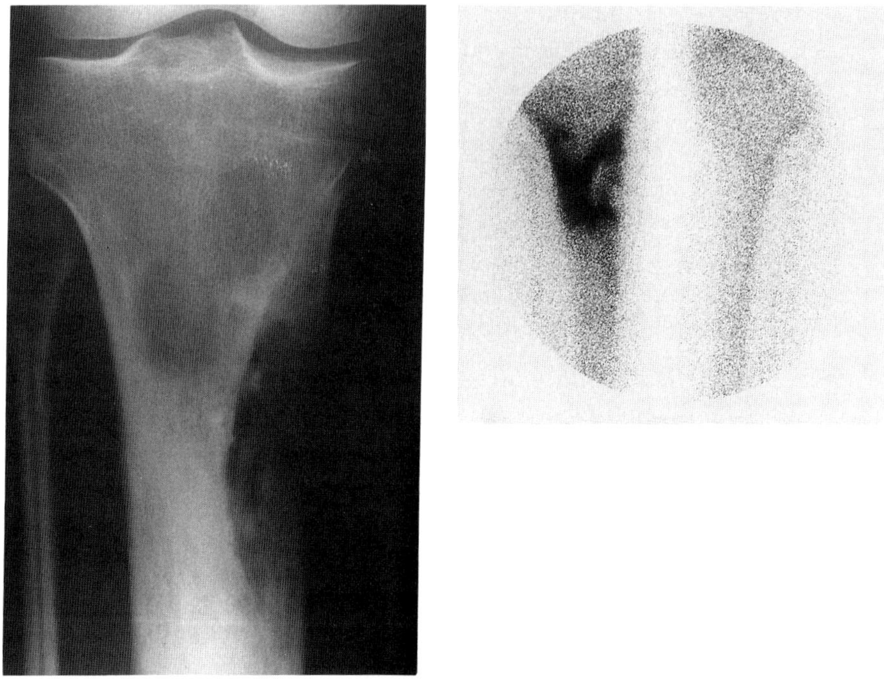

Figure 15-5. *(A) Chronic osteomyelitis of the proximal tibia with extensive eccentric destruction caused by squamous-cell carcinoma arising in a sinus. (B)* ^{99m}*Tc diphosphonate bone scan of the same lesion.*

Outcome of Management in Chronic Osteomyelitis

Suppression is perhaps a better concept than cure, because recurrences can occur very late (116). Follow-up in the literature is usually one or 2 years. One disease-free year may be considered as a possible cure and 5 years as a probable cure. An alternative approach is to use survival profiles, as has been done for the outcome of joint replacements.

The problem of comparison was discussed in the introduction to this chapter. Until agreement is reached on staging and until follow-up studies use uniform methodology, only broad generalizations about outcome are justified.

1. Antibiotic therapy alone may temporarily suppress chronic osteomyelitis in 70% to 80% of patients (58,117).

2. In general, hyperbaric oxygen therapy does not improve these results.
3. No convincing case has been made for the use of adjuvant immunotherapy.
4. The combination of antibiotic therapy with surgical management based on the principles of debridement, obliteration of dead space, and restoration of functional stability can achieve arrest of the disease after 2 years in 85% to 95% of patients with hematogenous and postoperative infection, and in 80% to 95% of patients with infected nonunions. The arrest rate at 2 years for individuals with normal host defenses may approach 100% (1).

Despite the complexity of chronic osteomyelitis and the consequent difficulties of establishing high-quality comparative studies, general adoption of a classification predictive of outcome, such as that of Cierny and Mader (1), or development of better classification (see Chapter 1) would be of real value, both in evaluation of new management protocols and in counseling individuals with the disease.

References

1. Cierny G, Mader JT. Adult chronic osteomyelitis: an overview. In: D'Ambrosia RD, Marier RL, eds. Orthopaedic Infections. Thorofare, NJ: Slack, 1989:31–48.
2. Kelly PJ, Fitzgerald RHJ, Cabanela ME, et al. Results of treatment of tibial and femoral osteomyelitis in adults. Clin Orthop 1990;259:295–303.
3. Waldvogel FA, Medoff G, Swartz MN. Osteomyelitis: a review of clinical features, therapeutic considerations and unusual aspects. N Engl J Med 1970;282:260–266.
4. Ogunjumo DO. Socio-economic implications of chronic pyogenic osteomyelitis in a developing community. R Soc Health J 1981;101:152–154.
5. Burri C. Post-traumatic osteomyelitis. Bern: Hans Huber, 1975.
6. Trendel H. Beitrage zur kenntnis der akuten infectiosen Osteomyelitis und ihrer Folgeerscheinungen. Beitr Z Klin Chir 1904;41:607–675.
7. Wilensky AO. Osteomyelitis: its pathogenesis, symptomatology and treatment. New York: Macmillan, 1934.
8. Gentry LO, Rodriguez Gomez G. Ofloxacin versus parenteral therapy for chronic osteomyelitis. Antimicrob Agents Chemother 1991;35:538–541.
9. Hall BB, Fitzgerald RHJ, Rosenblatt JE. Anaerobic osteomyelitis. J Bone Joint Surg [Am] 1983;65:30–35.

10. Nakata MM, Lewis RP. Anaerobic bacteria in bone and joint infections. Rev Infect Dis 1984;6(suppl 1):S165–S170.
11. Templeton WC, Wawrukiewicz A, Melo JC, Schiller MG, Raff MJ. Anaerobic osteomyelitis of long bones. Rev Infect Dis 1983;5:692–712.
12. Mackowiak PA, Smith JW. Polymicrobial infections in osteomyelitis. Rev Infect Dis 1983;5:167–168.
13. Leveuf J. Les lesions initiales de l'osteomyelite aigue. Rev Orthop 1947; 33:177–216.
14. Bohm E, Josten C. What's new in exogenous osteomyelitis? Pathol Res Pract 1992;188:254–258.
15. Frost HM. Pyogenic osteomyelitis. The normal bone spaces as a bacterial reservoir. Henry Ford Hosp Med Bull 1960;8:263–266.
16. Ginsburg I, Neeman N, Gallily R. Degradation and survival of bacteria in sites of allergic inflammation. In: Dumonde DC, ed. Infection and immunology in the rheumatic diseases. Oxford: Blackwell, 1976:43–59.
17. Gristina AG, Naylor PT, Myrvik QN. Mechanisms of musculoskeletal sepsis. Orthop Clin North Am 1991;22:363–371.
18. Gristina AG, Costerton JW. Bacterial adherence to biomaterials and tissue. The significance of its role in clinical sepsis. J Bone Joint Surg [Am] 1985;67:264–273.
19. Mayberry-Carson KJ, Tober-Meyer B, Smith JK, Lambe DW, Costerton JW. Bacterial adherence and glycocalyx formation in osteomyelitis experimentally induced with Staphylococcus aureus. Infect Immun 1984;43:825–833.
20. Herrmann M, Suchard SJ, Boxer LA, Waldvogel FA, Lew PD. Thrombospondin binds to Staphylococcus aureus and promotes staphylococcal adherence to surfaces. Infect Immun 1991;59:279–288.
21. Herrmann M, Vaudaux PE, Pittet D, Auckenthaler R, Lew PD. Fibronectin, fibrinogen and laminin act as mediators of adherence of clinical staphylococcal isolates to foreign material. J Infect Dis 1988;158:693–701.
22. Baltimore RS, Mitchell M. Immunologic investigation of mucoid strains of Pseudomonas aeruginosa. Comparison of susceptibility of opsonic antibody in mucoid and non-mucoid strains. J Infect Dis 1980;141:238–247.
23. Johnson GM, Lee DA, Regelmann WE, Gray ED, Peters G, Quie PG. Interference with granulocyte function by Staphylococcus epidermidis slime. Infect Immun 1986;54:13–20.
24. Gristina AG, Jennings RA, Naylor PT, Myrvik QN, Webb LX. Comparative in vitro antibiotic resistance of surface colonizing coagulase-negative staphylococci. Antimicrob Agents Chemother 1989;33:813–816.
25. Merritt K. Role of medical materials, both in implant and surface applications, in immune response and in resistance to infection. Biomaterials 1984;5:47–53.
26. Leake ES, Wright MJ, Gristina AG. Comparative study of the adherence of alveolar and peritoneal macrophages, and of blood monocytes to methyl methacrylate, polyethylene, stainless steel, and vitallium. J Reticuloendothel Soc 1981;30:403–414.

27. Petty W. The effect of methylmethacrylate on bacterial phagocytosis and killing by human polymorphonuclear leukocytes. J Bone Joint Surg [Am] 1978;60:752–757.
28. Petty W. The effect of methylmethacrylate on the bacterial inhibiting properties of normal human serum. Clin Orthop 1978;132:266–278.
29. Petty W. The effect of methylmethacrylate on chemotaxis of polymorphonuclear leukocytes. J Bone Joint Surg [Am] 1978;60:492–498.
30. Hunt TK. Surgical wound infections: an overview. Am J Med 1981;70: 712–718.
31. Niinikoski J, Hunt TK. Oxygen tensions in healing bone. Surg Gynecol Obstet 1972;134:746–750.
32. Hohn DC. Host resistance to infection: established and emerging concepts. In: Hunt TK, ed. Wound healing and wound infection: theory and surgical practice. New York: Appleton Century Crofts, 1980:264–279.
33. Perry CR, Pearson RL, Miller GA. Accuracy of cultures of material from swabbing of the superficial aspect of the wound and needle biopsy in the preoperative assessment of osteomyelitis. J Bone Joint Surg [Am] 1991; 73:745–749.
34. Hierholzer S, Hierholzer G. Nonspecific and specific host defense mechanisms in chronic post-traumatic bone infections. Unfallchirurg 1985;88: 255–262.
35. Schluter B, Bergmann U, Josten C, Walz M, Konig W. Impairment of specific host defense mechanisms in patients with chronic post-traumatic osteomyelitis. J Trauma 1991;31:68–73.
36. Burnet FM. Interactions of staphylococcus toxin, anatoxin, and antitoxin. J Pathol Bacteriol 1931:34:471–492.
37. Buchman J. The use of staphylococcus toxoid in the treatment of chronic osteomyelitis. JAMA 1937;108:1151–1156.
38. Ciotti M, Laus M, Romeo N, Savoini E. Complementary immunotherapy in the treatment of chronic osteomyelitis. Ital J Orthop Traumatol 1982; 8:437–444.
39. Karpas K, Capousek M, Charvat J. Use of immunoactive treatment in the therapy of chronic osteomyelitis. Acta Chir Orthop Traumatol Czech 1983; 50:378–382.
40. Foster TJ. Potential for vaccination against infections caused by Staphylococcus aureus. Vaccine 1991;9:221–227.
41. Winston DJ, Ho WG, Gale RP. Therapeutic granulocyte transfusions for documented infections. A controlled trial in ninety five infectious granulocytopenic episodes. Ann Intern Med 1982;97:509–515.
42. Matsumoto M, Matsubara S, Matsuno T, et al. Protective effect of human granulocyte colony-stimulating factor on microbial infection in neutropenic mice. Infect Immun 1987;55:2715–2720.
43. Smith TK. Prevention of complications in orthopedic surgery secondary to nutritional depletion. Clin Orthop 1987;222:91–97.
44. Greene KA, Wilde AH, Stulberg BN. Preoperative nutritional status of total

joint patients. Relationship to postoperative wound complications. J Arthroplasty 1991;6:321–325.
45. Tchervenkov JI, Latter DA, Psychogios J, Christou NV. The influence of long-term protein deprivation on in vivo phagocytic cell delivery to inflammatory lesions. Surgery 1988;103:463–469.
46. Lepantalo MJ, Haajanen J, Lindfors O, Paavolainen P, Scheinin TM. Predictive value of preoperative segmental blood pressure measurements in below-knee amputations. Acta Chir Scand 1982;148:581–584.
47. Resnick D, Niwayama G. Diagnosis of bone and joint disorders. Philadelphia: WB Saunders, 1981.
48. Kuhn JP, Berger PE. Computed tomographic diagnosis of osteomyelitis. Radiology 1979;130:503–506.
49. Dangman BC, Hoffer FA, Rand FF, O'Rourke EJ. Osteomyelitis in children: gadolinium-enhanced MR imaging. Radiology 1992;182:743–747.
50. Gandsman EJ, McCullough RW. Dynamic bone imaging in the differential diagnosis of skeletal lesions. Int J Radiol Appl Instrum 1990;17:533–541.
51. Patton JT. Imaging of bone and joint infections. Curr Opin Radiol 1991;3:713–718.
52. Merkel KD, Brown ML, Dewanjee MK, Fitzgerald RHJ. Comparison of indium-labeled-leukocyte imaging with sequential technetium-gallium scanning in the diagnosis of low-grade musculoskeletal sepsis. A prospective study. J Bone Joint Surg [Am] 1985;67:465–476.
53. Oyen WJ, Van Horn JR, Claessens RA, Slooff TJ, van der Meer JW, Corstens FH. Diagnosis of bone, joint, and joint prosthesis infections with In-111-labeled nonspecific human immunoglobulin G scintigraphy. Radiology 1992;182:195–199.
54. Graham GD, Lundy MM, Frederick RJ, Berger DE, O'Brien AW, Brown TJ. Predicting the cure of osteomyelitis under treatment: concise communication. J Nucl Med 1983;24:110–113.
55. Quinlan WR, Hall BB, Fitzgerald RH. Fluid spaces in normal and osteomyelitic canine bone. J Lab Clin Med 1983;102:78–87.
56. Fitzgerald RH. Antibiotic distribution in normal and osteomyelitic bone. Orthop Clin North Am 1984;15:537–546.
57. Norden CW. Experimental osteomyelitis. IV. Therapeutic trials with rifampin alone and in combination with gentamycin, sisomycin, and cephalothin. J Infect Dis 1975;132:493–499.
58. Norden CW, Fierer J, Bryant RE. Chronic staphylococcal osteomyelitis: treatment with regimens containing rifampin. Rev Infect Dis 1983;5(suppl 3): S495–S501.
59. Cole WG. The management of chronic osteomyelitis. Clin Orthop 1991; 264:84–89.
60. Bell SM. Oral penicillins in the treatment of chronic staphylococcus osteomyelitis. Lancet 1968;2:295–297.
61. Bell SM, Gatus BJ, Shepherd BD. Antibiotic prophylaxis for the prevention of late infections of prosthetic joints. Aust NZ J Surg 1990;60:177–181.

62. Finsterbush A, Weinberg H. Venous perfusion of the limb with antibiotics for osteomyelitis and other chronic infections. J Bone Joint Surg [Am] 1972;54:1227–1234.
63. Organ CHJ. The utilization of massive doses of antimicrobial agents with isolation perfusion in the treatment of chronic osteomyelitis. Intermediate term results. Clin Orthop 1971;76:185–193.
64. Smith-Petersen MN, Larson CB, Cochran W. Local chemotherapy with primary closure of septic wounds by means of drainage and irrigation cannulae. J Bone Joint Surg 1945;27:562–571.
65. Compere EL. Treatment of osteomyelitis and infected wounds by closed irrigation with detergent antibiotic solution. Acta Orthop Scand 1962; 32:324–333.
66. Clawson DK, Davis FJ, Hansen ST. Treatment of chronic osteomyelitis with emphasis on closed suction-irrigation technic. Clin Orthop 1973;96: 88–97.
67. Kawashima M, Torisu T, Kamo Y, Iwabuchi A. The treatment of pyogenic bone and joint infections by closed irrigation-suction. Clin Orthop 1980; 148:240–244.
68. Oguachuba HN. Use of instillation-suction technique in treatment of chronic osteomyelitis. Acta Orthop Scand 1983;54:452–458.
69. Perry CR, Pearson RL. Local antibiotic delivery in the treatment of bone and joint infections. Clin Orthop 1991;263:215–226.
70. Boda A. Septopal-chain exchange operation for the treatment of osteomyelitic cavities. Preliminary report on 10 cases. Arch Orthop Trauma Surg 1982;101:39–45.
71. Henry SL, Ostermann PA, Seligson D. The prophylactic use of antibiotic impregnated beads in open fractures. J Trauma 1990;30:1231–1238.
72. Tamada J, Langer R. The development of polyanhydrides for drug delivery applications. J Biomater Sci Polym Ed 1992;3:315–353.
73. Yu D, Wong J, Matsuda Y, Fox JL, Higuchi WI, Otsuka M. Self-setting hydroxyapatite cement: a novel skeletal drug-delivery system for antibiotics. J Pharm Sci 1992;81:529–531.
74. Rowling DE. The positive approach to chronic osteomyelitis. J Bone Joint Surg [Br] 1959;41:681–688.
75. Rowling DE. Further experience in the management of chronic osteomyelitis. J Bone Joint Surg [Br] 1970;52:302–307.
76. Swiontkowski MF. Surgical approaches in osteomyelitis. Use of laser doppler flowmetry to determine nonviable bone. Infect Dis Clin North Am 1990; 4:501–512.
77. Jenny G, Kempf I, Jaeger JH, Betar S, Gebauer G. The use of sulphan blue dye during surgical procedures for bone infection. Rev Chir Orthop 1977; 63:531–537.
78. Lidgren L, Torholm C. Intramedullary reaming in chronic diaphyseal osteomyelitis: a preliminary report. Clin Orthop 1980;151:215–221.
79. Ochsner PE, Gosele A, Buess P. The value of intramedullary reaming in the

treatmennt of chronic osteomyelitis of long bones. Arch Orthop Trauma Surg 1990;109:341–347.
80. Orr HW. Osteomyelitis in compound fractures and other infected wounds. St. Louis: Mosby, 1929.
81. Hazlett JW. The use of cancellous bone grafts in the treatment of subacute and chronic osteomyelitis. J Bone Joint Surg [Br] 1954;36:584–590.
82. De Oliveira JC. Bone grafts and chronic osteomyelitis. J Bone Joint Surg [Br] 1971;53:672–683.
83. Papineau LJ, Alfageme A, Dalcourt JP, Pilon L. Chronic osteomyelitis: open excision and grafting after saucerization. Int Orthop 1979;3:165–176.
84. Cabanela ME. Open cancellous bone grafting of infected bone defects. Orthop Clin North Am 1984;15:427–440.
85. Ger R. Muscle transposition for treatment and prevention of chronic post-traumatic osteomyelitis of the tibia. J Bone Joint Surg [Am] 59:784–791.
86. Fitzgerald RHJ, Ruttle PE, Arnold PG, Kelly PJ, Irons GB. Local muscle flaps in the treatment of chronic osteomyelitis. J Bone Joint Surg [Am] 1985;67:175–185.
87. Mathers SL, Nahai F. Clinical applications for muscle and musculocutaneous flaps. St. Louis: Mosby, 1982.
88. Anthony JP, Mathes SJ, Alpert BS. The muscle flap in the treatment of chronic lower extremity osteomyelitis: results in patients over 5 years after treatment. Plast Reconstr Surg 1991;88:311–318.
89. McCraw JB. The recent history of myocutaneous flaps. Clin Plast Surg 1980;7:3–7.
90. McCraw JB, Fishman JH, Sharzer LA. The versatile gastrocnemius myocutaneous flap. Plast Reconstr Surg 1978;62:15–23.
91. Ponten B. The fasciocutaneous flap: its use in softtissue defects of the lower leg. Br J Plast Surg 1981;34:215–220.
92. Tolhurst DE, Haeseker B, Zeeman RJ. The development of the fasciocutaneous flap and its clinical applications. Plast Reconstr Surg 1983; 71:597–606.
93. Taylor GI, Miller GD, Ham FJ. The free vascularized bone graft. A clinical extension of microvascular techniques. Plast Reconstr Surg 1975;55: 533–544.
94. Vitkus K, Vitkus M. Reconstruction of large infected tibia defects. Ann Plast Surg 1992;29:97–106.
95. Ilizarov GA, Kaplunov AG, Degtiarev VE, Lediaev VI. Treatment of pseudarthroses and ununited fractures, complicated by purulent infection, by the method of compression-distraction osteosynthesis. Ortop Travmatol Protez 1972;33:10–14.
96. Green SA. Osteomyelitis. The Ilizarov perspective. Orthop Clin North Am 1991;22:515–521.
97. Green SA, Jackson JM, Wall DM, Marinow H, Ishkanian J. Management of segmental defects by the Ilizarov intercalary bone transport method. Clin Orthop 1992;280:136–142.
98. Cattaneo R, Catagni M, Johnson EE. The treatment of infected nonunions

and segmental defects of the tibia by the methods of Ilizarov. Clin Orthop 1992;280:143–152.
99. Calhoun JH, Anger DM, Mader J. The Ilizarov technique in the treatment of osteomyelitis. Tex Med 1991;87:56–59.
100. Aronson J. Cavitary osteomyelitis treated by fragmentary cortical bone transportation. Clin Orthop 1992;280:153–159.
101. Martini M, Martini Benkeddache Y, Bekkechi T, Daoud A. Treatment of chronic osteomyelitis of the calcaneus by resection of the calcaneus. A report of twenty cases. J Bone Joint Surg [Am] 1974;56:542–548.
102. Crandall RC, Wagner WF. Partial and total calcanectomy. J Bone Joint Surg [Am] 1981;63:152–155.
103. Lerner RK, Esterhai JLJ, Polomono RC, Cheatle MC, Heppenstall RB, Brighton CT. Psychosocial, functional, and quality of life assessment of patients with posttraumatic fracture nonunion, chronic refractory osteomyelitis, and lower extremity amputation. Arch Phys Med Rehabil 1991; 72:122–126.
104. Green SA, Ripley MJ. Chronic osteomyelitis in pin tracks. J Bone Joint Surg [Am] 1984;66:1092–1098.
105. Christie J. Surgical heat injury of bone. Injury 1981;13:188–190.
106. Schatzker J. Horne JG, Sumner-Smith G. The reaction of cortical bone to compression by screw threads. Clin Orthop 1975;111:263–265.
107. Mainous EG, Boyne PJ, Hart GB. Elimination of sequestrum and healing of osteoradionecrosis of the mandible after hyperbaric oxygen therapy: report of case. J Oral Surg 1973;31:336–339.
108. Saighi-Bouaouina A, Daoud A, Martini M. Chronic haematogenous osteomyelitis of the tibia treated by operation. A survey of 122 cases. Int Orthop 1991;15:127–133.
109. Onuba O. Chronic osteomyelitis in children in Bulawayo, Zimbabwe. Trop Doct 1991;21:63–64.
110. Tudisco C, Farsetti P, Gatti S, Ippolito E. Influence of chronic osteomyelitis on skeletal growth: analysis at maturity of 26 cases affected during childhood. J Pediatr Orthop 1991:11:358–363.
111. Kyle RA, Bayrd ED. Amyloidosis: review of 236 cases. Medicine 1975; 54:271–299.
112. Gertz MA, Kyle RA. Secondary systemic amyloidosis: response and survival in 64 patients. Medicine 1991;70:246–256.
113. Park R. On the deformities and malformations resulting from acute infections in bone. Trans Am Orthop Assoc 1896;8:102–115.
114. Fitzgerald RHJ, Brewer NS, Dahlin DC. Squamous-cell carcinoma complicating chronic osteomyelitis. J Bone Joint Surg [Am] 1976;58:1146–1148.
115. Sedlin ED, Fleming JL. Epidermoid carcinoma arising in chronic osteomyelitic foci. J Bone Joint Surg [Am] 1963;45:827–838.
116. Gallie WF. First recurrence of osteomyelitis eighty years after infection. J Bone Joint Surg [Br] 1951;33:110–111.
117. Hierholzer G, Rehn J, Knothe H, Masterson J. Antibiotic therapy of chronic post-traumatic osteomyelitis. J Bone Joint Surg [Br] 1974;56:721–729.

CHAPTER 16

Conditions That Mimic Osteomyelitis

Multifocal bone lesions detected radiologically are rare in childhood but have diverse causes, including leukemia, neuroblastoma, histiocytosis X, Gaucher's disease, as well as infection (1). Because of an increasing number of nonstaphylococcal bone infections, atypical presentations are becoming more common and produce clinical appearances that can be confused with apparently noninfective disorders.

Chronic Multifocal Osteomyelitis

There are three general classes of nonspecific chronic osteomyelitis: (a) a sequel to acute osteomyelitis, (b) unifocal subacute or chronic osteomyelitis, and (c) chronic multifocal osteomyelitis. Many terms have been used to describe the multifocal form of chronic osteomyelitis, including chronic recurrent multifocal osteomyelitis, chronic symmetrical osteomyelitis, chronic multifocal cleidometaphyseal osteomyelitis, as well as multifocal forms of Garré's sclerosing osteomyelitis, plasma cell osteomyelitis, and tumorous osteomyelitis (2–5). Because the clinical, radiological, and pathological features of each disorder are essentially the same, it is likely that they are all part of the same disease and should be more simply considered together as chronic multifocal osteomyelitis. Similarly, condensing osteomyelitis of the clavicle and recurrent hyperostosis of the clavicle share many features of chronic multifocal osteomyelitis (6,7). There is sufficient evidence to support classification of this condition as a definite disease entity. Infantile cortical hyperostosis (i.e., Caffey's disease) and multifocal recurrent periostitis (8,9) are similar but differ from chronic multifocal osteomyelitis. They are periosteal diseases of unknown etiology that affect the diaphyses of long bones and the mandible, but there is little data to support an infective or endosteal origin.

The syndrome of chronic multifocal osteomyelitis, originally called subacute symmetrical osteomyelitis, was first described in 1972 in four children (10). The term *chronic recurrent multifocal osteomyelitis* was coined by Probst and colleagues in 1978 (11). In contrast to other forms of osteomyelitis, most children with chronic multifocal osteomyelitis are girls. They often have many months, even years, of malaise, painful lesions, arthralgia, and painful swelling of adjacent joints. Although references can be found for more cases, a recent review (12) indicated that of approximately 50 cases reported in the literature (13–22), only four occurred in adults. Disuse atrophy and diminished function of the involved regions are common. Onset is usually insidious, with mild or moderate pain, and symptoms may wax and wane for months or years. Deep tenderness is common, and the affected regions may be swollen.

Sometimes there are associated skin disorders. Pustular rashes, referred to as pustulosis palmoplantaris (PPP), may be noted in soles and palms (23–28); it has also been described in patients with severe acne (29). Some reports suggest that "bone pain" worsens when the pustular lesions are active. Chronic bowel disease was reported in 5 of 30 patients (30). White cell counts are normal, whereas the erythrocyte sedimentation rate is usually increased. C-reactive protein levels are not usually increased (6). Blood cultures are negative and cultures of the lesion rarely grow *Staphylococcus aureus*.

The etiology remains unknown. An autoimmune cause has been suggested, but detailed studies of the immune status of affected children have not supported this proposal (6). The most widely held view is that chronic multifocal osteomyelitis is infective despite the low frequency of organisms grown from biopsy specimens. The possibility (31) that a fastidious slow-growing bacterium, such as a *Mycoplasma* (32), is the most likely causative agent has not been excluded. One report (33) indicated that *Propionibacterium acnes* had been found in some bone and joint lesions. There is a reported molecular interaction between bone sialoprotein and staphylococcal cells, which supports the theory of osteotropism or chondrotropism of certain strains of staphylococci. In one patient (34), *S. epidermidis* was isolated from blood and also had a strong affinity for sialoprotein in laboratory testing.

Some investigators believe that the unusual condition of PPP is a manifestation of psoriasis vulgaris. Another group (35) reported two patients with psoriasis in the absence of PPP and speculated that the condition is a variant of the musculoskeletal manifestations of psoriasis. Following a multicenter study of 85 patients in France (36), the name SAPHO (*s*ynovitis, *a*cne, *p*ustulosis, *h*yperostosis, *o*steitis) was coined to represent the association.

Radiographs and isotope bone scans reveal number, distribution, and type of bone lesions. There may be five to ten skeletal lesions (24), as well as aggressive lesions or benign cavities. Aggressive lesions are most common in the narrow long bones (i.e., tibia, clavicle, fibula, femur, and radius), in order of decreasing frequency (10). Less commonly involved sites are the tubular bones of hands and feet, the sternum, the humerus, and the ribs. Characteristic lesions are well demarcated and osteolytic, with a pyramidal shape or a sinuous border located in the metaphysis of a tubular bone adjacent to the physis. In short tubular bones, the lesions are less typical, with irregular destruction and periosteal bone formation. They cannot be distinguished from pyogenic osteomyelitis. The base of the lesions can be from a few millimeters to the entire width of the metaphysis. Periosteal reaction is infrequent. Epiphyseal lesions are rare and, if present, are small. Metaphyseal and epiphyseal cavities may be well circumscribed, as in unifocal cases, but may also be diffuse. In the latter, tomograms show diffuse cavitation and sclerosis of the metaphysis and epiphysis, as well as irregularities of the growth plate. Figures 16-1 and 16-2 show typical radiographic appearances. Sclerosis on both sides of the sacroiliac joint may be seen. Less frequently, there may be an area of osteopenia, with no periosteal reaction or sclerotic margin. The lower limbs are likely to be affected more often than the upper. In the spine, affected vertebral bodies may collapse, leading to marked kyphosis. In a report of seven patients (37), vertebra plana was present in three, in whom reconstitution to normal vertebral height did not occur. The authors questioned the usual interpretation of such a vertebra in children, which is usually said to be due to eosinophilic granuloma.

Radioisotope bone scans with ^{99m}Tc-methylene diphosphonate regularly show increased uptake regardless of the appearance of the region

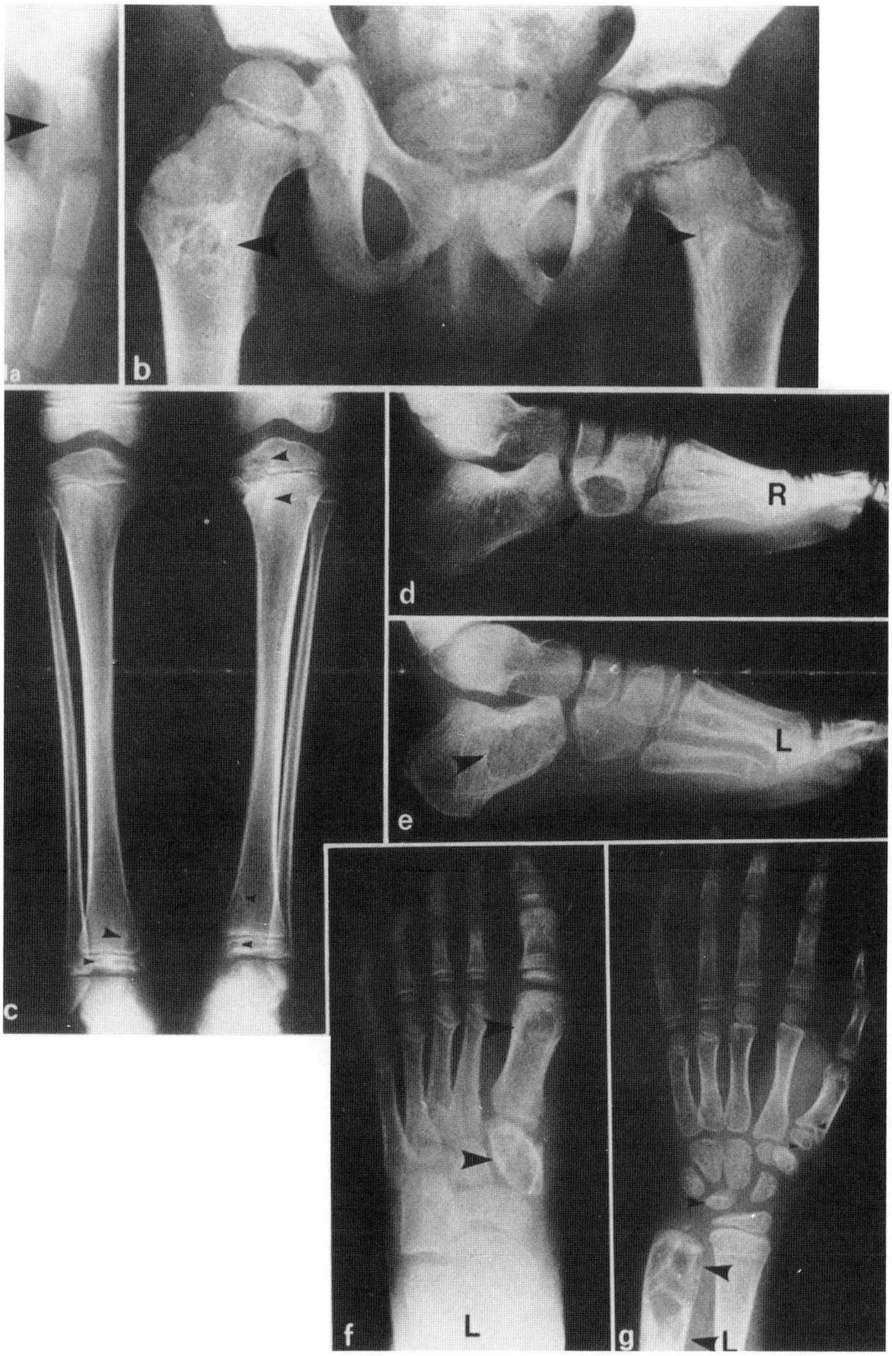

Figure 16-1. *The spectrum of radiographic appearances seen in chronic multifocal osteomyelitis. (a) Osteolytic changes in the sternum in a child aged 5 years and 9 months. At age 7 and 1 month, radiographs (b–e) show multifocal destructive bone changes at different stages of development or bone healing. Some months later, others (f,g) were detected.* (Reproduced by permission from Kozlowski K, Masel J, Harbison S, Yu J. Multifocal chronic osteomyelitis of unknown etiology. Pediatr Radiol 1983;13:130–136.)

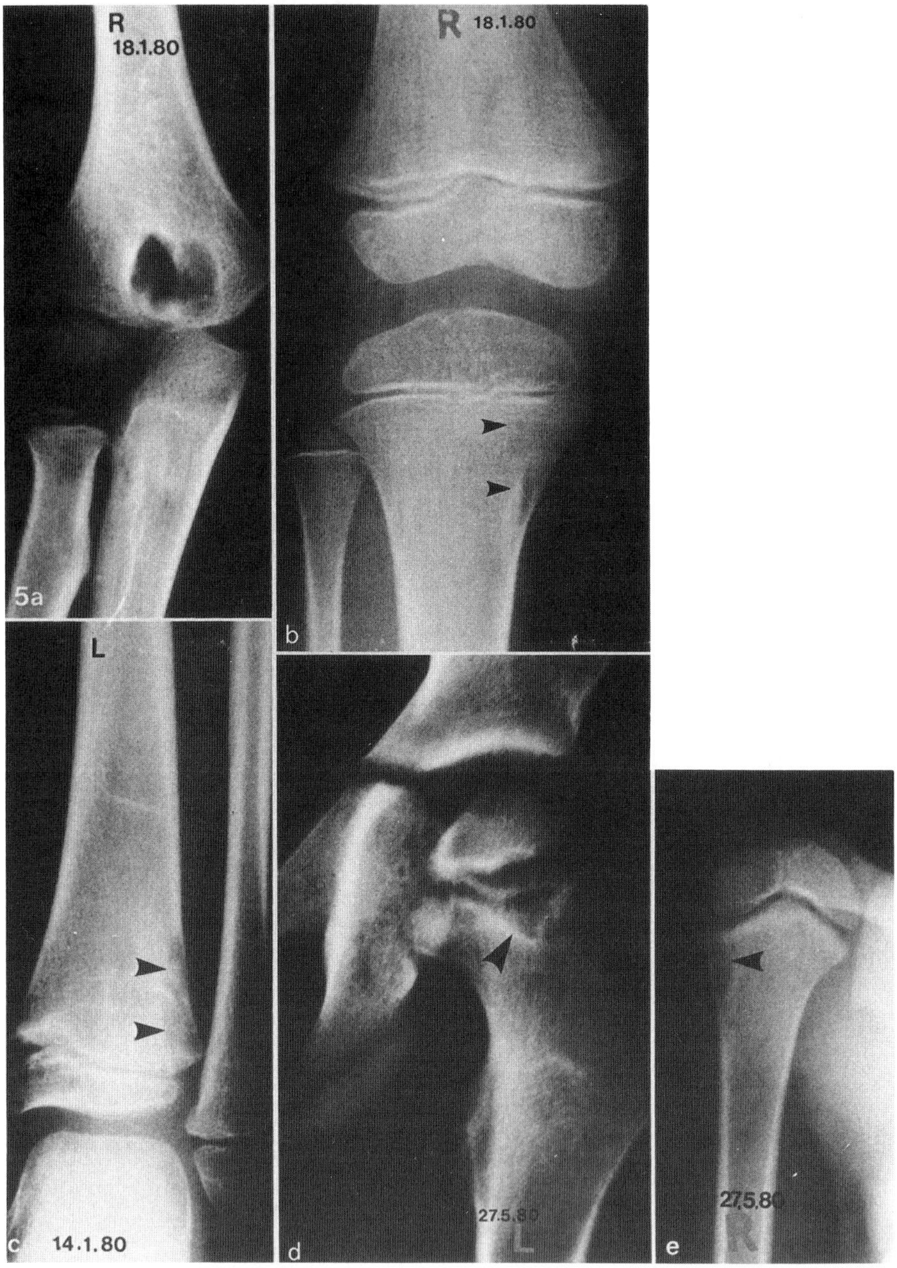

Figure 16-2. *Further examples of the spectrum of radiological lesions seen in chronic multifocal osteomyelitis from a boy aged 6 years. (a) A lytic lesion with well-defined sclerotic margins in the right lower humerus; (b,c) Smaller lytic areas with fairly well-defined margins in the right upper tibia and the left lower fibula. Eight months after onset of symptoms, radiographs showed additional metaphyseal lesions in the left upper femur (d) and the right upper humerus (e); these lesions were not associated with symptoms.* (Reproduced by permission from Kozlowski K, Masel J, Harbison S, Yu J. Multifocal chronic osteomyelitis of unknown etiology. Pediatr Radiol 1983;13:130–136.)

on plain radiographs. Not all show hyperemia on the radionuclide angiogram (38). The value of scintigraphy is as an early guide to the distribution of lesions in bone and to indicate which other sites may be subjected to conventional radiography if an initial site does not show characteristic features of this condition.

When histological examination of biopsy specimens had been performed, the findings within the same specimen were usually those of an acute, subacute, and chronic inflammation with a varying number of polymorphonuclear leukocytes, lymphocytes, plasma cells, histiocytes, and, occasionally, eosinophils. Granulation tissue was evident. Osteonecrosis was sometimes seen, but reactive bone formation at the periphery of inflammatory foci was common. There are no characteristic diagnostic features. Organisms are not usually detected. In vertebral biopsies from patients with vertebra plana, no histochemical features of eosinophilic granuloma have been recognized.

In Europe, histological diagnosis of chronic plasma cell osteomyelitis is commonly made for a form of osteomyelitis in children characterized by insidious or subacute onset of low-grade symptoms and mild to moderate inflammatory signs (39). In these patients, two types of radiological bone lesion could be separated. Most often seen was a sharply defined ("punched out") osteolytic area with different degrees of surrounding sclerosis; the other lesion was a sclerotic bone reaction without any osteolysis. Although Exner (39) believed that this was a distinct entity, we believe that its features place it within the category of chronic multifocal osteomyelitis.

To experienced physicians, clinical and radiological features of chronic multifocal osteomyelitis are usually characteristic, and a biopsy is not usually required to confirm diagnosis. However, a trephine biopsy of the most readily accessible lesion enables specimens to be obtained for bacteriological examination. A trephine can be guided into a cavity under the control of a computerized tomograph. Specimens should be cultured immediately for aerobic and anaerobic organisms and for specific organisms, such as mycobacteria and fungi. Special care should be taken to detect organisms with fastidious or slow growth. A histological search is also made for organisms.

Those few patients in whom *S. aureus* or other organisms are identified are likely to respond to antibiotic therapy (1). In most patients, cultures are negative and antibiotics are usually ineffective. Some authors suggest that a 6-week course of antistaphylococcal antibiotics be given as a therapeutic trial. We believe it is futile to continue if there is no clinical response and do not, in general, support empiric therapy if this entity is suspected.

Management of children with chronic multifocal osteomyelitis is often difficult because of persisting symptoms. Nevertheless, it is important to remember that chronic multifocal osteomyelitis is a self-limiting disease. In many patients, symptomatic care with simple analgesics is all that is necessary while waiting for spontaneous resolution of the lesions. Repeated biopsies and repeated courses of antibiotics are unwarranted.

One follow-up study of pediatric patients (40) confirmed that the appearance of the lesion in adulthood remains the same as that observed in childhood. Radiological appearance may change during the healing phase. Plain radiographs show diffuse increases in radiodensity, whereas computerized tomograms commonly show a mixture of multiple small cavities and widespread radiodensity. The lesions commonly spread across the full width of a metaphysis and the epiphysis. Progressive diaphyseal lesions of long tubular bones are similar to those that have in the past been described as Garré's osteomyelitis or chronic sclerosing osteomyelitis. (Garré's original report [41] preceded the discovery of x-rays.) Surgical cure of these radiographic abnormalities should not be attempted.

The disease process usually persists for many months or even years. It is important to be aware of this condition and to establish the diagnosis as chronic multifocal osteomyelitis. Unnecessary diagnostic procedures and prolonged use of antibiotics, steroid drugs, or chemotherapeutic agents can therefore be avoided.

Sternocostoclavicular Hyperostosis

When described in 1977, sternocostoclavicular hyperostosis was a rare condition characterized by persistent, pulling pain in the sternum, the clavicles, and the upper ribs exacerbated by cold and dampness (42). The differential diagnosis of persistent pain and swelling at the sternal end of the clavicle or the sternoclavicular joints includes Tietze's syndrome, aseptic necrosis, luxations, infections, and tumors. Sternocostoclavicular hyperostosis is usually associated with PPP. It occurs more frequently in the Far East than in the Western hemisphere (43) and is more common in women than in men. Pain intensity varies and is related to changes in weather and to common infections. It is probably now best classified as chronic multifocal osteomyelitis.

Condensing Osteitis of the Clavicle

Sclerosis of the medial end of the clavicle occurs in condensing osteitis of the clavicle, but the condition is unilateral and does not involve the sternoclavicular joint. It was first described in 1974 (44). A condition known as recurrent hyperostosis of the clavicles has also been described (45). These conditions are also best classified as part of the spectrum of chronic multifocal osteomyelitis.

Histiocytosis X (Eosinophilic Granuloma)

The term *histiocytosis X* was coined by Lichtenstein (46) in 1953 as a general designation for a malady that included eosinophilic granuloma of bone, Letterer-Siwe, disease and Hand-Schüller-Christian disease. We describe histiocytosis X localized to bone, either single or multiple, which is also known as eosinophilic granuloma.

Eosinophilic granulomas represent the pathological expression of an early, rapidly developing reaction to the etiological agent, whatever it might ultimately prove to be. An infective agent, possibly viral, seems to be a more plausible explanation than any other cause. Fever, weight loss, and night sweats may sometimes occur, and there may be spread to regional lymph nodes.

Eosinophilic granulomas may show one, several, or occasionally many destructive foci within the skeleton, as well as usually no apparent constitutional indications of illness or any discernible cutaneous, pulmonary, hypophyseal, or other extraskeletal involvement. Lichtenstein (47) regarded eosinophilic granuloma of bone (an apt pathological description) as a skeletal localization that is an indication of successful confinement of the etiological agent, which may account for its favorable outcome. There is a good prognosis for recovery in such patients, even if a number of skeletal lesions are present or subsequently appear, as occasionally occurs.

When determining a clinical diagnosis, a focus of eosinophilic granuloma may develop so rapidly and break through the cortex of the cortical bone so readily, that it is often mistaken for a primary malignant tumor or infection before biopsy. Despite such ominous behavior, such lesions often heal rapidly following curettage or low dose irradiation.

They may regress or disappear spontaneously (47), but extraskeletal manifestations may also follow lesions initially confined to bone.

Eosinophilic granulomas mainly occur in older children and adults, but infants are occasionally affected. In older adults, the eosinophilic granuloma may be asymptomatic. The most common sites affected are the limb bones, the skull, the vertebrae, and the pelvis. Flattening of vertebrae may occur as a compression fracture, and the spinal cord or a nerve root may be compressed. In children, this condition may develop insidiously without early detection. It produces the radiological feature of vertebra plana, which is not, as once thought, a form of ischemic necrosis of bone.

Metaplastic Ossification in Other Sites

Periosteal Ossification

Periosteal ossification may appear similar to the repair reaction that occurs in infection. Scurvy, hemophilia, and trauma may have an effect on periosteum, causing it to produce bone after hemorrhage in the region of periosteum, either lifting it from bone or adjacent to it.

Hypertrophic osteoarthropathy, which is associated mainly, but not exclusively, with pulmonary neoplastic or suppurative disease, shows widespread periosteal new bone apposition, which may be layered on phalanges, metacarpals, and metatarsals, as well as the distal portion of the long bones of the arm or leg. It is usually bilateral and more or less symmetrical. The soft tissues over the bones and joints are warm and tender. The condition is often associated with clubbing of fingers and toes. The mechanism of production of the syndrome is unknown but is thought to be related to increased vascularity. The pathological findings are edema, infiltration of the periosteal connective tissue by lymphocytes and plasma cells, followed by bone formation. The new bone is at first cancellous and highly vascular and later becomes more compact as it becomes incorporated into the original cortex. Clinical presentation may mimic infection.

Skeletal Changes in Certain Blood Diseases

Hemophilia

More than half of all hemophiliacs bleed into their joints. The knee is most often involved, but hips, ankles, and elbows are frequently affected. Rapidly developing hemarthrosis is likely to be painful and disabling, and causes overlying warmth. If the diagnosis of hemophilia has not been previously made, the condition may mimic a joint infection. Osteoarticular destruction may occur. The combination of bone destruction and bone repair may produce bizarre radiographs that can be confused with chronic osteomyelitis in some patients.

Chronic Hemolytic Anemias

In chronic hemolytic anemia, the skeletal changes (in children) may be pathognomonic and are often among the most characteristic features. The principal conditions are sickle-cell anemia, thalassemia, and spherocytic anemia. In response to increased destruction of erythrocytes, the bone marrow becomes markedly hyperplastic. Within young growing bones, this marrow overgrowth causes widening of the medullary cavities and pressure atrophy of cortical and cancellous bone, which are reflected radiographically in distinctive patterns. Sickle-cell anemia is characterized by symptoms of anemia, arthritic manifestations (e.g., aching pains in the joints or elsewhere in the extremities commonly ascribed to rheumatism), chronic leg ulcers, and acute attacks of pain. The bones may in fact be infected in this condition, because the osteomyelitis that occurs is commonly due to *Salmonella* species, as well as the site of sepsis in the diaphysis. Noninfectious manifestations may involve the metacarpals and the proximal phalanges, with cortical thinning and widening of the diameter of the bone. Usually, there is no difficulty in determining that the diagnosis is not due to infection, but the combination of pain in an extremity, tenderness of bone, and radiological changes in bone of rarefaction and bone production can sometimes mimic a bone infection.

Gaucher's Disease

Gaucher's disease is a hereditary metabolic disturbance characterized by accumulation of cerebrosides (kerasin and phrenosin) in reticuloendothelial cells. There are three distinct forms; all have autosomal recessive inheritance and deficient acid β-glucuronidase activity. Type I disease is the most common form and occurs predominantly in Ashkenazi Jews. It has a variable severity and age of onset, although half the patients present in the first decade of life. Vague symptoms of weakness, fatigue, and weight loss are present. Abdominal discomfort is common, and liver enlargement is seen in approximately 75% of patients. Almost all have an enlarged spleen. Abnormalities in blood count may be seen. The bone symptomatology includes pain and limitation of movement, usually of the hips and the knees. Vascular infarction can lead to acute symptoms that mimic osteomyelitis. Pathological fracture occurs in 5% to 10% of children but rarely in adults. Hips, ribs, and vertebrae are usually involved.

Radiographically, the most frequent sites of skeletal involvement are femora, spine, hips, shoulders, tubular bones, and pelvis. The lower extremities are more often involved than the upper. The femur often has a characteristic appearance, with ischemic necrosis at the proximal end and an "Erlenmeyer flask" deformity at the distal end. The basic processes of bone involvement are similar to those of other diseases in which there is proliferation of bone marrow or infiltration of bone marrow with abnormal cells. There may be loss of bone density, simulating osteoporosis. Bone trabeculae are resorbed, particularly in the spine, and the remaining trabeculae stand out in relief to give a picture of altered or coarsened bone trabecular pattern. Reparative processes may reinforce this picture and lead to areas of increased bone density. Patchy destructive areas may occur in a geographic or "moth-eaten" pattern, giving a picture very similar to osteolytic metastases. Margination of these lesions varies. Local or patchy sclerosis may also occur.

The combination of bone necrosis and repair phenomena produces radiological appearances that can be similar to those that follow bone infection. Complete examination of patients reveals the enlarged spleen and liver, which may be the clue to this diagnosis in a (usually) Jewish patient. However, a cautionary word was sounded in one report (48), in which it was found that in 11 of 49 patients with Gaucher's disease who had a so called crisis, five proved to have acute hematogenous osteomyelitis; as a consequence of delay in diagnosis, outcome was unsatisfactory. There is no clear discussion in the literature that addresses the issue of how to distinguish osseous crises in Gaucher's disease from osteomyelitis. One indicator to infection in the presence of Gaucher's disease is the change from a "hollow appearance" in the bone on radionuclide scans with ^{99m}Tc-MDP to a less hollow appearance. This feature can be enhanced if both ^{99m}Tc-MDP and radiogallium scans are done simultaneously, and if the activity from the ^{99m}Tc is subtracted from the radiogallium scan. Radiogallium excess might indicate osteomyelitis, even in the absence of clinical signs (49). Magnetic resonance imaging possibly has a role, with the combination of an inflammatory signal from surrounding musculature and marrow signal abnormalities. Abnormal marrow in patients with Gaucher's disease produces a lower signal intensity, with longer T1 and shorter T2 values.

Osteitis Pubis

In 1924, Beer (50) described a syndrome of pubic pain with characteristic radiological changes occurring after suprapubic operations. Such suprapubic pain, with radiological changes, has since been recognized in a number of other clinical situations, not all of which are associated with infection. The condition is rare following surgery, particularly because suprapubic prostatectomy is uncommonly performed. Patients undergoing urological or gynecological surgery are most at risk. Some cases follow vaginal parturition with or without surgical intervention. In such patients, a putative portal of entry is apparent. The fact that gram-negative organisms predominate in the postoperative group (51) lends strength to the local source of organisms near the pubis. Hematogenous osteomyelitis in the pubis does occur, often detected by radionuclide scanning for undiagnosed pain in the groin.

Another population of patients, with similar symptoms but without signs of infection, also develop radiological changes in bone. These changes sometimes appear without any clinical symptoms or signs, particularly in professional football players (52). However, symphyseal pain in athletes is common, suggesting that repeated minor or even greater activity-related trauma may produce clinical features and radiological signs identical with infective osteitis pubis.

Clinical features include pubic region pain radiating to the adductor region of one or both thighs, exacerbated by exercise and relieved by rest. If severe, the person may be unable to walk or have a characteristic waddling gait. Sneezing, coughing, micturition, and defecation may exacerbate the pain; tenderness over one or both pubic bones (which are quite easily accessible to the examining finger), symphyseal pain on pelvic compression, and symphyseal clicking also occur.

Plain radiological appearances (53,54) usually do not appear for approximately one week after an initiating cause can be identified, which is similar to acute osteomyelitis in any site. It is not possible to say how long it takes for radiological changes to become obvious after noninfective causes. There may be patchy osteoporosis of peri-symphyseal bone (see Figure 10-2); patchy periosteal reaction; reactive sclerosis, mainly subchondral with irregularity and usually widening of the symphysis (Figure 16-3); and instability indicated on stress films (52). The lesions may arrest naturally or as a result of treatment in three ways: resolution, persistence of sclerosis and symphyseal irregularity, or fusion.

Noninfective osteitis pubis is usually a self-limiting condition that resolves over a period of months or years. In contrast, the clinical course of osteomyelitis is progressive, with increasing bone destruction and widening of the symphysis seen on radiographs (55). A rational approach to management is to distinguish the infective cases from those more likely to have a mechanical cause for symptoms. The first group should be treated for acute osteomyelitis, whereas the others should be managed expectantly with analgesic medication and restriction of activity. This approach can sometimes cause clinical concern if the awareness of such entities is unknown. Post-traumatic osteolysis of the pubic bone can simulate a malignant lesion (56), particularly if a history of trauma (often weeks or even months previously) is not elicited by the physician. The term *pubic osteolysis* has been placed on yet another condition with similar symptoms and signs, but in which the radiological features are those of bone destruc-

A B

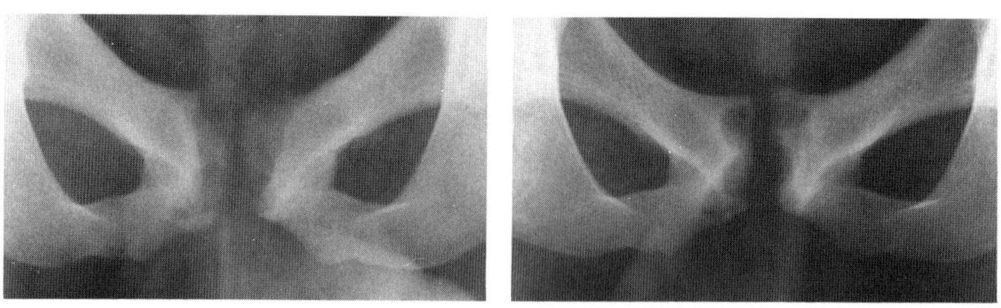

Figure 16-3. *(A) A well-established case of osteitis pubis (due to* Escherichia coli*). Note the loss of a considerable amount of bone on each side of the pubic symphysis and the adjacent osteopenia. (B) When the infection is controlled (by antibiotics or surgery on some occasions), some bone repair occurs; the margins of the infected area have increased density due to bone production, but the irregular margins of bone adjacent to the symphysis persist.*

tion in the pubis, with maintenance of the normal configuration of the pubic symphysis (57). This condition is also self-limiting and does not require antibiotic treatment or surgical debridement.

References

1. Kozlowski K, Masel J, Harbison S, Yu J. Multifocal chronic osteomyelitis of unknown etiology. Pediatr Radiol 1983;13:130–136.
2. Cole WG. The management of chronic osteomyelitis. Clin Orthop 1991; 264:84–89.
3. Bjorksten B, Boquist L. Histopathological aspects of chronic recurrent multifocal osteomyelitis. J Bone Joint Surg [Br] 1980;62:376–380.
4. Cyrlak D, Pais MJ. Chronic recurrent multifocal osteomyelitis. Skeletal Radiol (Berlin) 1986;15:32–39.
5. Gamble JG, Rinsky LA. Chronic recurrent multifocal osteomyelitis: a distinct clinical entity. J Pediatr Orthop 1986;6:579–584.
6. Pelkonen P, Ryoppy S, Jaaskaleinen J, Rapola J, Repo H, Kaitila I. Chronic osteomyelitis-like disease with negative bacterial cultures. Am J Dis Child 1988;142:1167–1173.
7. Chigira M, Maehara S, Nagase M, Ogimi T, Udagawa E. Sternocostoclavicular hyperostosis. A report of nineteen cases with special reference to etiology and treatment. J Bone Joint Surg [Am] 1986;68:103–112.
8. Kozlowski K, Anderson R, Tink A. Multifocal recurrent periostitis. Forschr Rontgenstr 1981;135:597–602.
9. Kozlowski K, Hochberger O. Rare forms of chronic osteomyelitis (multifocal recurrent periostitis and chronic symmetric osteomyelitis—report of 3 cases). Aust Radiol 1984;28:152–155.
10. Giedion A, Holthusen W, Masel LF, Vischer D. Subacute and chronic "symmetrical" osteomyelitis. Ann Radiol 1972;15:329–342.
11. Probst FP, Bjorksten B, Gustavson K-H. Radiological aspect of chronic recurrent multifocal osteomyelitis. Ann Radiol 1978;21:115–125.
12. Rahav G, Sacks TG, Bar-Zvi J. Chronic recurrent multifocal osteomyelitis: report of a case. Clin Infect Dis 1992;14:587–588.
13. Willert H-G, Enderle A. Multifocale symmetrische chronische osteomyelitis. Arch Orthop Unfall-Chir 1977;89:109–113.
14. Meller Y, Yagupsky P, Elitsur Y, Inbar-Ianay I, Bar-Zvi J. Chronic multifocal symmetrical osteomyelitis. Am J Dis Child 1984;138:349–351.
15. Murray SD, Kehl DK. Chronic recurrent multifocal osteomyelitis. J Bone Joint Surg [Am] 1984;66:1110–1112.
16. Wiener MD, Newbold RG, Merten DF. Chronic recurrent multifocal osteomyelitis. Am J Radiol 1986;146:87–88.
17. Gustavson K-H, Wilbrand HF. Chronic symmetric osteomyelitis. Acta Radiol (Diagn) (Stockh) 1974;15:551–557.

18. Kornreich HK, Bernstein BH, King KK, et al. The rheumatic presentation of osteomyelitis. Arthritis Rheum 1979;22:631.
19. Girardet J-P, Sambucy F, Douillet P, Faure C, Fontaine J-L, Laplane R. Osteomyelite symetrique subaigue. Arch Fr Pediatr 1979;36:418–422.
20. Solheim LF, Paus B, Liverud K, Stoen B. Chronic recurrent multifocal osteomyelitis—a new clinical-radiological syndrome. Acta Orthop Scand 1980;51:37–41.
21. Case 28-1986, Case records of the Massachusetts General Hospital. N Engl J Med 1986;315:178–185.
22. King SM, Laxer RM, Manson D, Gold R. Chronic recurrent multifocal osteomyelitis. A non-infectious inflammatory process. Pediatr Infect Dis 1987;6:907–914.
23. Benhamou CL, Chamot AM, Kahn MF. Synovitis-acne-pustulosis-hyperostosis-osteomyelitis syndrome (SAPHO). A new syndrome among the spondyloarthropathies? Clin Exp Rheumatol 1988;6:109–112.
24. Huaux J-P, Esselinckx W, Rombouts J-J, et al. Pustulotic arthroosteitis and chronic recurrent multifocal osteomyelitis in children. Report of three cases. J Rheumatol 1988;15:95–100.
25. Paller AS, Pachman L, Rich K, Esterly NB, Gonzalez-Crussi F. Pustulosis palmaris et plantaris: its association with chronic recurrent multifocal osteomyelitis. J Am Acad Dermatol 1985;12:927–930.
26. Bergdahl K, Bjorksten B, Gustavson K-H, Liden S, Probst F. Pustulosis palmoplantaris and its relation to chronic recurrent multifocal osteomyelitis. Dermatologica 1979;159:37–45.
27. Kawai K, Doita M, Tateishi H, Hirohata K. Bone and joint lesions associated with pustulosis palmaris et plantaris. A clinical and histological study. J Bone Joint Surg [Br] 1988;70:117–122.
28. Bjorksten B, Gustavson K-H, Eriksson B, Lindholm A, Nordstrom S. Chronic recurrent multifocal osteomyelitis and pustulosis palmoplantaris. J Pediatr 1978;93:227–231.
29. Bookbinder SA, Fenkse NA, Clement GB, Espinoza LR, Germain BF, Vasey FB. Clavicular hyperostosis and acne arthritis. Ann Intern Med 1982;97: 615–616.
30. Kahn MF. Letter to Editor. J Bone Joint Surg [Am] 1990;72:305–306.
31. Speer DP. Chronic multifocal symmetrical osteomyelitis. Am J Dis Child 1986;138:340.
32. Hummell DS, Anderson SJ, Wright PF, Cassell GH, Waites KB. Chronic recurrent multifocal osteomyelitis: are mycoplasmas involved? N Engl J Med 1987;317:510–511.
33. Edlund E, Johnsson U, Lidgren L, et al. Palmo-plantar pustulosis and sternocostoclavicular arthro-osteitis. Ann Rheumatol Dis 1988;47:809–815.
34. Ryden C, Yacoub A, Hirsch G, Wendel M, Oldberg A, Ljungh A. Binding of bone sialoprotein to Staphylococcus epidermidis isolated from a patient with chronic recurrent multifocal osteomyelitis. J Infect Dis 1990;161: 814–815.

35. Laxer RM, Shore AD, Manson D, King S, Silverman ED, Wilmot DM. Chronic recurrent multifocal osteomyelitis and psoriasis—a report of a new association and review of related disorders. Semin Arthritis Rheum 1988; 17:260–270.
36. Chamot AM, Benhamou CL, Kahn MF, Beraneck L, Kaplan G, Prost A. Le syndrome acne pustulose hyperostose osteite (SAPHO). Resultats d'une enquete nationale. Rev Rheumatol 1987;54:187–196.
37. Yu L, Kasser JR, O'Rourke E, Kozakewich H. Chronic recurrent multifocal osteomyelitis. J Bone Joint Surg [Am] 1989;71:105–112.
38. Mortensson W, Edeburn G, Fries M, Nilsson R. Chronic recurrent multifocal osteomyelitis in children. Acta Radiol 1988;29:565–570.
39. Exner GU. Plasmacellular osteomyelitis in children, clinical and radiological features. Follow up. Z Kinderchir 1980;31:262–275.
40. Jurik AG, Helmig O, Ternowitz T, Moller BN. Chronic recurrent multifocal osteomyelitis. A follow-up study. J Pediatr Orthop 1988;8:49–58.
41. Garre G. Uber besondere Formen und Folgezustande der akuten infectiosen Osteomyelitis. Bruns Beitr Klin Chir 1893;10:241–257.
42. Kohler H, Uehlinger E, Kutzner J, West TB. Sternocostoclavicular hyperostosis: painful swelling of the sternum, clavicles, and upper ribs. Ann Intern Med 1977;87:192–194.
43. Wetzel R, Gondolph-Zink B, Puhl W. Pustular osteoarthropathy and its differential diagnosis. Int Orthop 1991;15:101–104.
44. Brower AC, Sweet DE, Keats TE. Condensing osteitis of the clavicle: a new entity. Am J Roentgen Radium Ther Nucl Med 1974;121:17–21.
45. Keipert JA, Campbell PE. Recurrent hyperostosis of the clavicles: an undiagnosed syndrome. Aust Pediatr J 1970;6:97–104.
46. Lichtenstein L. Histiocytosis X: integration of eosinophilic granuloma of bone, "Letterer-Siwe disease", and "Schuller-Christian disease" as related manifestations of a single nosological entity. Arch Pathol 1953;56:84–102.
47. Lichtenstein L. Diseases of bone and joints, ed 2. St. Louis: CV Mosby, 1975:196–203.
48. Bell RS, Mankin HJ, Doppelt SH. Osteomyelitis in Gaucher disease. J Bone Joint Surg [Am] 1986;68:1380–1388.
49. Sziklas JJ, Negrin JA, Rosshirt W, Rosenberg RJ, Spencer RP. Diagnosing osteomyelitis in Gaucher's disease. Clin Nucl Med 1991;16:487–489.
50. Beer E. Periostitis of symphysis and descending rami of pubes following suprapubic operations. Int J Med Surg 1924;37:224–225.
51. Bouza E, Winston DW, Hewitt WL. Infectious osteitis pubis. Urology 1978;12:663–669.
52. Harris NH, Murray RO. Lesions of the pubic symphysis in athletes. Br Med J 1974;4:211–214.
53. Alperin LJ, Bender MJ. Osteitis pubis. Am J Dis Child 1954;88:227–233.
54. Klinefelter EW. Osteitis pubis: review of literature and a report of a case. Am J Roentgenol 1950;63:368–371.
55. Rosenthal RE, Spickard WA, Markham RD, Rhamy RK. Osteomyelitis of

the symphysis pubis: a separate disease from osteitis pubis. J Bone Joint Surg [Am] 1982;64:123–128.
56. Hall FM, Goldberg RP, Kasdon EJ, Glick H. Post-traumatic osteolysis of the pubic bone simulating a malignant lesion. J Bone Joint Surg [Am] 1984;66:121–126.
57. McGuigan LE, Edmonds JP, Painter DM. Pubic osteolysis. J Bone Joint Surg [Am] 1984;66:127–129.

CHAPTER 17

Infection in Total Joint Replacement

Although many infections following total joint replacement are clearly blood-borne from distant sources, it is likely that the majority are a consequence of introduction, at operation, of organisms from room air (mainly shed from the skin of the operating team) or from the recipient's own skin. Strenuous attempts to reduce this risk by strict aseptic discipline, use of prophylactic antibiotics, and provision in the wound environment of ultraclean air and laminar airflow patterns have reduced reported infection rates over the last two decades. The combination of these precautions—and more recently, introduction, for reasons of personal protection as well as infection control, of exhaust ventilated suits—has made it possible to attain infection rates well under 1% in cemented and uncemented arthroplasty.

Progress has also been made in the management of infected joint prostheses, although major problems remain to be solved. Established infection was initially an absolute indication for permanent removal of all foreign material and conversion to excision arthroplasty or arthrodesis. Increasingly encouraging results of one- or two-stage exchange arthroplasty for established infection have since been reported. Joint replacement is now a very common operation; it is estimated that between one quarter and half a million procedures are performed each year worldwide. An infection rate of 0.5%, if universally attained, would still be followed by 1,250 to 2,500 new infections each year. Rigorous infection control remains the key to containing the problem.

Nomenclature

Early discussions of infection in joint replacement lacked a consistent nomenclature. Uniform definition of variables and outcome measures has not yet been achieved, although progress has been made. Until recently, survivorship analysis was rarely used to present the outcome of joint replacement; its use gives a clearer picture of the pattern of infections over time (1,2). A distinction has been made, on the basis of outcome, between infection with a significant cellulitic component precluding debridement, and infection in which the drainage of an infected hematoma predominates (3). In practice, cellulitis and a draining hematoma may coexist. In the early postsurgical period, surgeons like to distinguish between superficial (i.e., apparently confined to skin or superficial fascia) and deep infection; this distinction has also been associated with outcome (4). However, it is not always possible to be confident that the infection has been confined, or that it will remain so.

The classification of infection after joint replacement proposed by the Mayo Clinic group (5) has been widely used. Stage 1 infections are those that occur in the first 3 months after surgery. Stage 2 infections occur between 3 months and 2 years after surgery; the great majority occur within one year and must be considered to have been derived at surgery. Late infections (Stage 3) occur after 2 years. The proportion of infections that are hematogenous in origin increases with the duration of follow-up (6).

Epidemiology

Infecting Organisms

Extensive experience with replacement arthroplasty and its outcomes has been published from a number of specialist clinics (3,7,8). These data indicate that in joints becoming infected, gram-positive organisms, particularly staphylococcal species, are the most common isolates; *S. epidermidis* predominates in some, *S. aureus* in others. In early infection acquired from the urinary tract, gram-negative enteric species may be isolated. These patterns have implications for prophylaxis. In 70% to 80% of patients, a single pathogen only can be identified; the remaining cases are approximately equally divided between mixed and sterile cultures (9).

Reported infection rates vary between centers. Variation in the employment of rigorous prophylactic measures, as a result of surgical or bureaucratic indifference, may have a part (10). For individual surgeons, the difference between a low and a very low infection rate may be hard to identify unless special efforts are made (11). However, differences between, and sampling variability within, populations presenting for surgery are probably also important. Declining rates of infection in consecutive cohorts of arthroplasty recipients have been reported (1,2). Overall, reported deep infection rates, although mostly less than 2.5%, continue to range over an order of magnitude below that level (Figure 17-1). There can be little doubt that both surveillance and reporting bias occur and that rates are higher in some centers.

Sources of Infection

It is now widely accepted that a main source of infection after joint replacement is wound contamination by bacteria derived from operating room air (mainly through dispersal of desquamated skin from the surgical team) and from the patient's own skin (12–15). Therefore, strategies to reduce the number of contaminated particles are an important component of prophylactic efforts.

Hematogenous infection of implants also occurs, and a number of

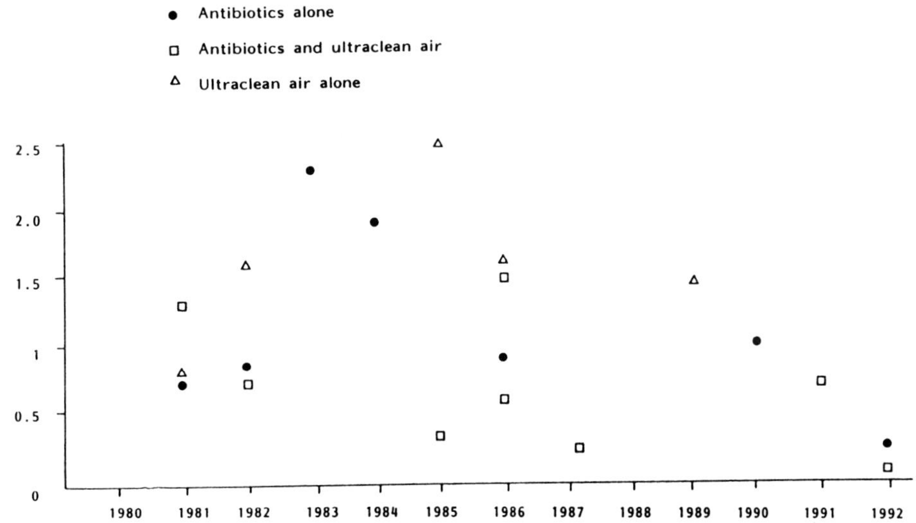

Figure 17-1. *Deep infection rates in cohorts of total hip arthroplasty (n ≥ 300) 1980 to 1992.*

collected series have been published (6,16,17). Some early and intermediate infections may be nosocomially acquired from vascular access sites (18), which are certainly a major cause of bacteremia, now increasingly important, with *S. epidermidis* species (19). Other well-documented sources of hematogenous spread include abscesses in various sites; skin ulcers of varying etiology; and chest, wound, and urinary tract infections. As the incidence of operatively acquired infections decreases, the proportion of infections from hematogenous seeding increases. In patients with multiple joint replacements, hematogenous infection of one joint is associated with an 18% risk of a subsequent infection in another (20). The affinity of *S. aureus* for the musculoskeletal system is emphasized by its dominance in hematogenous infection, despite the wide range of possible sources. Experimental studies (17,21) suggest that infection of a joint implant from bacteremia is most easily achieved in the early postoperative period. Thus, whenever a significant risk of hematogenous spread of pathogens exists, appropriate antibiotic prophylaxis is indicated.

Prophylaxis Against Prosthetic Infection

An infected joint implant is a personal tragedy for the afflicted individual. For the health care system, costs (estimated at four to six times that of a successful primary intervention [22,23]) justify substantial expenditure on prophylaxis. Approaches to reducing infection rates include careful host assessment and modification; use of vaccination, antiseptics, and aseptic discipline; augmentation of host defenses with antibiotic prophylaxis (either local or systemic); sterilization of air particles by ultraviolet light; and reduction of particle content of the operating room air.

Host Assessment and Optimization

Considerable energy has been directed toward understanding the effects of implant materials on host defenses (24–26). Host factors that alter the effectiveness of the immune response or that increase the probability of persistent but dormant bacterial colonies in bone or periarticular tissues have been reported as risk factors for the development of infection after joint replacement. These factors include previous local surgery (2,27,28), previous sepsis (2,27,29), remote infection at the time of surgery (30), diabetes mellitus (31), sickle-cell disease (32), and, possibly, rheumatoid arthritis (33,34). However, previous sepsis need not preclude successful joint arthroplasty (35,36).

Systemic factors that may influence the host's ability to mount an adequate response to infection and surgery should be identified and modified if possible. The program could include patient education, cessation of smoking, and relevant adjustment of medication. If immunosuppressive drugs can be temporarily discontinued, infection rates in susceptible patients (37) may be reduced. Stabilization of diabetes may be particularly helpful in prosthetic surgery. Assessment of glycosylated hemoglobin has been recommended for diabetics in whom penile prosthetic surgery is planned (38) because it appears to predict high risk of infection. Relevance of this observation to joint replacement has not been reported. Dental and periodontal sepsis should be excluded (39). Anergic cellular immune responses have been associated with significantly increased infection rates in hip replacement surgery (40). Whether this finding reflects specific abnormalities of T-cell function or simply a poor nutritional state is unresolved. Nutritional deficiency is quite common in older patients. Considerable work needs to be done to establish conclusively the appropriate indicators of clinically significant malnutrition and the effect of nutritional supplementation on a range of postsurgical outcomes, including infection. Emerging information, however, points to an association between nutritional status and wound outcomes in joint replacement. Lymphocyte counts of less than 1,500 cells/mm^3 and albumin levels of less than 3.5 g/dL are associated with greater frequency of wound complications (41).

Vaccination

Vaccination against *S. aureus* infection was under active investigation in the decade prior to the introduction of antibiotics, the success of which halted most research into staphylococcal vaccines until recently. Two reports, neither from controlled studies, indicate that the introduction of preoperative vaccination has been associated with a subsequent reduction in infection rates after joint replacement (42,43). In principle, augmentation of host defenses this way might be useful for some joint replacement recipients, but controlled studies of modern vaccines are required.

Preparation of the Skin

Routine preoperative skin disinfection over a period of 12 to 24 hours has long been practiced in many orthopedic units. It is effective in reducing contamination of the superficial layers of the skin, but has little effect on the deeper layers, thus allowing recontamination to occur quite rapidly (44). In one study, skin contamination of the wound was reduced from 15% to 1.6% following use of an iodophor-impregnated adhesive drape (45). The value of conventional nonimpregnated adhesive drapes during surgery, although they are widely used, is in doubt: Their use is associated with greater numbers of surface organisms during surgery (46), they have no confirmed impact on infection rates, and use contributes to operating room and disposal costs (47).

Operating Room Discipline

Discipline in the operating room is fundamentally important to reduce infection rates in prosthetic surgery. Aseptic techniques should be of the highest standards. The importance of shedding of potential pathogens by members of the surgical team and others in the operating room has been clearly established (48). A strong correlation exists between the number of colony forming units (CFUs) and the number of individuals entering and leaving the operating room. Strategies to improve operating room discipline have demonstrated effectiveness (49).

During long procedures, consideration should be given to changing frequently handled items to avoid the possibility of introduction of contamination. Surgical suction apparatus may also concentrate organisms from the air at its tip (50).

Antibiotic Prophylaxis

As early experience with total joint replacement began to indicate an unacceptably high infection rate, many surgeons introduced antibiotic prophylaxis (51,52), for which principles had been established in the early 1960s (53). A number of controlled clinical studies of varying size and quality (11,54–57) testify to the effectiveness of antibiotic prophylaxis, both alone and in combination with other techniques, in reducing the incidence of infection after joint replacement. Some issues, however, remain unresolved.

Choice of Antibiotic

The agent chosen should be effective against the expected pathogens, have a pharmacodynamic profile that will ensure adequate antimicrobial activity at the site of surgery throughout the procedure, have minimum toxicity or allergenicity, and carry a low risk of inducing resistant bacterial strains.

Many surgeons select narrow-spectrum agents effective mainly against staphylococcal species, which is a rational policy in view of the profile of infecting organisms. Penicillins were used initially; use of cephalosporins is now widespread. Increasingly, *S. epidermidis* species are resistant to penicillins and to some cephalosporins, and a regular review of sensitivity patterns must guide prophylactic choice. Also, a significant percentage of gram-negative infections have been reported (14,58). Most early gram-negative infections are derived from the urinary tract; therefore, the choice of prophylaxis in patients with a history of recurrent urinary infection should ensure appropriate protection.

Considerable confusion has been generated by reports of widely differing abilities of antibiotic agents to penetrate bone. These differences appear to reflect methodological variations: In practice, what matters is the concentration in the bone extracellular space at the interface with the prosthesis, which is directly proportional to the blood level (59). Regional perfusion below a tourniquet can provide very high local tissue antibiotic levels (60), but infection rates following use of this technique have not been reported.

Route of Antibiotic Administration

Alternatives to systemic antibiotic administration have been explored. Buchholz introduced the use of antibiotic-impregnated polymethylmethacrylate (AIPMMA) in 1969. The topic has been reviewed (61,62), and many experimental studies have been published (63–65). Pharmacodynamic studies indicate that elution of antibiotic from the bone cement provides bactericidal concentrations in wound exudate and at the prosthesis-bone interface over a period of weeks to months, with serum concentrations below 3 μg/mL with the quantities of cement normally used (65). Levels found after use of low-viscosity cement are somewhat higher, presumably as a consequence of a larger surface area in the cured cement mantle (66).

Experimental and clinical studies indicate that use of antibiotic-impregnated cement alone is effective in the prophylaxis of deep infection after joint replacement (61,67,68). In one study (68), which found AIPMMA to be more effective than systemic therapy in prophylaxis against deep infection, the infection rate in the systemic group was high by contemporary standards. A recent, small study found no significant difference in efficacy (67). The value of using both techniques over either alone has not yet been established.

Pulsed irrigation with saline is frequently used to effect mechanical rinsing of bone surfaces during joint replacement surgery. This technique may reduce antibiotic concentration in the periprosthetic zone at implantation, particularly if a tourniquet is in use (69). Many surgeons have used intraoperative irrigation with antibiotic solution. Experimental studies suggest that this approach may be valuable in heavily contaminated wounds (70). Contamination of clean operative wounds increases with duration of the procedure (71). We have been able to find only three comparative clinical studies addressing the use of antibiotic irrigation (72–74), but their methodology was inadequate for any conclusions to be drawn.

Timing and Duration of Antibiotic Prophylaxis

Although wound sampling studies indicate that the rate of contamination of a surgical wound increases toward the end of the procedure (71), a potential risk exists from the time of skin incision. Antibiotics should be administered to achieve levels above the expected minimum inhibitory concentration (MIC) for likely pathogens throughout the operation. After intravenous injection, adequate levels in the extracellular space are attained within 10 minutes (75). Pneumatic tourniquet application should be delayed to allow this equilibration to occur. Administration of a second dose of antibiotic at tourniquet release increases three-fold the concentration of antibiotic in the tissue fluid bathing a recently implanted total knee replacement (76).

Short prophylactic programs of 24 hours' duration or less appear as effective as longer programs, and have obvious advantages with regard to cost and risk of complication (54). Single-dose prophylaxis is an attractive concept. One recent study of prophylaxis in a range of implant operations found one dose less effective than five (77). Bactericidal levels of antibiotic may not have been present throughout surgery in every patient (78). Other studies (79,80) showed no difference but lacked power to confirm that single-dose intraoperative prophylaxis is as effective as a three-dose regimen. Single-dose prophylaxis therefore cannot yet be recommended.

Some surgeons believe that antibiotic prophylaxis should be continued until suction drains are removed. Colonization of drains by skin organisms can occur (81), but overt infection develops in only 10% of patients with positive drain tip culture. Further studies to address the role of drains and vascular catheter access sites in postoperative bacteremia after joint replacement are required.

Risk of Antibiotic Prophylaxis

The emergence of resistant strains is a well-established complication of the widespread use of antibiotic prophylaxis (82). Other risks are more immediate. Administration of a single dose of a semisynthetic penicillin has been estimated to carry a 0.04% risk of anaphylaxis, a 5% risk of skin sensitivity (83), and a 0.01% risk of initiating *Clostridium difficile* enteritis (84). Cephalosporins are estimated to carry a risk of pseudomembranous colitis 40 times that of penicillins (84).

Sterilization of Operating Room Environment

Use of ultraviolet chemotherapy (UVC) at 254 nm to sterilize the air in operating rooms has been described for several decades (85,86). Despite low potential risk to properly protected staff and strong evidence of efficacy in clean orthopedic surgery, its use has not become widespread. Attention has recently focussed instead on ultraclean air provision. Recently, an extensive reinvestigation of UVC was described (87): Contamination of the surgical environment compared favorably with that achieved in an ultraclean air enclosure. This appears to be an extremely cost-effective option (88).

Reduction of Air Particle Numbers in the Operating Environment

Reduction of air particle numbers in the operating environment may be achieved by the combination of modern ventilation approaches with ultrafiltration, directional air flow, and reduction of shedding by the operating team, using impermeable clothing or suit ventilation. Conventional positive pressure turbulent ventilation operating theaters contain up to 10^4 CFUs/m^3 (11). For prosthetic surgery, standards for operating room air handling, which aim for particle counts

Table 17-1. Air Conditions and Antibiotic Use in Joint Arthroplasty*

Conditions	No Studies	No. Patients	Deep Infection Rate	95% Confidence Interval
Ultraclean air/no antibiotic	8	2,986	0.0154	0.0110–0.0198
Ultraclean air/antibiotic	8	4,233	0.0066	0.0042–0.0091
Routine air/no antibiotic	15	5,896	0.0461	0.0409–0.0514
Routine air/systemic antibiotics	17	7,064	0.0137	0.0110–0.0164

*This interim analysis excludes data from the randomized trials (11,90) shown in Figure 17-2. It shows pooled data from cohort studies of outcome of joint arthroplasty published between 1972 and 1989.

of less than five CFU/m^3, have been determined (89). These standards specify rates of air change and filtration efficiency. The ability of laminar airflow systems derived for industrial use to lower particle numbers even further has encouraged their introduction into prosthetic surgical practice (33). They are expensive and have been aggressively marketed.

Are these measures reflected in a lowering of infection rates? Charnley (12), the dominant figure in the introduction of joint replacement, strongly supported their use. Other early investigations were less convincing (13). The controversy led to the mounting of a large multicenter study (11) in Europe, which offered strong support for a direct association between the number of contaminated particles in the air and subsequent proven prosthetic infections. As a consequence, many ultraclean air systems have been installed. The European study has been the subject of some criticism over its methodology, because antibiotic prophylaxis was not randomized (those who received it did so either because they were considered to be at high risk or because of policy in some participating centers). Further analysis indicated that the effects of ultraclean air and antibiotics appeared distinct and additive. It is hard to conceive of a systematic bias that would account for the strength of the protective effect of clean air in these patients, and, until recently, this study provided the best evidence of the utility of ultraclean air laminar flow systems. Provisional data from a randomized study of a horizontal laminar flow system in joint replacement recipients, all of whom received antibiotics, have been published (90). Data indicate only a small additional protective effect from ultraclean air. Figure 17-1 plots the deep infection rates using different prophylactic strategies reported in follow-up studies of total joint replacement recipients over the period 1980 to 1992. Table 17-1 shows rates and 95% confidence limits from pooled data. Figure 17-2 shows the relative risks and 95% confidence limits derived from the two randomized clinical trials. Typically, the effect in well-executed randomized studies appears smaller than in cohort studies. In summary, it appears that ultraclean air systems do offer protection against infection in total joint replacement, but that the benefit is probably small when antibiotic prophylaxis is also used.

Prophylaxis Against Hematogenous Infection

It is conclusively established that hematogenous infection of an implant can occur from remote intercurrent bacterial infection (16) or after genitourinary (57) and gastrointestinal (91) endoscopic surgery.

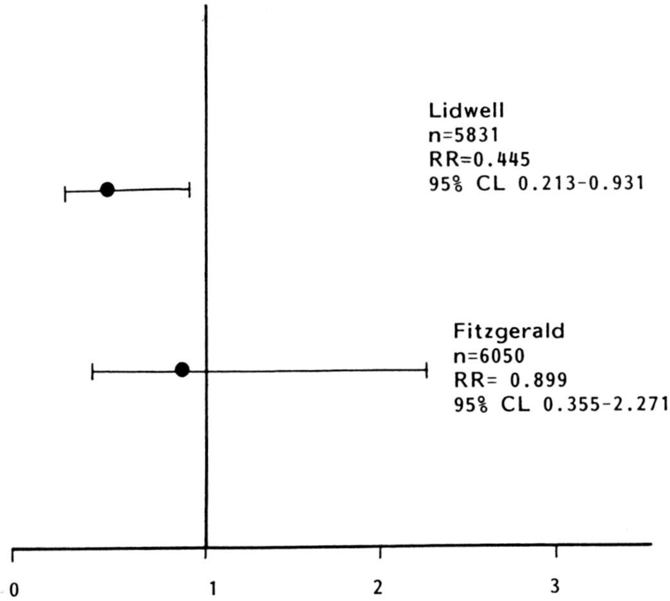

Figure 17-2. *Randomized trials of ultraclear air environment in total joint replacement with antibiotic prophylaxis (relative risk ± 95% confidence interval).*

Immunosuppressed patients and individuals with polyarthritis may be particularly at risk. More than half these infections occur more than 2 years after implantation (1,2), but the perioperative period also carries risks. Many units supply patients undergoing total joint replacement with a card advising prompt antibiotic treatment of intercurrent infection.

Urinary Tract Sepsis and Total Joint Replacement

Cases have been described in which arthroplasty was clearly infected from the urine (57,92). Bacteriuria has been reported in up to 28% of women and 8% of men presenting for total joint replacement (93,94). Tha majority of these infections are asymptomatic. Bacteriuria should be identified and eradicated prior to surgery, preferably during a presurgical evaluation performed days before the scheduled admission, to allow treatment. A single-dose regimen will usually sterilize the urine unless an anatomical abnormality or a long-standing pathology of the genitourinary tract is present. If—for example, in the management of intracapsular fracture of the hip—surgery cannot be delayed, antibiotic prophylaxis should include an agent effective against the organisms in the urine (almost always gram-negative enteric bacteria).

Despite preoperative management of bacteriuria, urinary tract infections will develop in a proportion of treated patients postoperatively, but the bacteria involved may be different (95). Although those with urinary tract infections have been reported to have a higher incidence of postoperative infection of total joint replacement, the correlation between the organisms infecting the urine and the joint is poor (92).

The incidence of bacteriuria increases with the duration of indwelling catheterization (96). In experimental models, a recently implanted artificial joint is susceptible to hematogenous infection (17). Many orthopedic surgeons therefore prefer postoperative intermittent catheterization, if required, to routine perioperative catheterization. Some use suprapubic drainage if required. An alternative has been to catheterize routinely for 24 hours to minimize the risk of bladder distension with subsequent urinary tract dysfunction and infection (95). Advocates of routine catheterization point out that up to half of all total hip replacement recipients require catheterization for urinary obstruction in the early postoperative period. Decision analysis based on plausible assumptions and published incidence data, however, supports a policy of catheterizing only those individuals who become overtly obstructed following total hip replacement (97). In a recent study, catheterization for 48 hours, when compared with intermittent catheterization as required, resulted in fewer late episodes of retention in women, but not in men, and infection rates were not significantly different (98). In a randomized study in elderly hip fracture patients, however, normal voiding returned more quickly after intermittent catheterization begun at the onset of retention (99). Overall infection rates were not significantly different. Provided that good technique is employed and indwelling catheterization longer than 24 to 48 hours is avoided, either protocol appears acceptable. Administration of the alpha-blocker, prazosin, may reduce the risk of postoperative retention in patients undergoing total hip replacement (100).

Prophylaxis for Dental Work

It has been recommended that all joint replacement patients undergoing dental work should have prophylactic antibiotics (101). We and others have argued (97,102,103), using available data and reasonable assumptions, that this approach may be unnecessary and may be associated with an unacceptable level of antibiotic-induced adverse effects if penicillins are used. Modeling indicates cost-effectiveness of administration of erythromycin (104) or cephalexin (105) for higher risk patients. Unfortunately, there is a paucity of data to confirm these predictions. In the presence of overt or imminent dental sepsis, however, or in immune-compromised patients, prohylaxis is strongly recommended against the probable or proven oral pathogen.

Infection Surveillance for Joint Replacement

Because the incidence of hematogenous infection of prosthetic joints increases with time after implantation, a complete surveillance program would require some form of lifetime follow-up. In practice, this follow-up is difficult, expensive, and subject to ascertainment bias. As a measure of the performance of a hospital or surgical team, acquisition of data on Stage 1 and 2 infections is relevant and more readily achieved. It requires careful planning (106) and a commitment on the part of the individual surgeon or clinic to evaluate all prosthetic joint patients at 2 years. Within each institution, all early infections and therapeutic responses should be recorded. Apparent "superficial" infections require particularly careful long-term follow-up. Patients undergoing prosthetic implantation should be categorized according to infection risk, and risk minimization policies should be reviewed annually in light of these data. Antimicrobial sensitivity patterns should also be scrutinized regularly to allow updating of prophylactic regimens.

Although impractical for all units, some long-term studies need to be mounted to establish more accurately the real risks of hematogenous infection and to reduce reliance on modeling in decision-making.

Diagnosis of Infected Joint Replacement

In overt infection, a confident clinical diagnosis can be readily made at any stage. Most Stage 1 infections are in this category, but some doubt may exist. Among hematological investigations, C-reactive protein appears to have a higher predictive value than the erythrocyte sedimentation rate (ESR) or the white blood cell count (107,108). Ultrasound may demonstrate the location of an infected hematoma or abscess (109) and guide diagnostic aspiration. We believe that scintigraphy currently has no important role in this clinical context.

Low-grade chronic infection may present as pain only and be difficult to distinguish from aseptic loosening. The need to do so prior to revision surgery depends on whether uninfected and infected loose implants are managed differently. Policies involving one-stage exchange may require a less exhaustive evaluation because no important decisions depend critically on preoperative confirmation of infection.

If two-stage exchange arthroplasty is contemplated, evaluation protocols involving history, physical examination, hematological screening, imaging, and aspiration (110) are widely used. Ultimately, identification of an organism or a biopsy confirming chronic infection is required for diagnosis. An ESR persistently increased to more than 30 to 35 mm/hr or C-reactive protein levels more than 20 mg/L are suggestive of infection (111–113).

In established infection, radiological changes are often difficult to distinguish from those of aseptic loosening. Appearances characteristic of active infection include change from the previous examination and periosteal new bone formation. Scalloped cortical erosions are indicative of infection but may also be associated with accumulation of sterile polyethylene or methylmethacrylate debris.

As an aid to clinical decision-making in the context of painful, loose, possibly infected joint prostheses, scintigraphic techniques are widely used but have proved somewhat disappointing. Reports in the imaging literature claim a broad range of sensitivity and specificity values for both ^{99m}Tc bone scanning and techniques that localize concentrations of inflammatory cells around the implant. Cell concentration and metabolic activity are continuous variables, the interpretation of which is subject to bias. Claims of test efficacy are also affected by the case mix of the patients presented for evaluation. Thus, any sensitivity/specificity pair contains an arbitrary element that introduces uncertainty into interpretation of the available literature.

In summary (114), ^{99m}Tc bone scanning alone cannot usefully distinguish septic and aseptic painful loose prostheses. ^{99m}Tc/^{67}gallium scanning has a high reported specificity, indicating that its positive results correlate well with confirmation of infection at aspiration or biopsy, but it has a low sensitivity. Thus, it cannot rule out those without the disease, which leaves physicians no closer to arriving at a management decision. ^{111}Indium-labeled leukocyte scans appear to have better sensitivity but poorer specificity than ^{99m}Tc/^{67}gallium studies (115). Newer techniques, which include scanning with leukocyte monoclonal antibodies (116), ^{111}indium immunoglobulin labeling (117), and ^{99m}Tc leukocyte labeling (118), await more evaluation.

Microbiological Diagnosis

Superficial sinus cultures are poor predictors of the active organism (119) and generally overstate the incidence of polymicrobial infections. Aspiration of a putatively infected joint, for which ultrasonography may aid needle placement (120), should be performed. Again, a wide range of sensitivity and specificity values has been reported for this investigation (114,121,122). Definitive isolation of a microorganism can be achieved from deep-tissue specimens obtained at surgery in more than 80% of patients. Histopathological analysis of frozen sections from the prosthetic interface at surgery may confirm the presence of acute inflammation, even if cultures are negative (123). Because anaerobic organisms may be implicated in approximately 10% of patients, specimens should be handled with that possibility in mind. Outcome studies indicate that the infecting organism may be an important predictor of the result.

Management of Infected Joint Arthroplasty

An algorithm for the management of infected joint arthroplasty is shown (Figure 17-3). Experience indicates that a useful distinction may be made between acute postsurgical infection of a joint replacement and established chronic infection. Briefly, the results of aggressive soft-tissue debridement with antibiotic therapy in early postsurgical infections in both hip (3) and knee (124,125) replacement are sufficiently good for it to be the recommended approach unless cellulitis is very extensive. Antibiotics may be administered either systemically or by implantable pump (126).

In established infection, in contrast, implant removal is generally a prerequisite for long-term control of infection. The overall objective is to provide, or to preserve, a stable, pain-free joint with adequate

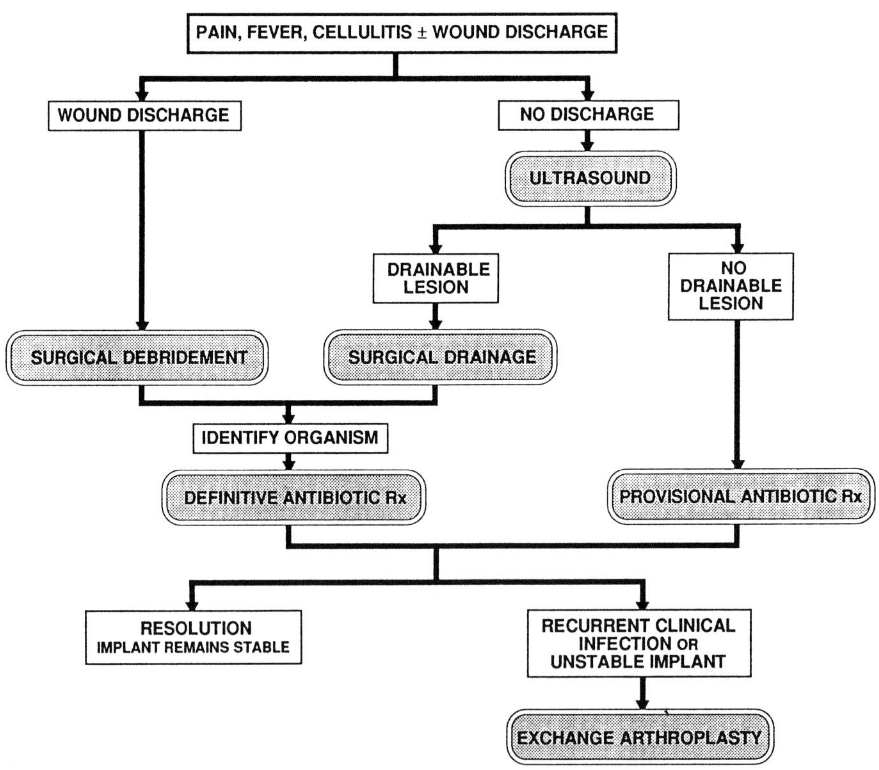

Figure 17-3. *Algorithm for management of infected total joint replacement.*

function for the individual's needs. The majority of those with long-standing prosthetic joint infection have significant pain and functional loss. These deficits, and the risks of intermittent exacerbations of infection, justify surgical reconstruction; the goal is exchange arthroplasty with eradication of infection. The cure, however, should not be worse than the disease, and there are some individuals with proven infection whose disease can be suppressed and symptoms minimized by use of systemic antibiotic therapy alone, although the long-term success rate is poor (127). We prefer intermittent administration in response to flares of infection. Agents suitable for once-daily injection, such as teicoplanin, have been used in this context for ambulant therapy (128). Although no randomized studies have been published, we advise against long-term prophylaxis in view of its cost, side effects, and lack of proven ability to prevent recurrence. No randomized studies of antibiotic suppression compared with exchange arthroplasty have been reported.

Management of Early Acute (Stage 1) Infections

Fitzgerald and colleagues (3) reviewed the outcome of management of acute prosthetic hip infections. In the presence of significant cellulitis that effectively precluded debridement of the infected area and subsequent wound closure, they recommended antibiotic administration and subsequent exchange arthroplasty if indicated. However, in the presence of a draining, infected hematoma without cellulitis, they urged thorough surgical debridement, irrigation, and antibiotics. Using this approach, they were able to save 70% or more implants. A similar picture emerges for total knee replacement. Factors associated with successful retention of the prosthesis are early and adequate debridement, aggressive antibiotic therapy, and infections that are apparently more superficial in nature (4,124,125).

Recently, delivery of high concentrations of antibiotic via implantable pumps has been used with very promising success in acute prosthetic infections (126) (85% success at 30 months in a series of 20 patients). Currently, these pumps are very expensive, and further evaluation of this technique is needed.

Successful arthroscopic debridement has been described in acutely infected knee replacements (129), but it seems to have limited potential in the postoperative period and further evaluation is required.

Management of Intermediate and Late (Stage II and III) Infections

Essentially, options for management of intermediate and late infections are one- or two-stage exchange arthroplasty or, if these procedures are not indicated, salvage procedures, such as excision arthroplasty or arthrodesis. The principles of management of established infection are listed in Table 17-2; they are essentially identical to those described for chronic osteomyelitis in Chapter 15.

A general assessment, with careful attention to correctable conditions that might compromise the outcome (similar to that undertaken before primary implantation of a joint prosthesis) should be performed.

Eradication of infection and successful reconstruction are unlikely, in principle, to succeed unless tissue oxygenation is adequate. Fitzgerald and Jones (130) found a high incidence of infection in heavily scarred, multiply operated patients and recommended consideration of soft-tissue replacement. Factors evaluated should include history of flares of infection, sinus activity, and healing and breakdown of scars. A history of recurrent skin breakdown is an indication for soft-tissue reconstruction. The anatomy of sinuses should be clarified by sinography. Although it may be difficult to identify definite signs of infection on radiological examination, surgical planning clearly requires careful assessment of the quality of bone and the position and extent of the implant, associated cement, and reactive changes in the surrounding bone.

Antibiotics may be administered systemically, locally in AIPMMA, or by implantable local infusion (131). Given the apparent inability of current antimicrobial agents to eradicate bacteria established on the surface of implants, the role of systemic antibiotics in the context of

Table 17-2. Principles of Management of Infected Total Joint Replacement

1. Microbiological diagnosis
2. Assessment and modification of the host
3. Anatomical definition of local disease
4. Antiobiotic therapy
5. Surgical debridement of implant, cement, scar, and granulation
6. Obliteration of debridement cavity
7. Restoration of functional stability

exchange arthroplasty may be considered prophylactic against reinfection, rather than therapeutic. Some advocates of one-stage exchange arthroplasty do not use them, but rely on local elution of antibiotics from the impregnated cement mass (9); however, systemic antibiotics appear as effective in clinical practice. There are no authoritative data on the most appropriate duration of administration. Most clinics use protracted periods of therapy, either empirically determined or based on stabilization of laboratory examinations (e.g., ESR and C-reactive protein levels) at normal values.

Details of surgical technique may be found in texts on operative surgery and are not described herein. Successful debridement requires removal of implant, cement, scar tissue, dead bone, and granulation. In a severely scarred area, soft-tissue replacement may be indicated. Surgery and postoperative management are difficult, complicated, and expensive with regard to time and resources. A case can be made for special units devoted to revision arthroplasty.

The space left by surgical debridement is most effectively filled by another implant. One-stage exchange also rapidly fulfills the final principle of restoration of function and stability. It has been practiced widely in Europe, in some centers in the United States, and elsewhere (9,132–134), usually using AIPMMA.

When there has been massive bony destruction after removal of an infected joint replacement, successful use of both bulk and morselized allografts has been described (135). Published experience remains small, and bulk allografts should be used with caution.

In two-stage exchange arthroplasty, the temporary dead space left after removal of the implant may be filled with a muscle flap (136), beads (137,138), or shaped block spacers of AIPMMA.

Initially, results of exchange arthroplasty appeared poor (139). Published results for both one- and two-stage exchange arthroplasty in the hip and knee (9,132–136,140–145), however, indicate that, although inferior to primary joint replacement and revision for aseptic loosening, very worthwhile results can be obtained. The outcome of some categories of infection (e.g., with *Pseudomonas aeruginosa*) appears to be less satisfactory (9).

In the elbow, infection rates are higher than in hip and knee, and the results of reimplantation are thus far less satisfactory (146). For less commonly implanted prostheses, significant data are not yet available.

Results of excision arthroplasty of the hip for infection are controversial (147–150). Functional results are poor, and infection may persist, requiring further reconstruction with muscle flaps (139,151). Hip excision is now recommended only when exchange arthroplasty is inappropriate (e.g., in nonambulatory patients with significant sepsis, individuals with major bone loss associated with infection, and perhaps in some gram-negative infections).

If exchange arthroplasty in the knee fails, the preferred surgical option is arthrodesis, which can be achieved in approximately 80% of patients (152,153). Above-knee amputation has been the outcome in some severe infections following total knee replacement (153), which may be compatible with continued ambulation in some individuals. More proximal amputation following failed total hip replacement requires crutch walking at all times and is a major difficulty for elderly patients.

Exposure of a prosthesis following sloughing of a skin flap is a special case of prosthetic infection that may be successfully salvaged by use of muscle or fasciocutaneous flaps (154,155) to reconstitute a well-vascularized, soft-tissue prosthetic environment.

Conclusion

Although advances in our understanding of the biology of persisting chronic implant infection offer some hope that we may be able to control it with drug therapy, the most productive approach in the short term will be to aim for universal application of preventive strategies that are now well established. These strategies include careful preoperative evaluation, appropriate antibiotic prophylaxis, optimal operating room discipline and environment, good operative technique, and careful postoperative management. Perhaps most important is evaluation of these measures by thorough, high-quality infection surveillance and outcome audit.

References

1. Ahnfelt L, Herberts P, Malchau H, Andersson GB. Prognosis of total hip replacement. A Swedish multicenter study of 4,664 revisions. Acta Orthop Scand 1990;238(suppl):1–26.

2. Schmalzried TP, Amstutz HC, Au MK, Dorey FJ. Incidence of deep sepsis in total hip arthroplasty. Survivorship analysis over 17 years from one hospital. J Arthroplasty 1991;6(suppl):S47–S51.
3. Fitzgerald RHJ, Nolan DR, Ilstrup DM, Van Scoy RE, Washington JA, Coventry MB. Deep wound sepsis following total hip arthroplasty. J Bone Joint Surg [Am] 1977;59:847–855.
4. Rasul AT, Tsukayama D, Gustilo RB. Effect of time of onset and depth of infection on the outcome of total knee arthroplasty infections. Clin Orthop 1991;273:98–104.
5. Coventry MB. Treatment of infections occurring in total hip surgery. Orthop Clin North Am 1975;6:991–1003.
6. Schmalzried TP, Amstutz HC, Au MK, Dorey FJ. Etiology of deep sepsis in total hip arthroplasty. The significance of hematogenous and recurrent infections. Clin Orthop 1992;280:200–207.
7. Mulier JC, Vandepitte J, Stuyck J, Burssens A, Vermaut G, Van Ruymbeke J. Long-term study of the perioperative infection rate in 1,007 total hip replacements using prophylactic cefamandole and other precautions. Arch Orthop Trauma Surg 1987;106:135–139.
8. Marotte JH, Frottier J, Cazalet G, Lord G, Blanchard JP, Guillamon JL. Preventive antibiotic therapy and postoperative infection in orthopedic surgery: 1,983 total hip prostheses. Rev Chir Orthop 1985;71:79–86.
9. Buchholz HW, Elson RA, Engelbrecht E, Lodenkamper H, Rottger J, Siegel A. Management of deep infection of total hip replacement. J Bone Joint Surg [Br] 1981;63:342–353.
10. Wilson NI. A survey, in Scotland, of measures to prevent infection following orthopaedic surgery. J Hosp Infect 1987;9:235–242.
11. Lidwell OM, Lowbury EJ, Whyte W, Blowers R, Stanley SJ, Lowe D. Infection and sepsis after operations for total hip or knee-joint replacement: influence of ultraclean air, prophylactic antibiotics and other factors. J Hygiene Lond 1984;93:505–529.
12. Charnley J. Postoperative infection after total hip replacement with special reference to air contamination in the operating room. Clin Orthop 1972; 87:167–187.
13. Franco JA, Baer H, Enneking WF. Airborne contamination in orthopedic surgery. Evaluation of laminar air flow system and aspiration suit. Clin Orthop 1977;122:231–243.
14. Lidwell OM, Lowbury EJ, Whyte W, Blowers R, Stanley SJ, Lowe D. Bacteria isolated from deep joint sepsis after operation for total hip or knee replacement and the sources of the infections with Staphylococcus aureus. J Hosp Infect 1983;4:19–29.
15. Ayliffe GA. Role of the environment of the operating suite in surgical wound infection. Rev Infect Dis 1991;13(suppl 10):S800–S804.
16. Blomgren G. Hematogenous infection of total joint replacement. An experimental study in the rabbit. Acta Orthop Scand 1981;187(suppl):1–64.
17. Maderazo EG, Judson S, Pasternak H. Late infections of total joint prosthe-

ses. A review and recommendations for prevention. Clin Orthop 1988;229: 131–142.
18. Friedman RJ. Infection in total joint arthroplasty from distal intravenous lines. A case report. J Arthroplasty 1988;3(suppl):S69–S71.
19. Stillman RI, Wenzel RP, Donowitz LC. Emergence of coagulase negative staphylococci as major nosocomial bloodstream pathogens. Infect Control 1987;8:108–112.
20. Murray RP, Bourne MH, Fitzgerald RHJ. Metachronous infections in patients who have had more than one total joint arthroplasty. J Bone Joint Surg [Am] 1991;73:1469–1474.
21. Southwood RT, Rice JL, McDonald PJ, Hakendorf PH, Rozenbilds MA. Infection in experimental hip arthroplasties. J Bone Joint Surg [Br] 1985; 67:229–231.
22. Henderson PJ, Gillespie WJ. Costs of prophylaxis against infection for joint replacement. NZ Med J 1989;102:388.
23. Persson U, Montgomery F, Carlsson A, Lindgren B, Ahnfelt L. How far does prophylaxis against infection in total joint replacement offset its cost? Br Med J 1988;296:99–102.
24. Petty W. The effect of methylmethacrylate on bacterial phagocytosis and killing by human polymorphonuclear leukocytes. J Bone Joint Surg [Am] 1978;60:752–757.
25. Petty W. The effect of methylmethacrylate on the bacterial inhibiting properties of normal human serum. Clin Orthop 1978;132:266–278.
26. Petty W. The effect of methylmethacrylate on chemotaxis of polymorphonuclear leukocytes. J Bone Joint Surg [Am] 1978;60:492–498.
27. Surin VV, Sundholm K, Backman L. Infection after total hip replacement. With special reference to a discharge from the wound. J Bone Joint Surg [Br] 1983;65:412–418.
28. Canner GC, Steinberg ME, Heppenstall RB, Balderston R. The infected hip after total hip arthroplasty. J Bone Joint Surg [Am] 1984;66:1393–1399.
29. Jerry GJJ, Rand JA, Ilstrup D. Old sepsis prior to total knee arthroplasty. Clin Orthop 1988;236:135–140.
30. Carpiniello VL, Cendron M, Altman HG, Malloy TR, Booth R. Treatment of urinary complications after total joint replacement in elderly females. Urology 1988;32:186–188.
31. Vannini P, Ciavarella A, Olmi R, et al. Diabetes as pro-infective risk factor in total hip replacement. Acta Diabetol Lat 1984;21:275–280.
32. Acurio MT, Friedman RJ. Hip arthroplasty in patients with sickle-cell haemoglobinopathy. J Bone Joint Surg [Br] 1992;74:367–371.
33. Charnley J, Eftekhar N. Postoperative infection in total prosthetic replacement arthroplasty of the hip-joint. With special reference to the bacterial content of the air of the operating room. Br J Surg 1969;56:641–649.
34. Lidwell OM. Air, antibiotics and sepsis in replacement joints. J Hosp Infect 1988;11(suppl C):18–40.
35. Kim YY, Ko CU, Ahn JY, Yoon YS, Kwak BM. Charnley low friction arthro-

plasty in tuberculosis of the hip. An eight- to 13-year follow-up. J Bone Joint Surg [Br] 1988;70:756–760.
36. Kim YH. Total arthroplasty of the hip after childhood sepsis. J Bone Joint Surg [Br] 1991;73:783–786.
37. Bridges SLJ, Lopez Mendez A, Han KH, Tracy IC, Alarcon GS. Should methotrexate be discontinued before elective orthopedic surgery in patients with rheumatoid arthritis? J Rheumatol 1991;18:984–988.
38. Bishop JR, Moul JW, Sihelnik SA, Peppas DS, Gormley TS, McLeod DG. Use of glycosylated hemoglobin to identify diabetics at high risk for penile periprosthetic infections. J Urol 1992;147:386–388.
39. Field EA, Martin MV. Prophylactic antibiotics for patients with artificial joints undergoing oral and dental surgery: necessary or not? Br J Oral Maxillofac Surg 1991;29:341–346.
40. Dubois G. The use of multi-test IMC in pre-operative assessment of the risk of infection after hip prosthetic surgery. Rev Chir Orthop 1984;70:371–376.
41. Greene KA, Wilde AH, Stulberg BN. Preoperative nutritional status of total joint patients. J Arthroplasty 1991;6:321–325.
42. Kluge K, Grasshoff H, Weise EM, Weickert H. Perioperative antibiotic prophylaxis in allo-arthroplasty. Beitr Orthop Traumatol 1990;37:207–210.
43. Liechti R, Weber BG. Study of prophylaxis of operative infection using a staphylococcal vaccine. Chirurg 1973;44:269–272.
44. Brown E, Wenzel RP, Hendley JO. Exploration of the microbial anatomy of human skin using plasmid pattern profiles of coagulase-negative staphylococci: search for the reservoir of the resident skin flora. J Infect Dis 1989;160:644–650.
45. Fairclough JA, Johnson D, Mackie I. The prevention of wound contamination by skin organisms by the pre-operative application of an iodophor impregnated plastic adhesive drape. J Int Med Res 1986;14:105–109.
46. Katthagen BD, Zamani P, Jung W. Effect of surgical draping on bacterial contamination in the surgical field. Z Orthop Ihre Grenzgeb 1992;130: 230–235.
47. Belkin NL. Barrier materials. Their influence on surgical wound infections. AORN J 1992;55:1521–1528.
48. Ritter MA, Marmion P. Exogenous sources and controls of microorganisms in operating room. Orthop Rev 1987;16:224–232.
49. Borst M, Collier C, Miller D. Operating room surveillance: a new approach in reducing hip and knee prosthetic wound infections. Am J Infect Control 1986;14:161–166.
50. Strange Vognsen HH, Klareskov B. Bacteriologic contamination of suction tips during hip arthroplasty. Acta Orthop Scand 1988;59:410–411.
51. Benson MK, Hughes SP. Infection following total hip replacement in a general hospital without special orthopaedic facilities. Acta Orthop Scand 1975;46:968–978.
52. Ericsson C, Lidgren L, Lindberg L. Cloxacillin in the prophylaxis of postoperative infections of the hip. J Bone Joint Surg [Am] 1973;55:808–813.

53. Burke JF. The effective period of preventive antibiotic action in experimental incisions and dermal lesions. Surgery 1961;50:161–168.
54. Hill C, Flamant R, Mazas F, Evrard J. Prophylactic cefazolin versus placebo in total hip replacement. Report of a multicentre double-blind randomised trial. Lancet 1981;1:795–796.
55. Pollard JP, Hughes SP, Scott JE, Evans MJ, Benson MK. Antibiotic prophylaxis in total hip replacement. Br Med J 1979;1:707–709.
56. Schulitz KP, Winkelmann W, Schoening B. The prophylactic use of antibiotics in alloarthroplasty of the hip joint for coxarthrosis. Arch Orthop Trauma Surg 1980;96:79–82.
57. Klenerman L, Seal D, Sullens K. Combined prophylactic effect of ultraclean air and cefuroxime for reducing infection in prosthetic surgery. Acta Orthop Belg 1991;57:19–24.
58. Irvine R, Johnson BLJ, Amstutz HC. The relationship of genitourinary tract procedures and deep sepsis after total hip replacements. Surg Gynecol Obstet 1974;139:701–706.
59. Fitzgerald RH. Antibiotic distribution in normal and osteomyelitic bone. Orthop Clin North Am 1984;15:537–546.
60. Hoddinott C, Lovering AM, Fernendo HC, Dixon JH, Reeves DS. Determination of bone and fat concentrations following systemic cefamandole and regional cefuroxime administration in patients undergoing knee arthroplasty. J Antimicrob Chemother 1990;26:823–829.
61. Buchholz HW, Elson RA, Heinert K. Antibiotic-loaded acrylic cement: current concepts. Clin Orthop 1984;190:96–108.
62. Bayston R, Milner RD. The sustained release of antimicrobial drugs from bone cement. An appraisal of laboratory investigations and their significance. J Bone Joint Surg [Br] 1982;64:460–464.
63. Petty W, Spanier S, Shuster JJ. Prevention of infection after total joint replacement. Experiments with a canine model. J Bone Joint Surg [Am] 1988;70:536–539.
64. Elson RA, Jephcott AE, McGechie DB, Verettas D. Bacterial infection and acrylic cement in the rat. J Bone Joint Surg [Br] 1977;59:452–457.
65. Wahlig H, Dingeldein E. Antibiotics and bone cements. Experimental and clinical long-term observations. Acta Orthop Scand 1980;51:49–56.
66. Lindberg L, Onnerfalt R, Dingeldein E, Wahlig H. The release of gentamicin after total hip replacement using low or high viscosity bone cement. A prospective, randomized study. Int Orthop 1991;15:305–309.
67. McQueen MM, Hughes SP, May P, Verity L. Cefuroxime in total joint arthroplasty. Intravenous or in bone cement. J Arthroplasty 1990;5:169–172.
68. Josefsson G, Gudmundsson G, Kolmert L, Wijkstrom S. Prophylaxis with systemic antibiotics versus gentamicin bone cement in total hip arthroplasty. A five-year survey of 1,688 hips. Clin Orthop 1990;253:173–178.
69. MacMillan M, Petty W, Hendeles L. Effect of irrigation and tourniquet application on aminoglycoside antibiotic concentrations in bone. J Orthop Res 1988;6:311–316.

70. Rosenstein BD, Wilson FC, Funderburk CH. Use of bacitracin irrigation to prevent infection in post-operative skeletal wounds. An experimental study. J Bone Joint Surg [Am] 1989;71:427–430.
71. McLauchlan J, Smylie HG, Logie JR, Smith G. A study of the wound environment during total hip arthroplasty. Postgrad Med J 1976;52:550–557.
72. Maguire WB. The use of antibiotics, locally and systemically, in orthopaedic surgery. Med J Aust 1964;2:412–414.
73. Nachamie BA, Siffert RS, Bryer MS. A study of neomycin installation into orthopedic wounds. JAMA 1968;204:687–689.
74. Bertheusen KJ, Larsen P. Prophylactic irrigation of wounds with neomycin. Ugeskr Laeg 1980;142:685–686.
75. Bannister GC, Auchincloss JM, Johnson DP, Newman JH. The timing of tourniquet application in relation to prophylactic antibiotic administration. J Bone Joint Surg [Br] 1988;70:322–324.
76. Richardson JB, Roberts A, Robertson JFR, John PJ, Sweeney G. Timing of antibiotic administration in knee replacement under tourniquet. J Bone Joint Surg [Br] 1993;75:32–35.
77. Gatell JM, Garcia S, Lozano L, Soriano E, Ramon R, San Miguel JG. Perioperative cefamandole prophylaxis against infections. J Bone Joint Surg [Am] 1987;69:1189–1193.
78. Chambers ST, Gillespie WJ. Perioperative cefamandole prophylaxis against infections. J Bone Joint Surg [Am] 1988;70:950.
79. Wymenga A, van Horn J, Theeuwes A, Muytjens H, Slooff T. Cefuroxime for prevention of postoperative coxitis. One versus three doses tested in a randomized multicenter study of 2,651 arthroplasties. Acta Orthop Scand 1992;63:19–24.
80. Ritter MA, Campbell E, Keating EM, Faris PM. Comparison of intraoperative versus 24 hour antibiotic prophylaxis in total joint replacement. A controlled prospective study. Orthop Rev 1989;18:694–696.
81. Sorensen AI, Sorensen TS. Bacterial growth on suction drain tips. Prospective study of 489 clean orthopedic operations. Acta Orthop Scand 1991;62: 451–454.
82. Archer GL. Alteration of cutaneous staphylococcal flora as a consequence of antimicrobial prophylaxis. Rev Infect Dis 1991;13(suppl 10):S805–S809.
83. Norden CW. Prevention of bone and joint infections. Am J Med 1985;78: 229–232.
84. Aronsson B, Mollby R, Nord CE. Antimicrobial agents and Clostridium difficile in acute enteric disease: epidemiological data from Sweden, 1980–1982. J Infect Dis 1985;151:476–481.
85. Goldner JL, Moggio M, Beissinger SF, McCollum DE. Ultraviolet light for the control of airborne bacteria in the operating room. Ann NY Acad Sci 1980;353:271–284.
86. Lowell JD, Kundsin RB, Schwartz CM, Pozin D. Ultraviolet radiation and reduction of deep wound infection following hip and knee arthroplasty. Ann NY Acad Sci 1980;353:285–293.

87. Berg M, Bergman BR, Hoborn J. Ultraviolet radiation compared to an ultra-clean air enclosure. Comparison of air bacteria counts in operating rooms. J Bone Joint Surg [Br] 1991;73:811–815.
88. Berg-Perier M, Cederblad A, Persson U. Ultraviolet radiation and ultra-clean air enclosures in operating rooms. U-V protection, economy, and comfort. J Arthroplasty 1992;7:457–463.
89. McQuarrie DG, Glover JL, Olson MM. Laminar airflow systems. Issues surrounding their effectiveness. AORN J 1991;51:1035–1048.
90. Fitzgerald RHJ. Total hip arthroplasty sepsis. Prevention and diagnosis. Orthop Clin North Am 1992;23:259–264.
91. Norfleet RG. Infective endocarditis and infections of orthopedic and vascular prostheses following gastrointestinal endoscopy and dilation. Gastrointest Endosc 1990;36:546–547.
92. Wroblewski BM, del Sel HJ. Urethral instrumentation and deep sepsis in total hip replacement. Clin Orthop 1980;146:209–212.
93. Bailey RR, Peddie BA, Gorrie SI, Hume C, Gillespie WJ. Prevalence of asymptomatic bacteriuria in patients presenting for total hip or knee replacement. NZ Med J 1988;101:60.
94. Glynn MK, Sheehan JM. The significance of asymptomatic bacteriuria in patients undergoing hip/knee arthroplasty. Clin Orthop 1984;185:151–154.
95. Michelson JD, Lotke PA, Steinberg ME. Urinary-bladder management after total joint-replacement surgery. N Engl J Med 1988;319:321–326.
96. Stamm WE. Catheter-associated urinary tract infections: epidemiology, pathogenesis, and prevention. Am J Med 1991;91:65S–71S.
97. Gillespie WJ. Infection in total joint replacement. Infect Dis Clin North Am 1990;4:465–484.
98. Lampe HI, Sneller ZW, Rijnberg WJ. Urination problems following total hip arthroplasty: insertion or not of an indwelling catheter? Ned Tijdschr Geneeskd 1992;136:827–831.
99. Skelly JM, Guyatt GH, Kalbfleisch R, Singer J, Winter L. Management of urinary retention after surgical repair of hip fracture. Can Med Assoc J 1992;146:1185–1189.
100. Petersen MS, Collins DN, Selakovich WG, Finkbeiner AE. Postoperative urinary retention associated with total hip and total knee arthroplasties. Clin Orthop 1991;269:102–108.
101. Cioffi GA, Terezhalmy GT, Taybos GM. Total joint replacement: a consideration for antimicrobial prophylaxis. Oral Surg Oral Med Oral Pathol 1988;66:124–129.
102. Norden CW. Antibiotic prophylaxis in orthopedic surgery. Rev Infect Dis 1991;13(suppl 10):S842–S846.
103. McGowan DA, Hendrey ML. Is antibiotic prophylaxis required for dental patients with joint replacements? Br Dent J 1985;158:336–338.
104. Tsevat J, Durand Zaleski I, Pauker SG. Cost-effectiveness of antibiotic prophylaxis for dental procedures in patients with artificial joints. Am J Public Health 1989;79:739–743.

105. Jacobson JJ, Schweitzer SO, Kowalski CJ. Chemoprophylaxis of prosthetic joint patients during dental treatment: a decision-utility analysis. Oral Surg Oral Med Oral Pathol 1991;72:167–177.
106. Surin VV. Effect of different surveillance methods on statistics of postoperative wound infections. J Hosp Infect 1988;11:116–120.
107. Choudhry RR, Rice RP, Triffitt PD, Harper WM, Gregg PJ. Plasma viscosity and C-reactive protein after total hip and knee arthroplasty. J Bone Joint Surg [Br] 1992;74:523–524.
108. Waleczek H, Kozianka J, Everts H. C-reactive protein in the early diagnosis of postoperative infection following bone surgery. Chirurg 1991;62: 866–870.
109. Graif M, Schwartz E, Strauss S, Mouallem M, Schecter M, Morag B. Occult infection of hip prosthesis: sonographic evaluation. J Am Geriatr Soc 1991;39:203–204.
110. Cuckler JM, Star AM, Alavi A, Noto RB. Diagnosis and management of the infected total joint arthroplasty. Orthop Clin North Am 1991;22: 523–530.
111. Levitsky KA, Hozack WJ, Balderston RA, et al. Evaluation of the painful prosthetic joint. Relative value of bone scan, sedimentation rate, and joint aspiration. J Arthroplasty 1991;6:237–244.
112. Thoren B, Wigren A. Erythrocyte sedimentation rate in infection of total hip replacements. Orthopedics 1991;14:495–497.
113. Aalto K, Osterman K, Peltola H, Rasanen J. Changes in erythrocyte sedimentation rate and C-reactive protein after total hip arthroplasty. Clin Orthop 1984;184:118–120.
114. Evans BG, Cuckler JM. Evaluation of the painful total hip arthroplasty. Orthop Clin North Am 1992;23:303–311.
115. Pring DJ, Henderson RG, Keshavarzian A. Indium-granulocyte scanning in the painful prosthetic joint. AJR 1986;147:167–172.
116. Sciuk J, Brandau W, Vollet B, et al. Comparison of technetium 99m polyclonal human immunoglobulin and technetium 99m monoclonal antibodies for imaging chronic osteomyelitis. First clinical results. Eur J Nucl Med 1991;18:401–407.
117. Oyen WJ, van Horn JR, Claessens RA, Slooff TJ, van der Meer JW, Corstens FH. Diagnosis of bone, joint, and joint prosthesis infections with In-111-labeled nonspecific human immunoglobulin G scintigraphy. Radiology 1992;182:195–199.
118. Copping C, Dalgliesh SM, Dudley NJ, et al. The role of ^{99m}Tc-HMPAO white cell imaging in suspected orthopaedic infection. Br J Radiol 1992; 65:309–312.
119. Mackowiak PA, Jones SR, Smith JW. Diagnostic value of sinus-tract cultures in chronic osteomyelitis. JAMA 1978;239:2772–2775.
120. Foldes K, Gaal M, Balint P, et al. Ultrasonography after hip arthroplasty. Skeletal Radiol 1992;21:297–299.
121. Lopitaux R, Levai JP, Raux P, Hermet R, Grenier Gaudin A, Sirot J. Value

of puncture-arthrography in the diagnosis of infection of total hip arthroplasty. Rev Chir Orthop Reparatrice Appar Mot 1992;78:34–37.
122. Roberts P, Walters AJ, McMinn DJ. Diagnosing infection in hip replacements. The use of fine-needle aspiration and radiometric culture. J Bone Joint Surg [Br] 1992;74:265–269.
123. Wymenga AB, Van Dijke BJ, van Horn JR, Slooff TJ. Prosthesis-related infection. Etiology, prophylaxis and diagnosis. Acta Orthop Belg 1990;56: 463–475.
124. Hartman MB, Fehring TK, Jordan L, Norton HJ. Periprosthetic knee sepsis. The role of irrigation and debridement. Clin Orthop 1991;273:113–118.
125. Burger RR, Basch T, Hopson CN. Implant salvage in infected total knee arthroplasty. Clin Orthop 1991;273:105–112.
126. Perry CR, Hulsey RE, Mann FA, Miller GA, Pearson RL. Treatment of acutely infected arthroplasties with incision, drainage, and local antibiotics delivered via an implantable pump. Clin Orthop 1992;281:216–223.
127. Tsukayama DT, Wicklund B, Gustilo RB. Suppressive antibiotic therapy in chronic prosthetic joint infections. Orthopedics 1991;14:841–844.
128. Davey PG, Rowley DR, Phillips GA. Teicoplanin—home therapy for prosthetic joint infections. Eur J Surg 1992;567(suppl):23–25.
129. Flood JN, Kolarik DB. Arthroscopic irrigation and debridement of infected total knee arthroplasty. Arthroscopy 1988;4:182–186.
130. Fitzgerald RHJ, Jones DR. Hip implant infection. Treatment with resection arthroplasty and late total hip arthroplasty. Am J Med 1985;78: 225–228.
131. Perry CR, Pearson RL. Local antibiotic delivery in the treatment of bone and joint infections. Clin Orthop 1991;263:215–226.
132. Goksan SB, Freeman MA. One-stage reimplantation for infected total knee arthroplasty. J Bone Joint Surg [Br] 1992;74:78–82.
133. Harris WH. One-staged exchange arthroplasty for septic total hip replacement. AAOS Instr Course Lect 1986;35:226–228.
134. Wroblewski BM. One-stage revision of infected cemented total hip arthroplasty. Clin Orthop 1986;211:103–107.
135. Berry DJ, Chandler HP, Reilly DT. The use of bone allografts in two-stage reconstruction after failure of hip replacements due to infection. J Bone Joint Surg [Am] 1991;73:1460–1468.
136. Meland NB, Arnold PG, Weiss HC. Management of the recalcitrant total-hip arthroplasty wound. Plast Reconstr Surg 1991;88:681–685.
137. Hovelius L, Josefsson G. An alternative method for exchange operation of infected arthroplasty. Acta Orthop Scand 1979;50:93–96.
138. Lindberg LT. Septopal chains in operations to exchange infected total hip arthroplasties. Reconstr Surg Traumatol 1988;20:47–54.
139. Hunter GA. The results of reinsertion of a total hip prosthesis after sepsis. J Bone Joint Surg [Br] 1979;61:422–423.
140. Wilson MG, Kelley K, Thornhill TS. Infection as a complication of total knee-replacement arthroplasty. J Bone Joint Surg [Am] 1990;72:878–883.

141. Wilde AH, Ruth JT. Two-stage reimplantation in infected total knee arthroplasty. Clin Orthop 1988;236:23–35.
142. Grogan TJ, Dorey F, Rollins J, Amstutz HC. Deep sepsis following total knee arthroplasty. Ten-year experience at the University of California at Los Angeles Medical Center. J Bone Joint Surg [Am] 1986;68:226–234.
143. Johnson DP, Bannister GC. The outcome of infected arthroplasty of the knee. J Bone Joint Surg [Am] 1986;68:289–291.
144. Rand JA, Bryan RS, Morrey BF, Westholm F. Management of infected total knee arthroplasty. Clin Orthop 1986;205:75–85.
145. Windsor RE, Insall JN, Urs WK, Miller DV, Brause BD. Two-stage reimplantation for the salvage of total knee arthroplasty complicated by infection. J Bone Joint Surg [Am] 1990;72:272–278.
146. Wolfe SW, Figgie MP, Inglis AE, Bohn WW, Ranawat CS. Management of infection about total elbow prosthesis. J Bone Joint Surg [Am] 1990;72: 198–211.
147. Kantor GS, Osterkamp JA, Dorr LD, Fischer D, Perry J, Conaty JP. Resection arthroplasty following infected total hip replacement arthroplasty. J Arthroplasty 1986;1:83–89.
148. Bourne RB, Hunter GA, Rorabeck CH, Macnab JJ. A six-year follow-up of infected total hip replacements managed by Girdlestone's arthroplasty. J Bone Joint Surg [Br] 1984;66:340–343.
149. McElwaine JP, Colville J. Excision arthroplasty for infected total hip replacements. J Bone Joint Surg [Br] 1984;66:168–171.
150. Petty W, Goldsmith S. Resection arthroplasty following infected total hip arthroplasty. J Bone Joint Surg [Am] 1980;62:889–896.
151. Collins DN, Garvin KL, Nelson CL. The use of the vastus lateralis flap in patients with intractable infection after resection arthroplasty following the use of a hip implant. J Bone Joint Surg [Am] 1987;69:510–516.
152. Figgie HE, Brody GA, Inglis AE, Sculco TP, Goldberg VM, Figgie MP. Knee arthrodesis following total knee arthroplasty in rheumatoid arthritis. Clin Orthop 1987;224:237–243.
153. Rand JA, Bryan RS. The outcome of failed knee arthrodesis following total knee arthroplasty. Clin Orthop 1986;205:86–92.
154. Gault DT, Quaba A. Is flap cover of exposed metalwork worthwhile? A review of 28 cases. Br J Plast Surg 1986;39:505–509.
155. Greenberg B, La Rossa D, Lotke PA. Salvage of jeopardized total knee prosthesis. The role of the gastrocnemius muscle flap. Plast Reconstr Surg 1989;83:85–89.

CHAPTER 18

Infectious Arthritis

Every hour that an acute suppurative process continues within a joint is of urgent significance to prognosis. —D. C. Paterson, 1970 (1)

This statement does not exaggerate the sense of urgency required when confronted by either the certainty, probability or even the possibility of this affection. —G. C. Lloyd-Roberts, 1979 (2)

Infectious arthritis encompasses the terms *septic arthritis, pyogenic arthritis, suppurative arthritis, purulent arthritis,* and *pyarthrosis,* and implies that the patient has an inflammation involving a joint, from which an infecting micro-organism is either detected or presumed to be the cause of the inflammation.

Because the inside of a joint is lined either by synovium or articular cartilage, these tissues first manifest the effects of the infective inflammation. The inflammatory response is seen in the synovium, whereas the potential destructive effects of the process affect the articular cartilage.

Although not documented in precise terms, the different clinical patterns of infective arthritis are probably determined by the invasive and toxic characteristics of the causative "germ" and the way in which the synovium responds to the presence of the micro-organism. The clinical picture is therefore determined by the interplay of the two factors, and not only by the micro-organism.

Identification of causative organisms, if successful, merely provides a guide to the choice of which antibiotic drugs should be used to kill bacteria in the joint. The antibiotics restore the balance between host and parasite in favor of the host.

Introduction of antibiotics has changed the natural history of septic arthritis, and reports of patients managed before antibiotic use (3–5) are of little relevance except to point out the sequelae of inadequate management.

Hunter (6), in 1743, described the macroscopic features of joint infection and its unpleasant sequelae of amputation or premature death. Brodie (7) (1819) wrote of the difficulties of draining a septic joint and the ultimate inadequacy of arthrotomy in chronic joint infection. Following Lister's introduction of antisepsis, surgeons began to think in terms of supplementing arthrotomy with medication. Until comparatively recently, arthrotomy of a septic joint, either through a purulent swelling or through the site of easiest access to the joint, represented the entire treatment of pyarthrosis (8).

Almost every conceivable antiseptic has, at some time or another, been injected into joint cavities, but almost invariably the result has been disappointing or even harmful. Questions about the technique of arthrotomy—such as whether drainage should be instituted for a long period, whether the joint should be closed or left open, whether it should be immobilized or moved—have evoked considerable argument over many years. Early in World War II, sulfonamides were administered systemically and also into joints at arthrotomy; later, penicillin was used in the same way.

Now that the life of patients is rarely at stake and the infected limb almost never requires removal, therapeutic endeavors must be directed to restoration and maintenance of normal function. Many opinions regarding the treatment of septic arthritis are based on theory and there is a surprising paucity of accurate clinical reviews (1). Accumulated data from the Mayo Clinic (9) identified 103 children over a 30-year period, thus indicating the relative rarity of the condition.

Occurrence

Acute septic arthritis is uncommon. Recent reports (1,10–13) describe 52 cases in 16 years, 17 cases in 11 years, 96 cases in 8 years, and 50 cases in 4 years. In one series (11), 36% of children were less than 2 years of age. In another (13), 14 of 45 patients (31%) were less than 2 years of age, and 22 (48%) were less than 3 years of age. There may be a relatively low incidence between the ages of 3 and 6 months (10). The joint most commonly involved is the hip in infants and the knee in older children. These joints account for the majority of infectious arthritis sites in all age groups. Despite the fact that the joints of the lower limb are most often involved, any synovial joint can be infected, and in approximately 10% of patients, more than one joint is involved. The sex incidence suggests a male predominance, although less marked than in osteomyelitis. A second peak of incidence occurs in the elderly.

Pathology and Microbiology

It is pertinent to think about how micro-organisms enter a joint. Although the diagnosis of infectious arthritis is proven by detecting organisms inside the lumen of a joint, their route to that lumen is not always clear.

If the joint has been penetrated externally by accidental trauma or iatrogenic introduction of a needle or other instrument at elective surgery, a portal for the entry of organisms is established. The very low incidence of sepsis following needle puncture for the instillation of medication or arthroscopy and surgical manipulation (even through multiple portals stretched for relatively long periods) makes one think about the ability of a joint to avoid infection. In contrast, when there has not been a breach of the joint capsule, entry of organisms into the joint is either through the articular surface (presumably by extension of adjacent osteomyelitis [14]) or by escape from synovial capillaries, presuming a pre-existing bacteremia or septicemia. Transphyseal spread can occur in infants. In those joints in which the metaphyseal portion of the bone is intracapsular, especially the hip and shoulder, direct spread from a metaphyseal abscess may occur. The nature of synovial cells, which have a part in articular cartilage nutrition, joint lubrication, and maintenance of synovial fluid dynamics, is that a significant proportion (type B cells) are phagocytes. Therefore, for an infection to become established within a joint, there must be a major imbalance between the normal synovial cell function and the effects of the invading micro-organisms. How such organisms escape from within capillary lumens in sufficient numbers to initiate a clinical infection is not known.

Virulence of the infecting organism and resistance of the host determine whether suppuration ensues. Infancy, trauma, or prior arthropathy appear to reduce the resistance to spread of infection. In any acute joint disease, infection must be suspected.

As Lloyd-Roberts put it, "pus and articular cartilage are incompatible" (15). The inflammatory process in acute septic arthritis starts within the synovium. Intracapsular inflammation, with synovial proliferation and an exudate or transudate of fluid, may distend the joint capsule, causing laxity, subluxation, or dislocation. Containment of suppuration within the joint, by virtue of thick anatomical barriers, results in increased intra-articular pressure and conditions for destruction of articular cartilage. How this process occurs is discussed in Chapters 2 and 3.

Acute bacterial arthritis may be caused by a wide variety of microorganisms, depending on the age of the patient. The most common causative organism of acute septic arthritis in all age groups is *Staphylococcus aureus*. This statement has been challenged (16), as it may relate to hospital-acquired infections in infants under the age of 3 months, but it may be that the most common cause of community-acquired infectious arthritis is streptococcal. The pertinence of this controversy means that in any one geographical area, it is important to monitor the causative bacteria so that appropriate choice of antibiotics for treatment can bc made before their identification has been confirmed in the laboratory. Many other organisms have been isolated from septic joints. In infants under one year of age, a diverse group of organisms have been identified as causative agents, including group B streptococci, gram-negative bacilli, and *S. aureus*. In 1966, attention was drawn to the increasing importance of *Hemophilus influenzae* type b as a cause in infants and children (11); this finding was reinforced in another country (17) in 1970 and has been confirmed around the world since then in the age group between 6 months and 2 years. It is important to remember this observation when choosing antibiotics before the results of bacterial culture and antibiotic sensitivity are known. Other causative organisms reported include *Streptococcus pyogenes, Streptococcus pneumoniae, Escherichia coli, Proteus* sp., *Salmonella* sp., *Serratia marcescens* (18), *Clostridium welchii* (19), *Clostridium septicum* (20), *Neisseria* sp., *S. albus,* and *Bacteroides* sp. (21). However, organisms are not grown from all patients. Cultures of synovial fluid fail to grow organisms in a substantial number of patients in whom there is a clinical diagnosis of septic arthritis. A summary (11) of previous reports (10, 22–24) found that the causative organism was unknown in 71 of 250 patients (28%). Another study (13) did not find a bacterial cause in 19 of 45 patients with a clinical diagnosis of acute septic arthritis. Twenty-six joint aspirates produced organisms 16 times (62%), and in 19 patients treated with arthrotomy, pus was found on 18 occasions and organisms were grown from 15 (84%).

Several reasons have been proposed for the inability to obtain bacteriological proof of infection, including prior use of antibiotics, inadequate anaerobic cultures, standard of microbiological laboratories, changing patterns of the organisms involved and their cultural characteristics (e.g., *Hemophilus influenzae*), and failure to obtain blood for culture or to perform arthrocentesis sufficiently frequently. This situation persists despite significant advances in microbiology laboratory techniques. It may be that some fastidious organisms are not detected. One Israeli laboratory (25) adopted the practice of culturing synovial fluid in BACTEC 460 aerobic blood culture bottles in addition to solid media; they found a dramatic change in the spectrum of detected micro-organisms. In particular, the incidence of detection of *Kingella kingae* was increased. Cultures of blood from patients in whom this organism was detected in synovial fluid did not grow the bacteria, which became the second most common cause of septic arthritis in children in their population. They argued that the use of blood culture methods for synovial fluid might dilute substances in the joint fluid that have a detrimental effect on the growth of the organism on solid media, and suggested that blood culture methods should also be used for synovial fluid to raise the yield of organisms detected.

The most frequent etiological agent in adults under the age of 30 years is *Neisseria gonorrhoeae*. Beta-hemolytic streptococci are relatively uncommon agents in septic arthritis and have been reported as the cause identified in 3% to 17% of all cases of septic arthritis (26). Lancefield group A streptococcus is the most common beta-hemolytic streptococcus causing septic arthritis. Group B, group C, and group G streptococci also cause infection in joints. Group G streptococci are probably the second most common beta-hemolytic streptococci causing septic arthritis. A review of 56 patients (25) described the clinical features. Although group B streptococci are an uncommon cause of septic arthritis in adults, the organism is not benign and may produce an aggressive polyarthritis (27,28). Group C streptococcal arthritis is uncommon, and 10 patients have been reviewed recently (29). There are several organisms that are categorized in this group, including those known as "*S. milleri.*" Despite the sensitivity of streptococci to penicillin G, arthrolavage appears to have been required in approximately half the reported patients. It has been recommended (30) that when streptococci are isolated from a patient with septic arthritis, they should always be grouped. The presence of group G organisms should lead to a search for an underlying disease.

Unusual organisms are more likely to appear when there has been penetration of the joint by a foreign body, retention of a foreign body within a joint, systemic disease altering the immunological status of the patient, treatment with corticosteroids, or in patients who self-inject themselves with various substances under unsterile conditions. After a penetrating injury to a joint, the symptoms of infectious arthritis appear after 6 to 48 hours. *Clostridium perfringens* pyarthrosis may be present without gas appearing on radiographs or foul-smelling joint fluid and may exist in conjunction with aerobic organisms (31). It does not typically cause myonecrosis or articular degeneration.

Bacterial Arthritis in Infancy and Childhood

Clinical Features

Infectious Arthritis in Infancy

The importance of pyarthrosis in infants was recognized by Smith in 1874 (32), and it has subsequently been known as "Tom Smith's arthritis." It is not a common condition, and the sequel of delay in diagnosis or inadequate treatment can be crippling.

There are significant differences between infection occurring in infancy and in older children. Neonatal disease is more frequent, more deceptive in presentation, and more devastating (2).

In infants, several days' delay in diagnosis of septic arthritis of the hip is a frequent finding (23). The major features are those of septicemia. There may be irritability, apprehension, failure to feed or gain weight, muscle "spasm," dislike of being handled, temperature instability, tachycardia, anemia, and the presence of associated infection. "Pseudoparalysis" of a limb is an important and common sign but may be overlooked. Sometimes the parent draws attention to the lack of movement of a limb. Localization of the infective process in a joint, particularly the hip joint, is frequently not obvious, and subtle changes in posture are important. The baby may look deceptively healthy, with a "pyrexia of unknown origin." The traditional clinical signs of inflammation may be lacking. When infection in an infant is suspected, great care must be taken in clinical examination: All bones should be palpated and all joints should be moved. In any infant with septicemia, involvement of the hip joint must be suspected. Sepsis in the shoulder joint of infants may also not be obvious to cursory clinical examination.

Infectious Arthritis in Children

In contrast to infants, children with septic arthritis usually present with an acute fulminating disease. Fever and tachycardia are common, as are moderate to severe pain uniformly about the involved joint, evidence of joint effusion, muscle spasm, and reluctance to move the joint or even the whole limb. In such children, infection is usually suspected and local signs, together with history, localize the site of infection. The presence of a focus of infection elsewhere, such as otitis media, pneumonia, or a furuncle may reveal the source of the septicemia.

In acute septic arthritis in children, diagnosis in the crucial period to limit damage to articular cartilage can usually be made by clinical appraisal.

Conditions that can produce a similar clinical picture include the following: (a) Acute osteomyelitis that may present a sympathetic joint effusion adjacent to the involved metaphysis. The two conditions may occur together, particularly in hip, knee, or shoulder joints. In patients with acute osteomyelitis, gentle clinical examination usually allows some joint movement, whereas in patients with septic arthritis, muscle spasm usually prevents joint movement, which is nearly always very painful; (b) Rheumatoid arthritis, in which the initial manifestation may be monoarticular; (c) Traumatic synovitis, or joint effusion, in which a definite history of trauma is not always available, particularly in children with an "irritable" hip; (d) Cellulitis, which usually shows more local skin redness and edema than septic arthritis and a wider area of local tenderness. Lymphadenopathy usually accompanies cellulitis, and swelling is not circumferential; (e) Acute rheumatic fever, in which the symptoms tend to move from joint to joint. This condition can also occur during the septicemia of acute septic arthritis; (f) Hemophilia, which may present a diagnostic problem only as the first presentation of a coagulation disorder; (g) Henoch-Schönlein purpura, which may present with single or multiple arthralgia before cutaneous manifestations appear; (h) Legg-Calvé-Perthes' disease, which may present with hip or knee joint discomfort and restriction of movement by muscle spasm. If there is doubt on clinical or radiological examination, aspiration should be performed; and (i) Lyme disease.

Diagnostic and Laboratory Investigation

An algorithm (Figure 18-1) is provided as an approach to diagnosis and management.

Absolute diagnosis of infectious arthritis is made by demonstration of bacteria in synovial fluid or recovery of bacteria from synovial fluid culture. Aspiration of a suspected septic joint is a simple technique. In

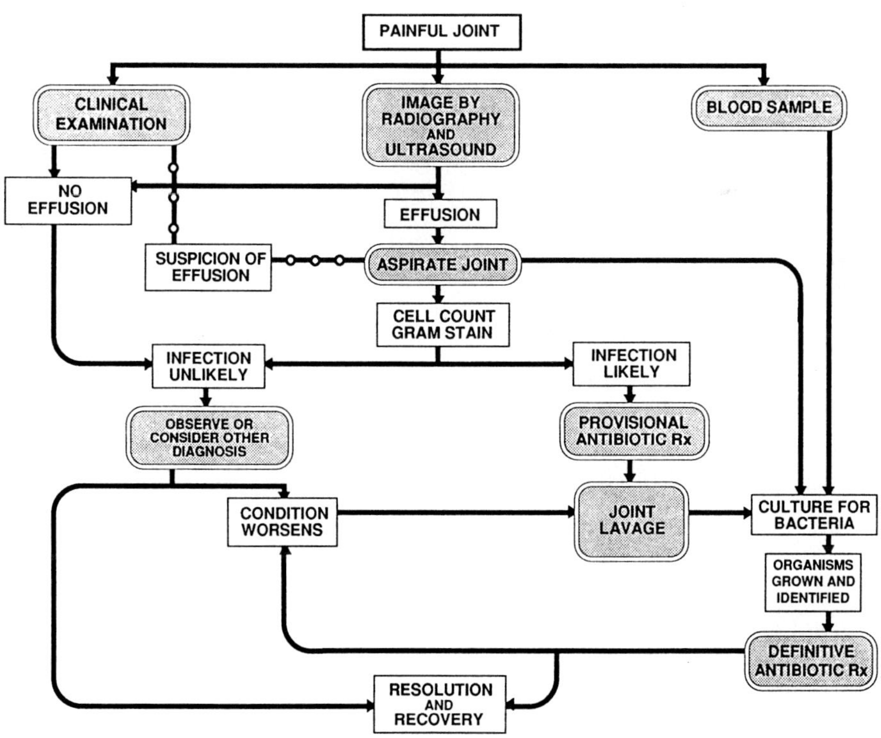

Figure 18-1. *Algorithm for investigation and management of infectious arthritis.*

a comparative study from two Australian cities, the aspiration rate of suspected septic joints in one was 93 of 184 patients (50%) and 36 of 110 patients (33%) in the other. Perhaps this finding reflects the different teaching of pediatric orthopedics in those medical centers. It also shows that an attempt at securing a diagnosis by the most direct method was not done as often as is advocated. Arthrocentesis should be performed with a wide-bore needle inserted into the joint through the site of easiest access, maximum tenderness, or fluctuation (if the pus is loculated). Puncture of the joint through an area of cellulitis should be avoided because of the risk of infecting a joint containing a sterile "sympathetic" effusion. Fluid obtained should not be assessed by its macroscopic appearance, because turbid fluid may not be infected and clear fluid may be teeming with organisms. In addition to bacteriological studies, cell counts of the fluid should be performed (33). Fluid from septic joints contains on average 100,000 cells/mm^3, with a range of 25,000 to 250,000 cells/mm^3. If there are more than 50,000 cells, of which more than 90% are polymorphonuclear leukocytes, infection is highly likely, even if organisms are not grown (34). However, it has recently been pointed out (35) that a significantly lower synovial fluid leukocytosis may be associated with culture-proven infection in immunocompromised patients, thus weakening its use as a diagnostic tool in this group of individuals.

Microscopy of gram-stained smears of a concentrated sediment of centrifuged joint fluid should also be done because the type of organism seen gives a good guide to the most effective choice of antibiotic before sensitivities are available.

Blood cultures should also be obtained before administration of antibiotics is begun. Any other septic areas in the body should be cultured. On occasion, the only clue to the cause of a septic arthritis has been obtained by culture of pathogens from cerebrospinal fluid or stool.

Radiographs of the affected site are usually quite helpful. Distension of the joint showing increased opacity, displacement of muscle surrounding the joint by the capsular distension, increased distance between the subchondral ends of bone, and even subluxation of the joint are frequently evident early in the course of the disease but are dependent on how peripheral the joint is (see Chapter 6).

Any doubt about the relevance of these radiological signs can be assessed by comparison with the opposite limb. In infants, because of the common delay in diagnosis, there may be evidence of erosion of the epiphysis or even its disappearance. Evidence of adjacent osteomyelitis should also be sought.

Ultrasound examination is now a useful tool in the detection of joint effusion, particularly in the hip, and because it can be done in real time, quickly, without moving the patient from bed, and is noninvasive, it is becoming an extension of regular clinical examination, both in hospitals and in office consulting rooms.

Management

In contrast to general agreement about management of a septic hip, there is much controversy aroused when other joints are involved.

There are two essential duties to perform: First, antibiotics must be given to diminish the systemic effects of sepsis; and second, the bacterial population and the concentration of chondrolytic products in a joint must be reduced. If unstable, a septic joint must be rested in a stable position, but clinical experience now seems to favor continuous passive motion early in treatment if the joint is stable. The major long-term sequel of infectious arthritis is degenerative osteoarthritis of the joint, which follows destruction of articular cartilage. The therapeutic principle that must be followed is that although antibiotics alone may control the infection, the health of the cartilage is dependent on drainage and lavage (36).

Choice of Antibiotics

Antibiotics used must be appropriate in type, dose, administration route, and duration. If the diagnosis of acute septic arthritis is suspected, antibiotics should not be administered before blood has been obtained for culture and aspiration of the joint has been performed. It takes approximately 48 hours before sensitivity of organisms to antibiotics can be determined; during that period, antibiotics should be given on a provisional or "best guess" basis. Knowledge of the natural history of the disease, age of the child, and type of organism (if seen) on a gram-stained smear of fluid aspirated from a joint are the best guides to the choice of the most appropriate antibiotic.

When a clinical diagnosis is made, an etiological agent is only found in approximately 60% of patients. In infants under 6 months of age, the most likely organisms are staphylococci or gram-negative enteric pathogens (11); between 6 months and 2 years of age, staphylococci or *Hemophilus influenzae;* and older than 2 years of age, staphylococci. Examination of a gram-stained smear of aspirates from children under 2 years of age could therefore be useful in determining whether the infecting organism was a staphylococcus, an enteric pathogen, or *H. influenzae.* Various recommendations—such as the combined use of methicillin and ampicillin as provisional therapy (37); or penicillin and a beta-lactamase–resistant drug given systemically, together with irrigation of the joint with penicillin, neomycin, and bacitracin (38)—have been made. These recommendations will vary, so use of provisional or "best guess" antibiotics should be based on age and smear findings.

In neonates, we recommend a third-generation cephalosporin or beta-lactamase–resistant penicillin in appropriate divided doses. In the age group 6 months to 2 years, ceftriaxone (75–100 mg/kg/day in divided doses every 12 hours) seems most appropriate. A sufficient number of patients with *H. influenzae* infectious arthritis resistant to ampicillin or amoxicillin have now been reported (39) to make these drugs less useful as provisional therapy. For children older than 2 years of age, an antistaphylococcal beta-lactamase–resistant drug alone can be administered (100–200 mg/kg/day in 4–6 divided doses).

All authors recommend the parenteral (preferably intravenous) route for initial administration of antibiotics. Obviously, when organisms have been cultured and their antibiotic sensitivity is known, the definitive antibiotic should be used in effective dosage. A careful study (11) pointed out the increasingly important etiological role of *H. influenzae* since the 1950s; this role may decline with the advent of widespread immunization against *H. influenzae* type b. As the natural history of the disease changes and as bacteria change their characteristics of antibiotic sensitivity, the most appropriate antibiotic to use initially will vary. Continuing studies to monitor microbiological data are mandatory to ensure that the most effective therapy will always be used.

Route of Antibiotic Administration

The major question regarding administration concerns the intra-articular route. An experimental study (40) in rabbits found that intra-articular administration of antibiotics produced sterility in the joint sooner than when given by the intramuscular route. In another experiment (41), irreversible joint damage occurred early in the course of suppurative arthritis, and sterilization of the joint, even by the intra-articular route, did not prevent this damage. It would appear that early institution of appropriate treatment is more important than the route of administration. Although removal of pus from the joint by aspiration is advocated (42), there is no need for intra-articular antibiotics, because adequate concentrations of antibiotic in the joint can be achieved by systemic administration. There is a paucity of good information regarding the transfer of antibiotics across synovium, particularly when inflamed. Attempts to compare joint levels following intra-articular, intramuscular, and intravenous administration of antibiotics (43–45) found that for most antibiotics (except erythromycin), the intravenous route was just as effective as the intramuscular route in producing intra-articular levels that were the same or even higher than those obtained by giving the antibiotic directly into the joint. The levels obtained with the normally recommended doses were greater than in vitro levels required to inhibit bacteria.

The pharmacodynamics of antibiotic penetration into joints has rarely been addressed (46). Evidence suggests that serum antibiotic concentration is the most important determinant of joint fluid penetration. Measurement of serum levels may be useful, but no studies have established appropriate levels needed. Intra-articular antibiotics are absorbed rapidly into the systemic circulation (47). In summary, there is no reason to use intra-articular antibiotics given the efficacy of intravenous administration.

Aspiration, Irrigation, or Arthrotomy

The basic aims of treatment are to sterilize the joint, evacuate the bacterial products and debris associated with infection, relieve pain, and prevent deformity. To achieve at least the second aim, we recommend surgical lavage of some type in all patients.

Until 20 years ago, much of the treatment of septic arthritis was derived from literature that contained opinions based on theory with a surprising paucity of clinical review (1). Using a strict routine based on four main principles—(a) immediate arthrotomy, (b) complete skin closure without drainage, (c) immobilization, and (d) antibiotics—surgeons in Adelaide, Australia, found that there were no failures if arthrotomy was performed within 5 days of onset of symptoms; if after

5 days, results were bad. This routine was a great improvement on previous outcomes. When arthrotomy was done within 5 days for childhood hip joint infection, there were no failures in 14 patients, compared with a high failure rate for late arthrotomy or other treatments. A logical extension of those findings would be to recommend early arthrotomy in all patients with acute septic arthritis.

Because such emphatic support had not been warranted by clinical experience from the Royal Hospital for Sick Children in Glasgow (48), however, the need for arthrotomy might be selective but not mandatory. There is little dispute about arthrotomy for septic hips in infants; perhaps in an older child, an infected hip can be treated by aspiration if the duration of symptoms is less than 4 days, and other joints could possibly be managed by aspiration.

Arthroscopy has become widely available and surgeons have become skilled in the technique. With such skill, joint lavage under arthroscopic vision can be performed in preference to arthrotomy if the facilities are available. Indeed, it has been stated (49) that compared with needle aspiration/irrigation or standard formal arthrotomy, arthroscopic evacuation of a septic joint provides significant joint distension and copious lavage. All preliminary reports show excellent results in both children and adults (50–53). Multiple needle aspiration has been compared with formal arthrotomy for pyarthrosis of the knee (54). If the history was longer than 3 days or if the causative organism was *S. aureus* or enteric gram-negative organisms, open drainage by arthrotomy was desirable. Although arthroscopically guided joint lavage may replace open arthrotomy, there seems little support for repeated needle aspiration to relieve pain and to remove inhibitors of bacterial killing (34). There is a strong case against repeated aspiration of joints (1) because the tension within the joint recurs, the procedure is painful, the results are uncertain, and pus is often thick and cannot be aspirated, even under tension. If a policy of arthrotomy for all septic arthritis is pursued, unnecessary arthrotomy occurs infrequently, and its effects are not noticeable in the incised joint.

Regarding treatment of the hip joint, there is no dissent. Knowing of the potential sequela of this condition (55), most authorities (1,15,56) advise surgical drainage as soon as possible if an aspirate of the joint reveals suppuration. Our preferred approach is drainage by a posterior incision making a wide hole in the capsule, with adequate irrigation and primary skin closure. This technique allows for dependent drainage. Following surgical drainage, splintage of the hip should be in abduction to prevent dislocation only if there is apparent instability at the time of surgery. Appropriate antibiotics should be administered systemically.

There should be no remorse if a hip is explored and pus is not found. The issues are formidable, and an occasional error is therefore justifiable and should be minimized if ultrasound imaging is available. If there is any doubt in the mind of the physician, clinical features should be the principal guide to intervention, not imaging.

Drainage

Institution of open drainage following arthrotomy is of historical interest only. Following adequate lavage of a joint at arthrotomy, closure of the skin without any form of drainage is adequate as long as the joint capsule is not closed (1). This is similar to the principle laid down by Trueta (57) for the treatment of acute osteomyelitis. Closed drainage systems using suction, with or without irrigation, are still used (58), but no comparison has been made of the end results after closed drainage or suction irrigation compared with primary skin closure and no drainage.

Duration of Treatment

The duration of immobilization and antibiotic therapy in acute septic arthritis is empirical. Various recommendations include: 6 weeks of immobilization and 6 weeks of antibiotic therapy (1) 2 to 3 weeks after patients became afebrile and joint effusion had ceased (37); systemic use of antibiotics by an intravenous route for 3 weeks and then orally for 3 weeks using the return to normality of the erythrocyte sedimentation rate (ESR) and clinical appearance as a guide (38); and 4 to 6 weeks of intravenous therapy for hip pyarthrosis followed by 3 months of oral therapy (59). Studies such as those performed by Blockey and Watson (60) regarding the duration of antibiotic therapy in acute hematogenous osteomyelitis have not been performed in patients with septic arthritis. The opinion of other surgeons from the same hospital with respect to infectious arthritis in children (48), however, was that at least 3 weeks of treatment should be given.

It is our view that an empirical period of antibiotic treatment of four weeks is adequate, as long as adequate blood levels have been maintained. Immobilization of the joint for this period no longer seems necessary, following wider acceptance of the advocacy by Salter and colleagues (61) of the technique of continuous passive motion following joint lavage. We do not advocate immobilization of joints after treatment for acute infection has commenced.

Outcome

Unfortunately, there is no clear statement of the current outcome after septic arthritis. It is generally accepted that prognosis after hip infection in neonates is poor, but for the other joints, the introduction of antibiotics has improved the prognosis. Factors predicting outcome in individual patients have not been defined.

Bad sequela of hip sepsis (55,56) include (a) destruction of the capital epiphysis with dislocation of the hip; (b) destruction of the capital epiphysis (the femoral neck remains in the acetabulum); (c) destruction of the growth plate (the femoral head remains in the acetabulum connected to the femoral neck by fibrous union); and (d) recovery with coxa magna, but no other deformity. In the preantibiotic era, complications of septic arthritis were frequent. A study of the end results in 113 patients with septic hips found only 7 in which a normal hip joint resulted following treatment (4). An additional 23 patients had a "functional hip joint" (i.e., 50% of the normal range of motion). Dislocation of the hip joint was common and was avoided by placing the leg in extension and abduction.

Sequestration of the head of the femur with spontaneous absorption (epiphysiolysis), or requiring removal, occurred in 43 patients. Although it is usually stated to be "aseptic necrosis" due to ischemia following increased intra-articular pressure, there is no good evidence for this classification, and transphyseal spread of osteomyelitis in infants is more likely. Following loss of the femoral head, some patients had normal range of motion but a marked Trendelenburg gait, and others had less than normal motion. Fibrous or bony ankylosis was a common sequel to loss of the femoral head. Methods of salvage and reconstruction after the various types of proximal femoral destruction have recently been reviewed (62).

Since the introduction of antibiotics, death no longer appears to follow acute septic arthritis. There are very few studies of outcome after septic arthritis in the antibiotic era. None are long term. Thirty nine of 52 patients had no disability through follow-up periods varying from a few months to 10 years (10). Thirteen patients showed one or more (a) limitation of motion, (b) osteomyelitis, or (c) dislocation of the hip. Another study (22) followed 15 patients with 21 involved joints for periods exceeding 10 years; 8 patients showed disturbances in growth (7 hips and 1 shoulder), and 10 of 19 hips had dislocated. All patients demonstrated destruction of the femoral capital epiphysis.

All complications had a direct relationship to the duration of joint symptoms prior to diagnosis and definitive treatment. Seventy-seven percent of all complications occurred in children who had symptoms for 7 or more days before establishment of diagnosis and treatment. Seventy-five percent of hip sepsis treated by aspiration, but only 47% treated by incision and drainage, showed dislocation. However, a translucent zone in the radiograph does not necessarily mean that part of the bone, epiphyseal cartilage, or growth plate is irreversibly destroyed (63). Clinical examination, occasionally augmented by arthrography, can usually confirm that cartilage or decalcified bone survived infection, particularly in the knee joint, in which the prognosis is far better than that of the hip joint. When there has been involvement of the growth plate, conventional treatment for shortening or deformity is indicated.

Although it has been said (24) that complete destruction of hip and shoulder joints can be expected in the premature and neonatal periods if incision and drainage are not accomplished within 48 to 72 hours of onset, this observation has not been confirmed by recent studies, in which the infecting agent was methicillin-resistant *S. aureus* in a neonatal intensive care unit (64). Nevertheless, the most important single factor for the preservation of a well-functioning joint is early diagnosis and adequate treatment.

The variability in presentation of this disease might be a function of immunological competence (65). In a retrospective study of 12 children known to have pyogenic arthritis in infancy, 6 still had hypofunction of the antibody-complement-phagocyte pathway. Furthermore, the extent of joint destruction was directly related to the presence of immunodeficiency.

To determine which factors affected prognosis, 38 patients with 39 involved septic hips were reviewed over a 21-year period (66). There were only two significant correlations with poor prognosis: the duration from clinical onset to initiation of therapy and the age of the child, especially if under 1 year of age. These findings were confirmed in another study of 45 hip joints in 43 infants and children. Four days seemed to be the delay in starting treatment that separated satisfactory from bad outcomes (67). Concomitant osteomyelitis of the femur produced a far worse prognosis than if the infection was confined to the synovium of the hip joint. If *S. aureus* was the causative organism, the prognosis was worse compared with other organisms.

In a recent unpublished study performed in Western Australia, outcome in 34 patients who had been treated for septic arthritis of infancy and childhood between 10 and 25 years previously was determined. None had any significant problem in the affected joint, and only those who were noted to have pus in the joint at the time of infection reported any late symptoms. The modes of therapy were not identical, but there was no difference in outcome related to type of treatment.

The term *postinfectious synovitis* has been used (68) to describe joints that were warm and tender, with accumulation of fluid within them, and had thickened synovium, in children without evidence of fever or other systemic disturbance. The one feature common to all patients in whom this syndrome developed was use of repeated injection of antibiotics into the affected joint; the syndrome was never observed in patients who did not receive instillation of antibiotics. Repeated arthrocentesis may increase the risk of superinfection.

Several classification and treatment schemes have been developed for deformities after hip sepsis (62,69,70). Patients with incongruent stable hips did worse than those with complete head destruction and dislocation. They concluded that for such painless hips, nonoperative treatment was indicated until adolescence, when an epiphysiodesis should be performed on the opposite side to correct leg length discrepancy. Techniques used by orthopedic surgeons to attempt to correct problems after infectious arthritis are many and varied and remain outside the scope of this book. Early mobilization of joints with septic arthritis is not a new concept, but it has not been widely practiced until recently (61). A recent study involving 14 children (71) who received antibiotic therapy, open arthrotomy, and suction drainage and were then subjected to continuous passive movement of the affected joint showed that the infection was eradicated in all children without recurrence. All were free from pain, had full range of movement in the affected joint, and normal gait 2 years after the acute pyarthrosis.

Bacterial Arthritis in Adults

Although bacterial arthritis is commonly hematogenously acquired, joints may be infected by bacteria entering from a penetrating wound, contiguous osteomyelitis, intra-articular injection, arthroscopy, or prosthetic joint surgery. The pathological changes appear to be the same regardless of the source of infection.

Joint effusions associated with disseminated gonococcal infection are often sterile and may involve immune or hypersensitivity mechanisms. This condition has been described as reactive arthritis rather than direct invasion with the organism. A component of gonococcal cell wall appears to act as the antigen to which synovium reacts. A review of the Mayo Clinic data for adult septic arthritis (72) found involvement of the knee in half, and the hip and shoulder each in one fourth the total patients.

Certain aspects of host–microbial interactions might explain why bacterial arthritis develops in certain persons, whereas most bacteremias do not result in a septic joint (73). Such factors include host phagocytic defects (e.g., chronic granulomatous disease, Chédiak-Higashi syndrome), impaired host defense mechanisms (e.g., hypogammaglobulinemia, cancer, chronic liver disease, immunosuppressive drugs), and rheumatoid arthritis, with granulation tissue in the involved joint.

In the population of human immunodeficiency virus (HIV)–infected individuals, particularly those with the acquired immunodeficiency syndrome, musculoskeletal infection may be more common than is widely recognized (74). Diagnosis is especially difficult in this group of patients because many will already have received a wide range of antimicrobial drugs prior to assessment. Even minimal joint swelling may indicate local infection in an immunocompromised individual. Tissue diagnosis is important because of the alternative possibilities of lymphoma or Kaposi's sarcoma; in some patients, malignant and infective lesions may coexist. The most commonly involved joint is the knee, and in the majority of patients, *S. aureus* or *S. pneumoniae* is the cause.

Opportunistic pathogens must also be suspected, and prompt appropriate treatment is often effective.

Nongonococcal Bacterial Arthritis

The organisms found are usually *S. aureus,* various species of streptococci, *E. coli,* and *Pseudomonas aeruginosa* (frequent in drug abusers). *H. influenzae* rarely affects adult joints. However, there are numerous isolated reports of large numbers of unusual bacteria as causes. *Borrelia burgdorferi* causes Lyme disease, which manifests as an arthritis.

Nongonococcal bacterial arthritis usually involves only one joint, most commonly the knee. Shoulder, hip, wrist, interphalangeal, and elbow joints may be affected. Most persons who suffer such infections have one or more underlying medical conditions, which may be risk factors. Cancer, hepatic cirrhosis, diabetes mellitus, rheumatoid arthritis, previous damage to joints, in-dwelling catheters, and intravenous drug addiction are risk factors. Approximately half the patients have a positive blood culture (75).

Mild fever is common, but rigors are rare. Peripheral blood leukocytosis is not always found. Synovial leukocyte count is usually greater than 50,000/mm^3. If the diagnosis is suspected and the synovial leukocyte count is lower than 50,000/mm^3, repeat arthrocentesis one day later usually shows an increased level. More than 90% are polymorphonuclear leukocytes.

Therapy requires antibiotic administration and arthrolavage. We have been impressed with continuous passive motion (as opposed to immobility by splintage), which results in rapid rehabilitation after arthrolavage. The initial choice of antibiotics will depend on the findings at examination of a gram-stained smear of joint fluid. This test should precede surgery, and antibiotic therapy should be initiated soon after. The choice of antibiotics will depend on the likelihood of certain infections. Any potential source of bacteremia should also be sampled. Antibiotics should be administered by vein in the first instance. Definitive drugs should be substituted for provisional antibiotics, in appropriate doses, once organisms and their sensitivities are known. Oral administration can be commenced when the patient is eating (usually within 48 hours of commencing effective treatment). Duration of therapy is empirical (e.g., 3–6 weeks). There is no indication for intra-articular administration of antibiotics.

A review of 18 patients with infectious arthritis of the shoulder (76) showed that nearly all had at least one serious associated disease and a delay in diagnosis. The ESR was always increased, but not necessarily body temperature or white blood cell count. After treatment, the functional result was usually poor. Arthrotomy appeared to offer a better result than repeated aspiration.

Sacroiliac joint infection is also uncommon; indeed, it is never certain whether the infection arises in the joint or in adjacent bone. Buttock, thigh, or lumbar pain are the usual symptoms, and most patients present within approximately 3 weeks of onset of pain, although longer delays in diagnosis are well recognized. Systemic signs of infection are usual. The ESR is usually increased. Radioisotope scanning frequently identifies a focus in the region of the sacroiliac joint, and computerized tomography is useful in identifying the extent of bone and joint involvement and soft-tissue extension of an abscess. Magnetic resonance imaging may show direction of fistulation of pus. Identification of causative organism may be achieved by culture of blood, but diagnostic aspiration is often difficult and should be done under computerized tomographic control. *S. aureus* is a frequent cause, and if therapy is to be given without bacteriological diagnosis, it should be directed at that organism. The role of surgery has not been determined; in the past, recommendations were given for nonoperative treatment (77). However, should the response to antibiotic administration not be obvious in 48 hours, then consideration should be given to surgical drainage or at least percutaneous insertion of a drainage catheter under radiological control.

Septic arthritis in the elderly population has been poorly described in the literature. The knee is most commonly involved (78) in patients over 60 years of age. Concurrent medical illness is found in the majority, with diabetes mellitus in one fourth. Two thirds had radiological evidence of pre-existing joint disease in the affected joint. Most were afebrile and had a normal blood white cell count at presentation. The ESR was elevated in all. Despite surgical treatment, the complication rate was high, with osteomyelitis developed in 38%, secondary osteoarthritis in 14%, and mortality due to sepsis in 19%. Septic arthritis in adults may be difficult to diagnose and carries a poor prognosis despite aggressive management.

Lancefield group B streptococcal arthritis is uncommon but warrants special mention. Although the organisms are usually quite sensitive to penicillin G, they may manifest aggressive behavior to joints, both normal and prosthetic, and involve multiple joints (27,28). Diabetes mellitus seems to be a risk factor. The most reliable method of diagnosis is by culture of joint fluid, but radioisotope scanning may reveal multiple affected joints in the same patient. This polyarticular involvement may be associated with a poor prognosis, including the need to remove prosthetic joints. The sites of infection are often central: acromioclavicular, sternoclavicular, manubriosternal, or lumbar intervertebral disk. Complete functional recovery may not occur because of permanent structural damage to the joints. This feature has not gained prominence in earlier literature on septic arthritis.

Septic arthritis due to group G beta-hemolytic streptococci has somewhat different features (26). Men are frequently affected (80%), and polyarticular infection occurred in approximately half the patients. The median age reported was 63 years, with a broad range. The most common joint affected was the knee, both unoperated or prosthetic. An extra-articular focus of infection could be detected in approximately half the patients, particularly cellulitis or endocarditis. Debilitating underlying conditions were not prominent.

Gonococcal Arthritis

Arthritis is the principal musculoskeletal complication of gonorrhea. Knee, wrist, ankle, and hand joints are commonly involved. Tenosynovitis occurs in approximately one third of patients. Osteomyelitis is rare (79,80) and, when present, has usually spread from an infected joint. The usual subject is a young and healthy adult. A migratory arthralgia, moving from joint to joint, is the clue to suspect a gonococcal cause. It is reported that septic arthritis will develop in 17% to 33% of patients with disseminated gonococcal infection, and *N. gonorrhoeae* is now the most common cause of infective arthritis in young adults under 30 years of age (81).

N. gonorrhoeae initially attaches to and penetrates genital mucosa. The incidence of disseminated gonococcal infection (DGI) with gonococcemia, which must precede isolation of the organism from a bone or joint infection, is estimated at 0.5% to 3% of all individuals with gonorrhea (82); *N. gonorrhoeae* can be recovered in blood or synovial culture from approximately half. Many cases of tenosynovitis and arthritis are reactive, and organisms cannot be isolated (82); however, in North America and in parts of the developing world, *N. gonor-*

rhoeae is the most common isolate in infectious arthritis in the sexually active population (83). In Europe, the incidence of septic gonococcal arthritis appears to be lower (84).

There are two distinct clinical presentations of arthritis in DGI (82). In the first, monoarthritis is recognized by a swollen, tender joint, with loss of function. Aspiration or biopsy usually reveals *N. gonorrhoeae*. The arthritis is often sterile, but leukocyte counts greater than 50,000/mm^3 are common. Gram-stained smears are positive in less than one fourth of patients with gonococcal arthritis. In the second, more common presentation, patients have a systemic illness characterized by migratory polyarthralgia, which settles into one or more joints and is associated with a pustular dermatitis and tenosynovitis that may occasionally be suppurative (85,86). The usual skin lesions are small papules on trunk or extremities, but bullae, vesicles, pustules, and purpura have been reported.

Investigation should include blood culture, aspiration, and culture of skin lesions and potentially infected mucosal sites, including urethra, cervix, pharynx, anus, or conjunctiva. If gonococcal arthritis is suspected, the microbiology laboratory should be alerted if possible swabs should be plated onto chocolate agar by the bedside. Serological tests for gonococcal infection are useful. Blood cultures are positive in less than 10% and are almost never positive simultaneously with joint culture.

Antibiotic management is the essential element of treatment. In many parts of the world, the incidence of penicillin-resistant strains of *N. gonorrhoeae* is sufficient to warrant the use of ceftriaxone for 7 to 10 days as the most effective initial treatment for DGI. If penicillin allergy is demonstrated, oral tetracycline or doxycycline may be substituted (82). In contrast to nongonococcal arthritis, arthrolavage is not usually needed for *N. gonorrhoeae* infections. Aspiration of involved joints and drainage of any suppurative collection are required. If a bacterial cause for arthritis is not determined, the therapeutic response to penicillin may be used as a further criterion to make a presumptive diagnosis of gonococcal infection.

Hemophilus Influenzae Infections

Although widely available immunization is likely to dramatically reduce the incidence of infection by *H. influenzae* type b, its importance as a musculoskeletal pathogen dictates a short description of the features. As well as suppurative disease, reactive arthritis occurs, as sequelae shared with other gram-negative pathogens that primarily lodge on mucosal surfaces (87). Infections caused by a range of other *Hemophilus* species have also been reported (88–91). The age-specific incidence of *H. influenzae* bacteremia varies in different societies with similar overall incidence; most episodes occur in the first few years of life. In Israel, contemporary data suggest that more than 90% of infections occur in children less than 2 years old. In Australia, the proportion is less than 50% (92,93). In the developed world it appears safe to assume that most infections occur in children less than 5 years of age, but both osteomyelitis and arthritis occur in older children (94) and in adults, in whom vertebral infections appear to be the most common manifestation (95–98). Risk of *H. influenzae* infection may be increased in patients with sickle-cell anemia (99,100), after splenectomy, and in HIV infection (101,102). Musculoskeletal sites account for approximately one-eighth of severe *H. influenzae* infections (103); these infections include septic arthritis (94,96), cellulitis (103), tenosynovitis (104,105), osteomyelitis (106), and soft-tissue abscesses (107). Only cellulitis has special features: it is characteristically raised, warm, reddish-blue in color, and is most often seen on the cheek in children. The risk of associated meningitis is substantial in individuals with *H. influenzae* bacteremia, even if local signs are present in the musculoskeletal system (103). Reactive arthritis in severe *H. influenzae* infection appears to have been generally recognized only in the last decade (108).

Other than the choice of antibiotic (109,110), the general principles of management are discussed in Chapter 7.

Meningococcal Infections

Joint symptoms occur and are quite common in meningococcal infection (111). Four types of presentation have been described (112), including arthritis associated with meningitis, isolated meningococcal purulent arthritis, and an arthritis-dermatitis syndrome resembling DGI, which appears to be becoming more common (113).

As in DGI, organisms may not always be isolated from blood or synovium in meningococcal arthritis-dermatitis syndrome. In monoarticular arthritis, which occurs mainly in infants (112), synovial cultures are regularly positive. Osteomyelitis has been described in children whose meningococcemia was complicated by disseminated intravascular coagulation (114–116). Examples of healed vertebral infection reported in the preantibiotic era (117) were attributed to direct spread from lumbar puncture; however, spondylitis can also occur following meningococcemia (118,119).

Penicillin is the drug of choice in meningococcal infections; chloramphenicol is an alternative when penicillin allergy is suspected.

Viral Arthritis

In patients with fever, rash, lymphadenopathy, and arthritis or arthralgia, a viral cause should be considered. Such a symptom complex is not uncommon. Arthropathy may be acute, subacute, or chronic in its mode of presentation. The most common viral diseases associated with arthropathy are rubella, hepatitis B, alphaviruses (Ross River virus in Australia, chikungunya in South East Asia, O'nyong-nyong in Kenya and Uganda), and parvovirus (in the United Kingdom). Epstein-Barr virus, associated with the symptoms of infectious mononucleosis, is commonly associated with an arthropathy. There is evidence of an immune complex mediation in a number of forms of viral arthritis. In some patients, the virus can be isolated from synovial fluid, but the specific role in joint pathology is not known.

Septic Bursitis

Septic bursitis, particularly on the extensor aspect of the knee and elbow, is a well-recognized clinical entity (120–122). Nonseptic bursitis due to gout, rheumatoid arthritis, or other causes, is more common than infective bursitis. In the infective cases, *S. aureus* is reponsible for more than 90%; hemolytic streptococci and anaerobes are also found (123). In half the patients there is an association with overlying skin lesions, and if magnification were used, a break in the integument might be seen more often. There is a history of previous trauma to the bursa or occupational irritation of the overlying skin in approximately 40% of patients. Constant features are peribursal cellulitis, edema, and bursal tenderness. About the knee, the involved bursa may be prepatellar (defined clearly by the bony margins of the patella), or infrapatellar (overlying the tubercule of the tibia). Fever is not a regular feature. An effusion may occur in the neighboring knee or elbow but is usually small and difficult to detect clinically. In patients with rheumatoid arthritis and an olecranon nodule with or without septic bursitis, there may also be infection in the elbow joint, which can be difficult to diagnose because of the surrounding inflammation and distorted anatomy (124).

Diagnosis is confirmed by aspiration, gram-stain, and culture of the bursal fluid. Although there are distinguishing features in the bursal fluid, such as cell count and fluid-to-serum glucose ratio (123), they are not usually required in diagnosis. Treatment involves administration of an appropriate antibiotic and rest of the region. If aspiration of the bursa is done for diagnostic purposes (this is not always necessary), the bursa can be drained at that time. Large collections of bursal fluid, as may be found in the olecranon bursa, should be drained by aspiration to allow the synovial lining of the bursa to appose and adhere. Operative surgical drainage by incision is rarely required.

Chronic bursal infection is seen in tuberculosis (125), atypical mycobacterial infection (126), brucellosis (127), fungal infections (128), and tertiary syphilis and yaws, in which firm periarticular nodules resembling those in rheumatoid arthritis may occur (129,130). These chronic lesions are usually amenable to appropriate chemotherapy.

References

1. Paterson DC. Acute suppurative arthritis in infancy and childhood. J Bone Joint Surg [Br] 1970;52:474–482.
2. Lloyd-Roberts GC. Septic arthritis in infancy. Aust Paediatr J 1979;15: 41–43.
3. Phemister DB. The effect of pressure on articular surfaces in pyogenic and tuberculous arthritides and its bearing upon treatment. Ann Surg 1924;80: 481–500.
4. Badgley CE, Yglesias L, Perham WS, et al. Study of the end results in 113 cases of septic hips. J Bone Joint Surg 1936;18:1047–1061.
5. Heberling JA. A review of two hundred and one cases of suppurative arthritis. J Bone Joint Surg 1941;23:917–921.
6. Hunter W. Of the structure and disease of articulating cartilages. Philos Trans R Soc Lond 1743;42:514–522.
7. Brodie BC. Pathological and surgical observations on diseases of joints. London: Longman, 1819.

8. Bick EM. Source book of orthopaedics, ed 2. Baltimore: Williams & Wilkins, 1948.
9. Morrey BF, Bianco AJ, Rhodes JH. Septic arthritis in children. Orthop Clin North Am 1975;6:923–934.
10. Borella L, Goodbar JE, Summitt RL, Clark GM. Septic arthritis in childhood. J Pediatr 1963;62:742–747.
11. Nelson JD, Koontz WC. Septic arthritis in infants and children: a review of 117 cases. Pediatrics 1966;38:966–971.
12. Wiley JJ, Fraser GA. Septic arthritis in childhood. Can J Surg 1979;22: 326–330.
13. Nade S, Robertson FW, Taylor TKF. Antibiotics in the treatment of acute osteomyelitis and acute septic arthritis in children. Med J Aust 1974;2: 703–705.
14. Alderson M, Emslie KR, Speers DJ, Nade S. Acute haematogenous osteomyelitis and septic arthritis—a single disease: an hypothesis based upon the presence of transphyseal blood vessels. J Bone Joint Surg [Br] 1986;58: 268–274.
15. Lloyd-Roberts GC. Orthopaedics in infancy and childhood. London: Butterworths, 1971.
16. Dan M. Septic arthritis in young infants: clinical and microbiologic correlations and therapeutic implications. Rev Infect Dis 1984;6:147–155.
17. Almquist EE. The changing epidemiology of septic arthritis in children. Clin Orthop 1970;68:96–99.
18. Martin CM, Merrill RH, Barrett ON. Arthritis due to Serratia. J Bone Joint Surg [Am] 1970;52:1450–1452.
19. Torg JS, Lammot TR. Septic arthritis of the knee due to Clostridium welchii. J Bone Joint Surg [Am] 1968;50:1233–1236.
20. Macy NJ, Lieber L, Haberman ET. Arthritis caused by Clostridium septicum. J Bone Joint Surg [Am] 1986;68:465–466.
21. Clarke HJ, Allum R. Anaerobic septic arthritis due to bacteroides: brief report. J Bone Joint Surg [Br] 1988;70:847–848.
22. Samilson RL, Bersani FA, Watkins MB. Acute suppurative arthritis in infants and children. Pediatrics 1958;21:798–804.
23. Obletz BE. Acute suppurative arthritis of the hip in the neonatal period. J Bone Joint Surg [Am] 1960;42:23–30.
24. Baitch A. Recent observations of acute suppurative arthritis. Clin Orthop 1962;22:157–166.
25. Yagupsky P, Dagan R, Howard CW, Einhorn M, Kassis I, Simu A. High prevalence of Kingella kingae in joint fluid from children with septic arthritis revealed by the BACTEC blood culture system. J Clin Microbiol 1992; 30:1278–1281.
26. Burkert T, Watanakunakorn C. Group G Streptococcus septic arthritis and osteomyelitis: report and literature review. J Rheumatol 1991;18:904–907.
27. Small CB, Slater LN, Lowy FD, Small RD, Salvati EA, Casey JI. Group B streptococcal arthritis in adults. Am J Med 1984;76:367–375.

28. Pischel KD, Weisman MH, Cone RO. Unique features of Group B streptococcal arthritis in adults. Arch Intern Med 1985;145:97–102.
29. Ortel TL, Kallianos J, Gallis HA. Group C streptococcal arthritis: case report and review. Rev Infect Dis 1990;12:829–837.
30. Rady M, Turner PG, Ross ERS. Group G streptococcal septic arthritis. Br J Clin Pract 1990;44:287–289.
31. McAllister CM, Zillmer D, Cobelli NJ. Clostridium perfringens and Staphylococcus epidermidis polymicrobial septic arthritis. Clin Orthop 1989;241: 245–247.
32. Smith T. On the acute arthritis of children. St Barts Hosp Rep 1874;10: 189–204.
33. Curtiss PH. Changes produced in the synovial membrane and synovial fluid by disease. J Bone Joint Surg [Am] 1964;46:873–888.
34. Ward J, Cohen AS, Bauer W. The diagnosis and therapy of acute suppurative arthritis. Arthritis Rheum 1960;3:522–535.
35. McCutchan HJ, Fisher RC. Synovial leukocytosis in infectious arthritis. Clin Orthop 1990;257:226–230.
36. Shaw BA, Kasser JR. Acute septic arthritis in infancy and childhood. Clin Orthop 1990;257:212–225.
37. Clawson DK, Dunn AW. Management of common bacterial infections of bones and joints. J Bone Joint Surg [Am] 1967;49:164–182.
38. Griffin PP. Bone and joint infections in children. Pediatr Clin North Am 1967;14:533–558.
39. Chang MJ, Controni G, Rodriguez WJ. Ampicillin-resistant Haemophilus influenzae Type B septic arthritis in children. Clin Pediatr 1981;20:139–141.
40. Bardenheier JA, Morgan HC, Stamp WG. Treatment and sequelae of experimentally produced septic arthritis. Surg Gynecol Obstet 1966;122: 249–254.
41. Orchard RA, Stamp WG. Early treatment of induced suppurative arthritis in rabbit knee joints. Clin Orthop 1968;59:287–294.
42. Schmid FR, Parker RH. Ongoing assessment of therapy in septic arthritis. Arthritis Rheum 1969;12:529–534.
43. Nelson JD. Antibiotic concentrations in septic joint effusions. N Engl J Med 1971;284:349–353.
44. Drutz DJ, Schaffner W, Hillman JW, et al. The penetrations of penicillin and other antimicrobials into joint fluid. J Bone Joint Surg [Am] 1967;49: 1415–1421.
45. Parker RH, Schmid FR. Antibacterial activity of synovial fluid during therapy of septic arthritis. Arthritis Rheum 1971;14:96–104.
46. Fraser GL. Treatment of nongonococcal bacterial septic arthritis. Drug Intell Clin Pharm 1981;151:531–535.
47. Schurman DJ, Kajiyama G. Antibiotic absorption from infected and normal joints using a rabbit knee joint model. J Orthop Res 1985;3:185–188.
48. Wilson NIL, DiPaola M. Acute septic arthritis in infancy and childhood. J Bone Joint Surg [Br] 1986;68:584–587.

49. Stanitski CL, Harwell JC, Fu FH. Arthroscopy in acute septic knees: management in paediatric patients. Clin Orthop 1989;241:209–212.
50. Jarrett MP, Grossman L, Sadler AH, Grayzel AI. The role of arthroscopy in the treatment of septic arthritis. Arthritis Rheum 1981;24:737–739.
51. Parisien JS. Arthroscopic management of pyarthrosis. Bull Hosp Joint Dis Orthop Inst 1987;47:52–57.
52. Skyhar MJ, Mubarak SJ. Arthroscopic treatment of septic knees in children. J Pediatr Orthop 1987;7:647–651.
53. Ivey M, Clark R. Arthroscopic debridement of the knee for septic arthritis. Clin Orthop 1985;199:201–206.
54. Lane JG, Falahee MH, Wojtys EM, Hankin FM, Kaufer H. Pyarthrosis of the knee: treatment considerations. Clin Orthop 1990;252:198–204.
55. Eyre-Brook AL. Septic arthritis of the hip and osteomyelitis of the upper end of the femur in infants. J Bone Joint Surg [Br] 1960;42:11–20.
56. Sharrard WJW. Paediatric orthopaedics and fractures. Oxford: Blackwell Scientific, 1971.
57. Trueta J. Studies of the development and decay of the human frame. Philadelphia: WB Saunders, 1968.
58. Compere EL, Metzger WI, Mitra RN. The treatment of pyogenic bone and joint infections by closed irrigation (circulation) with a non-toxic detergent and one or more antibiotics. J Bone Joint Surg [Am] 1967;49:614–624.
59. Stetson JW, DePonte RJ, Southwick WO. Acute septic arthritis of the hip in children. Clin Orthop 1968;56:105–116.
60. Blockey NJ, Watson JT. Acute osteomyelitis in children. J Bone Joint Surg [Br] 1970;52:77–87.
61. Salter RB, Bell RS, Keeley FW. The protective effect of continuous passive motion on living articular cartilage in acute septic arthritis. Clin Orthop 1981;159:223–247.
62. Choi IH, Pizzutillo PD, Bowen JR, Dragann R, Malhis T. Sequelae and reconstruction after septic arthritis of the hip in infants. J Bone Joint Surg [Am] 1990;72:1150–1165.
63. Lloyd-Roberts GC. Suppurative arthritis of infancy. J Bone Joint Surg [Br] 1960;42:706–720.
64. Ish-Horowicz M, McIntyre P, Nade S. Methicillin-resistant Staphylococcus aureus bone and joint infection in a neonatal intensive care unit. Pediatr Infect Dis J 1992;11:82–87.
65. Kuo KN, Lloyd-Roberts GC, Orme IM, et al. Immunodeficiency and infantile bone and joint infection. Arch Dis Child 1975;50:51–56.
66. Lunseth PA, Heiple KG. Prognosis in septic arthritis of the hip in children. Clin Orthop 1979;139:81–85.
67. Bennett OM, Namnyak SS. Acute septic arthritis of the hip joint in infancy and childhood. Clin Orthop 1992;281:123–132.
68. Argen RJ, Wilson CH, Wood P. Suppurative arthritis. Arch Intern Med 1966;117:661–666.
69. Hunka L, Said SE, MacKenzie DA, Rogala EJ, Cruess RL. Classification and

surgical management of the severe sequelae of septic hips in children. Clin Orthop 1982;171:30–36.
70. Wopperer JM, White JJ, Gillespie R, Obletz BE. Long term follow up of infantile hip sepsis. J Pediatr Orthop 1988;8:322–325.
71. Katz K, Goldberg I, Yosipovitch Z. Early mobilization in septic arthritis. Acta Orthop Scand 1990;61:161–162.
72. Kelly PJ. Bacterial arthritis in the adult. Orthop Clin North Am 1975;6: 973–982.
73. Goldenberg DL, Reed JI. Bacterial arthritis. N Engl J Med 1985;312: 764–771.
74. Hughes RA, Rowe IF, Shanson D, Keat ACS. Septic bone, joint and muscle lesions associated with human immunodeficiency virus infection. Br J Rheumatol 1992;31:381–388.
75. Goldenberg DL, Cohen AS. Acute infectious arthritis: a review of patients with non-gonococcal joint infections. Am J Med 1976;60:369–377.
76. Leslie BM, Harris JM, Driscoll D. Septic arthritis of the shoulder in adults. J Bone Joint Surg [Am] 1989;71:1516–1522.
77. Hodgson BF. Pyogenic sacroiliac joint infection. Clin Orthop 1989;246: 146–149.
78. Vincent GM, Amirault JD. Septic arthritis in the elderly. Clin Orthop 1990;215:241–245.
79. Tindall EA, Regan-Smith HG. Gonococcal osteomyelitis complicating septic arthritis. JAMA 1983;250:2671–2673.
80. Hurley PT, Salata RA, Hayden FG. Chronic gonococcal osteomyelitis. South Med J 1987;80:264–266.
81. Lee AH, Chin AE, Ramanujam T, Thadhani RI, Callegari PE, Freundlich B. Gonococcal septic arthritis of the hip. J Rheumatol 1991;18:1932–1933.
82. Hansfield HH. Neisseria Gonorrhoeae. In: Mandell GL, Douglas RG, Bennett JE, eds. Principles and practice of infectious diseases, ed 3. New York: Churchill Livingstone, 1990: 1613–1631.
83. Richens J. The diagnosis and management of common forms of arthritis in adults in Papua New Guinea. Papua New Guinea Med J 1991;34: 149–154.
84. Hook EW. Septic gonococcal arthritis is much more common in the USA than in the UK. Br J Rheumatol 1990;29:283.
85. Rosenfeld N, Kurzer A. Acute flexor tenosynovitis caused by gonococcal infection. A case report. Hand 1978;10:213–214.
86. DeHertogh D, Ritland D, Green R. Carpal tunnel syndrome due to gonococcal tenosynovitis. Orthopedics 1988;11:199–200.
87. Granfors K. Do bacterial antigens cause reactive arthritis? Rheum Dis Clin North Am 1992;18:37–48.
88. Chusid MJ, Schneider JP, Thometz JG, Dunne WM. Osteomyelitis and septic arthritis caused by Haemophilus influenzae, type f, in a young girl. Diagn Microbiol Infect Dis 1992;15:157–159.
89. Beauvais C, Berenbaum F, Spentchian M, Prier A, Kaplan G. Early diagnosis

of vertebral osteomyelitis due to a rare pathogen: Haemophilus parainfluenzae. J Rheumatol 1992;19:491–493.
90. Auten GM, Levy CS, Smith MA. Haemophilus parainfluenzae as a rare cause of epidural abscess: case report and review. Rev Infect Dis 1991;13: 609–612.
91. Houssiau FA, Huaux JP, Nagant de Deuxchaisnes C. Haemophilus aphrophilus: a rare pathogen in vertebral osteomyelitis. Ann Rheum Dis 1987;46:248–250.
92. Dagan R. A two-year prospective, nationwide study to determine the epidemiology and impact of invasive childhood Haemophilus influenzae type b infection in Israel. The Israeli Pediatric Bacteremia and Meningitis Group. Clin Infect Dis 1992;15:720–725.
93. McGregor AR, Bell JM, Abdool IM, Collignon PJ. Invasive Haemophilus influenzae infection in the Australian Capital Territory region. Med J Aust 1992;156:569–572.
94. Barton LL, Dunkle LM, Habib FH. Septic arthritis in childhood. A 13-year review. Am J Dis Child 1987;141:898–900.
95. Stephanian E, Coffey RJ, Segal R. Intervertebral disc space infection and osteomyelitis due to Hemophilus species: report of two cases and review. J Spinal Disord 1989;2:114–119.
96. van Linthoudt D, Stadler P, Humair L, Ott H. Adult septic arthritis with Hemophilus influenzae. Z Rheumatol 1987;46:198–200.
97. Beltrani VP, Echols RM, Vedder DK. Vertebral osteomyelitis caused by Haemophilus influenzae. J Infect Dis 1987;156:391–394.
98. Olk DG, Hamill RJ, Proctor RA. Haemophilus parainfluenzae vertebral osteomyelitis. Am J Med Sci 1987;294:114–116.
99. Powers D, Overturf G, Turner E. Is there an increased risk of Hemophilus influenzae septicaemia in children with sickle cell anaemia? Pediatrics 1983;71:927–931.
100. Webb DK, Serjeant GR. Haemophilus influenzae osteomyelitis complicating dactylitis in homozygous sickle cell disease. Eur J Pediatr 1990;149: 613–614.
101. Lawrence JM, Osborn TG, Paro R, Eaton C, Hyers TM, Moore TL. Septic arthritis caused by Hemophilus influenzae type B in a patient with HIV-1 infection. J Rheumatol 1991;18:1772–1773.
102. Fritz P, Bardin T, Vittecoq D. Septic arthritis due to Haemophilus influenzae in a patient with HIV infection. Clin Exp Rheumatol 1991;9: 91–93.
103. Todd JK, Bruhn FW. Severe Haemophilus influenzae infections. Am J Dis Child 1975;129:607–611.
104. Bansal S, Magnussen CR, Nnapodano RJ. Haemophilus influenzae tenosynovitis. Ann Rheum Dis 1979;38:561–562.
105. Mustafa MM, Lebel MH, McCracken GHJ. Tenosynovitis and transient arthritis associated with Haemophilus influenzae type b bacteremia. Pediatr Infect Dis J 1988;7:517–519.

106. Lebel MH, Nelson JD. Haemophilus influenzae type b osteomyelitis in infants and children. Pediatr Infect Dis J 1988;7:250–254.
107. San Joaquin VH, Kiball JB. Subscapular abscess due to Haemophilus influenzae type b. Pediatrics 1980;65:331–332.
108. Likitnikul S, McCracken GH, Nelson JD. Arthritis in children with bacterial meningitis. Am J Dis Child 1986;140:424–427.
109. Vallejo JG, Kaplan SL, Mason EOJ. Treatment of meningitis and other infections due to ampicillin-resistant Haemophilus influenzae type b in children. Rev Infect Dis 1991;13:197–200.
110. Kulhanjian J, Dunphy MG, Hamstra S, et al. Randomized comparative study of ampicillin/sulbactam vs. ceftriaxone for treatment of soft tissue and skeletal infections in children. Pediatr Infect Dis J 1989;8:605–610.
111. Pinals RS, Ropes MW. Meningococcal arthritis. Arthritis Rheum 1964;7: 241–258.
112. Fam AG, Tenenbaum J, Stein JL. Clinical forms of meningococcal arthritis: a study of five cases. J Rheumatol 1979;6:567–573.
113. Rompalo AM, Hook EW, Roberts PL, Ramsey PG, Handsfield HH, Holmes KK. The acute arthritis-dermatitis syndrome. The changing importance of Neisseria gonorrhoeae and Neisseria meningitidis. Arch Intern Med 1987;147:281–283.
114. Tochen ML. Bone lesions in a child with meningococcal meningitis and disseminated intravascular coagulation. J Pediatr 1977;91:342–343.
115. Patriquin HB, Trias A, Jecquier S, et al. Later sequelae of infantile meningococcemia in growing bones of children. Radiology 1981;141: 77–82.
116. Robinow M, Johnson F, Nanagas MT, et al. Skeletal lesions following meningococcaemia and disseminated intramuscular complications. A recognizable skeletal dystrophy. Am J Dis Child 1983;137:279–281.
117. Billington RW. Spondylitis following cerebrospinal meningitis. JAMA 1924; 83:683–686.
118. Freehafer AA, Huser DP, Saunders AP. Infection of the lower lumbar spine with Neisseria meningitidis. J Bone Joint Surg [Am] 1978;60:1001–1002.
119. Christopher GW. Meningococcal arthritis, bacteremia and osteomyelitis following arthroscopy. Clin Orthop 1982;171:127–130.
120. Thompson GR, Manshady BM, Weiss JJ. Septic bursitis. JAMA 1978; 240:2280–2281.
121. Ho G, Tice AD, Kaplan SR. Septic bursitis in the pre-patellar and olecranon bursae. Ann Intern Med 1978;89:21–27.
122. Ho G, Tice AD. Comparison of non-septic and septic bursitis. Arch Intern Med 1979;139:1269–1273.
123. Tollerud DL, Albano L, Bia FJ. Anaerobic septic bursitis. Arch Intern Med 1979;91:494.
124. Viggiano DA, Garrett JC, Clayton ML. Septic arthritis presenting as olecranon bursitis in patients with rheumatoid arthritis. J Bone Joint Surg [Am] 1980;62:1011–1012.

125. Rehm-Graves S, Weinstein AJ, Calabrese LH, et al. Tuberculosis of the greater trochanteric bursa. Arthritis Rheum 1983;26:77–81.
126. Winter FE, Runyon EH. Pre-patellar bursitis caused by Mycobacterium marinum. J Bone Joint Surg [Am] 1965;47:375–379.
127. Rotes-Querol J. Manifestaciones osteoarticulares en 174 casos consecutives de brucelosis. Rev Esp Rheum 1957;7:59–62.
128. Torstrick RF, Harrison K, Heckman JD, et al. Chronic bursitis caused by Phialphora richardsiae. J Bone Joint Surg [Am] 1979;61:772–774.
129. King AJ, Nicol C. Venereal diseases. London: Bailliere Tindall, 1975.
130. Qualls DM. Yaws. In: Jahss M, ed. Disorders of the foot. Philadelphia: WB Saunders, 1982:1420–1428.

CHAPTER 19

Lyme Disease

Predisposing Factors and Groups at Risk

Lyme disease is an illness that affects several systems of the body, primarily joints, heart, and nervous system. It was described in 1977 by Steere and colleagues (1), and the name *Lyme disease* was given because the first cases in children were described in Lyme, Connecticut. In a classic series of epidemiological studies, *Ixodes* ticks were identified as the vectors and *Borrelia burgdorferi* was isolated as the causative agent (2–4).

Lyme disease is now the most prevalent infection caused by vectors in the United States (5). Through 1988, almost 14,000 cases were reported, primarily from the northeast (Massachusetts to Maryland), the Midwest (primarily Wisconsin and Minnesota), and the far west (California and Oregon). The disease occurs worldwide (6,7). The greatest risk for acquisition of infection is probably when nymphal ticks feed during the summer, but the disease can occur in all seasons.

The white-tailed deer seems to be the preferred host for *Ixodes* ticks, but the ticks have been recovered from many other types of wild animals and birds (8). It is postulated that the increasing number of deer and their migration to new areas, as well as the increasing numbers of individuals living in suburbs and more rural areas, allows exposure to the tick and subsequent development of illness.

A recent study documents the potential for exposure to tick bites and subsequent development of Lyme disease. Eight recreational parks located in a Lyme disease–endemic area of southern New York state were studied for the presence of ticks in the summer of 1985 (9).

Ninety-two percent of the ticks collected were *Ixodes dammini,* the primary vector of Lyme disease in the northeast. Two of the three parks sampled, with the highest annual attendance, also had the highest population of ticks. It was concluded that recreational parks in Lyme disease–endemic areas represented a substantial human risk for tick bites; that control of the tick population would be extremely difficult; and that prevention of tick bites should be the goal in such areas (9). Emergence of Lyme disease in a previously unaffected mainland community in Massachusetts where deer were abundant and where *Ixodes* had recently been established was investigated (10). A nature preserve was adjacent to the community. The attack rate for a 7-year period was 35% among residents living within 5 km of the nature preserve and was greatest (66%) for those living closest to the preserve. Infections had a primary peak in June and a secondary peak in October, which corresponded to periods of increased transmission.

A double-blind, placebo-controlled trial of penicillin prophylaxis in patients bitten by ticks in an area endemic for Lyme disease was performed (11). The sample size was small, but symptoms of Lyme disease developed in only 1 of 29 patients in the placebo group. Similar results have been reported from West Germany (12). A larger sample size was studied in a double-blind, placebo-controlled trial in South Eastern Connecticut in an area in which Lyme disease is prevalent (13). Deer ticks from the bitten individuals were analyzed by polymerase chain reaction, and 15% were found to be infected with *B. burgdorferi.* Erythema migrans developed in only two individuals; both were in the placebo group. No individuals seroconverted without development of symptoms and there were no late findings of Lyme disease. The conclusion drawn from this study is that even in an endemic area for Lyme disease, the risk of infection after a recognized deer tick bite is too low to justify routine use of prophylactic antimicrobial treatment. Factors that have been associated with the development of Lyme disease after a deer tick bite include the likelihood that the tick is infected, the stage of development of the tick, and, probably most important, the length of time the tick is attached (14–16). In experimental studies, attachments of ticks for less than 48 hours is rarely associated with transmission of *B. burgdorferi,* in contrast to highly successful transmission when the ticks have been in place for at least 72 hours. As has been stressed elsewhere, prevention of Lyme disease is enhanced by appropriate use of repellents and protective clothing and most importantly by rapid removal of ticks as soon as possible.

Pathophysiology

In the earliest stages, *Borrelia burgdorferi* produces a skin rash called erythema migrans and systemic symptoms of fever and fatigue. As with syphilis, the organism may be seen at this stage, and specific antibodies are often lacking. The spirochete is spread days or weeks after inoculation via blood or lymph, to multiple body sites, including skin, muscles, central nervous system, and heart. During this stage, the organism can still be recovered from blood and may be seen in small numbers in specimens of certain tissues (e.g., myocardium, muscle, bone, liver, spleen, meninges, and brain). Immunoglobulin M (IgM) antibody responses usually peak between the third and sixth week of illness but may persist, followed by the development of specific IgG antibodies. Weeks to months after spread via the blood stream, central nervous system infections or cardiac involvement may develop; chronic arthritis is likely to occur months after initial onset and may last for years (8).

The histogenesis in Lyme disease is well described (17). Following infection, the spirochete disseminates via the blood stream; circulating immune complexes and immunoglobulins become elevated in the circulation, along with deposition of IgG in the synovium. T-cell lymphocytes seem to be a major responder in the central nervous system, whereas B cells, which differentiate into plasma cells, provide a major response in the deep skin soft tissues, such as myocardium and synovium. It is likely that visceral damage is caused by an interplay of these humoral and cellular elements, which may be responding to an ongoing presence of spirochetal antigen. Mild vasculitis and hypercellular vascular occlusion are often seen at multiple sites and may reflect secondary damage by immune cells and possibly immune complexes. Tissue necrosis is generally lacking, as are giant cells or granulomas or gummas (18).

The histopathology of the synovial lesions of Lyme arthritis has similarities to other chronic inflammatory processes, such as rheumatoid arthritis. The chronic lesions are reflected by varying degrees of hypertrophic proliferative synovitis consisting of aggregates of lymphocytes in the subsynovium, with mixtures of plasma cells, macrophages, and mast cells. Neutrophils are rarely found in the synovium in chronic Lyme arthritis. The synovial cells are hyperplastic and accompanied by villous hypertrophy. Vessels are prominent; deposits of fibrin and fibrinogen are frequently found on the surfaces of and within the stroma of villi (18). The synovial lesions of Lyme disease were compared with those of rheumatoid arthritis and found to be nearly identical (17). In both diseases, T cells, mainly the helper-induced subset, were distributed diffusely in subsynovial lining areas, often with nodular aggregates of intermixed T and B cells. IgD-bearing B cells were scattered throughout, and activated germinal center B cells were occasionally present. In addition to these aggregates, plasma cells, macrophages, endothelial venules, and a few dendritic macrophages were found. Both lesions are typical of a chronic hypersensitivity immune response to foreign antigen—presumably spirochetal antigen in Lyme disease (17). However, to date, successful efforts to identify either agent or antigen in synovial tissues have been only sporadically successful (19). It is postulated that the scarcity of organisms is reminiscent of the lesions of tertiary syphilis or tuberculoid leprosy and that in Lyme arthritis, the stimulus for the chronic synovial lesions is a small number of *B. burgdorferi* (17).

Chronic Lyme arthritis seems to have an immunogenetic basis involving major histocompatibility complexes. In initial studies of 10 patients with chronic Lyme arthritis, there was an increased frequency of DR2 and DR4 (20). In a much larger study, it was found that among patients with Lyme arthritis, the human leukocyte antigen (HLA)-DR4 specificity was present in 57% of those with chronic arthritis (12–48 months' duration), in 23% of those with arthritis of moderate duration (6–11 mo), and in only 9% of those with arthritis of short duration (1–5 mo) (21). A secondary association with the HLA-DR2 specificity was also noted (21). These HLA specificities appeared to act as independent, dominant markers of susceptibility for chronic arthritis. It was also observed that the presence of HLA-DR4 was significantly associated with the failure of treatment; of 22 patients with this HLA specificity who were treated with antimicrobial agents, treatment was effective in only two. Rheumatoid arthritis also has an increased association with the presence of HLA-DR4 (21).

Microbiology

In 1983, a newly recognized spirochete was recovered from the blood, skin lesions, or cerebrospinal fluid (CSF) in 3 of 56 patients with

Lyme disease and from 21 of 110 *Ixodes dammini* ticks in Connecticut (22). Those isolates appeared to have the same morphological and immunological characteristics. These studies, which also reported on antibody titers to this organism, confirmed the findings (suggested earlier by responses to antimicrobial therapy and by the epidemiology of the disease that the causative agent was a penicillin-sensitive organism, such as a spirochete.

B. burgdorferi, the agent of Lyme disease, belongs to the eubacterial phylum of spirochetes (23). *B. burgdorferi* is a fastidious, microaerophilic organism that grows best at 33°C in a complex liquid medium. The organism is more easily isolated from ticks than from patients; for practical purposes, isolation of the organism from clinical specimens is not a simple diagnostic tool. In hamster models, cross-immunity between some strains of spirochetes from the east coast of the United States was observed, but a similar cross immunity was not observed against strains from the west coast and Europe. Whether this diversity accounts for clinical variations of the disease in different geographic regions is unknown. A currently accepted system of subclassification of *B. burgdorferi* does not exist and would be helpful in terms of better understanding the immunological responsiveness to the organism, the variability in clinical presentations with different species from different geographic areas, and perhaps to clarify some of the inconsistencies in laboratory testing and serological responses.

Clinical and Laboratory Findings

The clinical picture of Lyme disease is generally one of distinct stages, with remissions and exacerbations. In the course unmodified by antibiotic therapy, patients first have erythema migrans, sometimes followed weeks to months later by either neurological or cardiac involvement, and then months or years later by arthritis. Although this schema is useful to review the course of the disease, all systems may be affected at any time in the illness. For the purposes of this text, we use one classification system (8,24).

Early Infection: Stage I (Localized Erythema Migrans)

Erythema chronica migrans (ECM) usually begins as a single red macule or papule. Multiple lesions may develop and, as the area of erythema expands, the lesions usually have red outer borders and partial central clearing. Although this is the classic lesion (Figure 19-1), many variations occur; the center of the lesion becomes much more red, indurated, or necrotic. Multiple secondary lesions of an annular variety develop in approximately half the patients within several days of the onset of ECM. These lesions resemble ECM, but are usually smaller, lack indurated centers, and are not related to previous tick bites. Both primary and secondary lesions usually fade within one month.

Skin involvement is often associated with systemic symptoms of fatigue, malaise, headache, fever, and chills. More severe symptoms, such as meningeal irritation, musculoskeletal pain, and lymphadenopathy, occur in less than half the patients. Fatigue and lethargy often persist, whereas the other signs and symptoms are usually intermittent and variable.

Early Infection: Stage II (Disseminated Infection)

B. burgdorferi spread to many sites in the body within days or weeks after inoculation. In this stage, the most frequent symptoms occur in the skin, the nervous system, or the musculoskeletal system. The secondary annular skin lesions occur in approximately half the patients and are generally smaller and less migratory than the primary ECM lesions. Severe headache and stiffness of the neck occur, but typically in short attacks that last only hours; CSF is usually normal in this stage. Migra-

A B

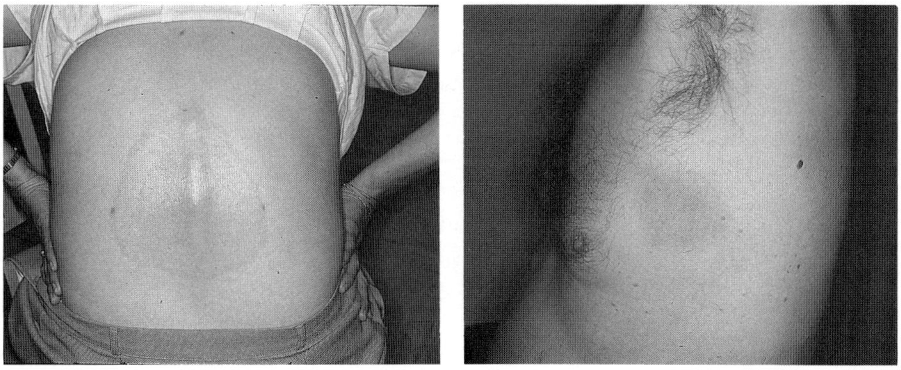

Figure 19-1. *(A,B) Lesions of erythema chronicum migrans.* (Courtesy of Dr. Gary Wormser.)

tory pain in joints, bursae, muscle, and bone are usually present for hours or days in a given location. In this stage, patients often appear quite ill and frequently have incapacitating malaise and fatigue.

After spread via the blood stream, the spirochete seems to entrench itself in certain areas of the body. The timing of this classification system seems less clear at this stage because systemic manifestations occur several weeks or months after the initial presentation.

It is estimated that frank neurological involvement develops in approximately 15% to 20% of patients in the United States several weeks or months after infection (8). Meningitis with cranial or peripheral neuropathy is one of the most common manifestations. Encephalitic signs, such as somnolence, poor memory, and changes in mood, may be found; radicular pain may also be among the first neurological findings. In patients with meningitis, the CSF usually has approximately 100 cells/cm^3, with a predominance of lymphocytes and an elevated protein level. *B. burgdorferi* has been cultured from spinal fluid in this stage. The most common cranial neuropathy is unilateral or bilateral facial palsy; asymmetrical motor, sensory, or mixed radiculoneuropathy of the limbs or trunk may also occur. Electromyographic (EMG) studies suggest axonal nerve involvement, with some demyelination. Any of these neurological abnormalities may last for weeks or months and can also recur or become chronic.

Less than 10% of patients (the range is 4%–8%) have cardiac involvement within several weeks after the onset of disease (8). Fluctuating degrees of atrioventricular block are the most common abnormalities, but myopericarditis and mild left ventricular dysfunction can also occur. Cardiac abnormalities are usually short lived (between 3 days and 6 weeks), and the arrhythmias do not usually require insertion of a pacemaker. Heart block usually resolves with appropriate antimicrobial therapy (i.e., penicillin or tetracycline).

From 2 weeks to 2 years after the onset of disease (mean, 6 months), approximately 60% of patients will have brief attacks of asymmetrical arthritis, primarily of the large joints (6). Synovial fluid aspiration reveals white counts ranging from 500 to 100,000/cm^3, and these cells are primarily polymorphonuclear leukocytes. Immune complexes are invariably present.

Late Infection: Stage III (Persistent Infection)

Chronic arthritis, defined as one year or more of continual joint inflammation, usually begins during the second and third year of illness;

episodes of arthritis become longer during the second and third years, lasting months rather than weeks, until they become "continuous." Usually one or a few large joints are affected; the most common is the knee. *B. burgdorferi* has been cultured from joint fluid (25,26). In severe cases, erosion of cartilage and bone occurs, which can progress, rarely, to permanent joint disability. The number of patients with recurrences decreases annually, and even patients with chronic Lyme arthritis are unlikely to have continuous inflammation of joints for more than several years (8). The entity of "chronic" or "tertiary" Lyme arthritis is described in more detail later.

Central and peripheral nervous system involvement with *B. burgdorferi* more than one year after the initial infection is now being recognized and better characterized. The most clearly defined late syndrome is progressive encephalomyelitis. A series of 48 patients from West Germany were found to have spastic paraparesis, bladder dysfunction, ataxia, and deficits of cranial nerves 7 or 8; some patients had cognitive impairment, including dementia (27). Intrathecal production of antibody to the spirochete was demonstrated (27). In the United States, more subtle syndromes of the central or peripheral nervous system have been described late in the illness (8). Patients with intermittent distal paresthesias or radicular pain with EMG evidence of axonal neuropathy have been found. More difficult to evaluate are patients who have less marked symptoms, such as sleepiness, amnesia, or behavior changes when other classic symptoms of Lyme disease have vanished. Part of the difficulty in evaluating the relation of these symptoms to Lyme disease is the lack of a test that uniformly indicates an active spirochetal infection in the central nervous system.

An example of a late manifestation in Lyme disease is acrodermatitis chronica atrophicans (24). This skin lesion, observed and described primarily in Europe, usually begins with bluish red discoloration and swollen skin on an extremity, often at the site of an earlier ECM lesion. The inflammatory phase gradually leads to skin atrophy; *B. burgdorferi* has been recovered from these lesions as late as 10 years after initial infection (28). In addition to the acrodermatitis, scleroderma-like skin lesions can also occur.

Laboratory Findings

Serology is generally the only practical laboratory aid. Early in the illness, nonspecific abnormalities, such as an elevated ESR and abnormal transaminase levels, may be found; these levels generally return to normal within several weeks. Laboratory tests are nonspecific and not helpful.

Diagnosis

Because culturing or visualizing *B. burgdorferi* in patient specimens is impractical, serology is currently the major tool in diagnosis. The enzyme-linked immunosorbent assay (ELISA) test is the preferred antibody assay (8). Within several weeks of infection, most patients with Lyme disease have elevated antibody titers to *B. burgdorferi*. False-negative test results occur usually in the first several weeks of disease; by capture IgM ELISA, approximately 90% of individuals will have an IgM response to the spirochete (8). False-positive test results have been reported in healthy subjects and in patients with syphilis, Rocky Mountain Spotted Fever, and autoimmune diseases (29,30).

Two important caveats regarding serological testing must be noted. First, testing for Lyme disease is not well standardized, and results may vary among laboratories (31,32). In one study, aliquots of serum from 9 patients were sent initially (and the same serum 2 weeks later) to 9 reference laboratories. Wide variability was observed, ranging from one laboratory detecting antibody in all 18 specimens to another detecting antibody in only 8 of 18 specimens. Equally disturbing was the fact that four-fold increases of titer within duplicate samples occurred three times; such a change is considered diagnostic of a positive serological test and infection. It is recommended that there be national reference material available to all laboratories and frequent national quality assurance programs to monitor performance. Second, up to 10% of patients in the United States will have asymptomatic infections due to *B. burgdorferi* (33). A tendency to attribute all symptoms to Lyme disease may lead to misdiagnosis in patients whose symptoms may be caused by other illnesses.

In a recent series, 17 patients who presented with acute Lyme disease and received prompt treatment with oral antibiotics were studied; these patients had evidence of fatigue, arthralgias, mild arthritis, headache, and peripheral neuropathy and were felt to have chronic Lyme disease (34). None had diagnostic levels of antibodies to *B. burgdorferi* by either ELISA or immunofluoresence assay. All patients had a strong T-cell proliferative response to whole *B. burgdorferi,* which was similar to that in 18 patients with chronic Lyme disease who had detectable antibodies. These T-cell responses were greater than that of a control group of healthy subjects. The authors postulated that the disorder in these seronegative patients reflects a dissociation between T-cell and B-cell immune responses, with the cell-mediated arm intact (34). They further speculated that early administration of antibiotics may have been responsible for the blunted humoral response (34). Although an important finding, it is unlikely that many patients who are seronegative will have access to testing of lymphoproliferative responses to *B. burgdorferi*. Thus, we are left with serological testing, imprecise as it is, as the major diagnostic tool; it should be ordered solely to confirm a diagnosis based on epidemiological and clinical evidence.

Therapy

Initial studies of treatment of the early stages of Lyme disease (i.e., erythema migrans) showed that patients treated with penicillin did better than untreated patients (35) and, subsequently, that tetracycline was superior to penicillin or erythromycin (36). It was also shown that patients with Stage II neurological abnormalities could be treated effectively with high-dose intravenous penicillin, but results were not as good in patients with arthritis (37).

Identification of *B. burgdorferi* as the etiological agent of Lyme disease allowed determination of antibiotic sensitivities. Johnson and colleagues (38), using broth dilution techniques, showed that *B. burgdorferi* was most susceptible to ceftriaxone (MBC, 0.04, μg/mL) and erythromycin (MBC, 0.05, μg/mL), and tetracycline (MBC, 0.8 μg/mL); penicillin G was less active (MBC, 6.4 μg/mL) (38). The same investigators used Syrian hamsters to determine the 50% curative doses in experimental models. Ceftriaxone and tetracycline had the highest activities, whereas erythromycin and penicillin G were significantly less effective (38).

Current recommendations for treatment are given in Table 19-1 (39). With early Lyme disease, oral doxycycline or amoxicillin appear to be the agents of choice. For patients with more serious neurological disease (not those with facial palsy alone and no abnormalities of the CSF), intravenous therapy is recommended, and the drug of choice appears to be ceftriaxone, which crosses the blood-brain barrier readily and can be administered once or twice a day (8). For patients

Table 19-1. Treatment of Lyme Disease*

	Drug	Adult Dosage	Pediatric Dosage[†]
Erythema Migrans	Doxycycline[‡] (*Vibramycin*, and others)	100 mg PO b.i.d.	
	or		
	Amoxicillin (*Amoxil*, and others)	250–500 mg PO t.i.d.	25–50 mg/kg/day divided t.i.d.
Alternative:	Cefuroxime axetil (*Ceftin*)	500 mg b.i.d.	250 mg b.i.d.
Neurological disease			
Bell's palsy	Doxycycline[‡]	100 mg PO b.i.d.	
	or		
	Amoxicillin	250–500 mg PO t.i.d.	25–50 mg/kg/day divided t.i.d.
More serious CNS disease[§]	Ceftriaxone (*Rocephin*)	2 grams/day IV	75–100 mg/kg/day IV
	or		
	Penicillin G	20–24 million units/day IV	300,000 units/kg/day IV

Cardiac disease			
Mild	Doxycycline[‡]	100 mg PO b.i.d.	
	or		
	Amoxicillin	250–500 mg PO t.i.d.	25–50 mg/kg/day divided t.i.d.
More serious[‖]	Ceftriaxone	2 grams/day IV	75–100 mg/kg/day IV
	or		
	Penicillin G	20–24 million units/day IV	300,000 units/kg/day IV
Arthritis[§]			
Oral	Doxycycline[‡]	100 mg PO b.i.d.	
	or		
	Amoxicillin	500 mg PO t.i.d.	50 mg/kg/day divided t.i.d.
Parenteral	Ceftriaxone	2 grams/day IV	75–100 mg/kg/day IV
	or		
	Penicillin G	20–24 million U/day IV	300,000 units/kg/day IV

*Recommendations are based on limited data and should be considered tentative. The duration of treatment is not well established for any indication; it is usually based on severity of disease and rapidity of response. Clinicians generally recommend 10 to 30 days for oral drugs and 14 to 21 days for intravenous treatment.

† Should not exceed adult dosage.

‡ Or tetracycline HCl (*Achromycin*, and others), 250–500 mg q.i.d. Neither doxycycline nor any other tetracycline should be used for children less than eight years old or for pregnant or lactating women.

§ In late disease, the response to treatment may be delayed for several weeks or months.

‖ A temporary pacemaker may be necessary.

Reproduced by permission from Med Lett 1992;34:95–97.

with allergies to ceftriaxone or penicillin, tetracyclines or chloramphenicol may be acceptable, but there is little data in this regard. Optimal treatment of Stage III joint or neurological abnormalities is not well defined. In one study of patients with established Lyme arthritis, treatment with intramuscular penicillin G benzathine was significantly better than placebo, but only 35% of patients responded (26). In that same study, only 55% of patients receiving intravenous penicillin were cured. In another study of 23 patients with late neurological and arthritic manifestations of Lyme disease, the authors reported that intravenous ceftriaxone was significantly better than intravenous penicillin (40).

The role of corticosteroids in the treatment of Lyme disease is also unclear. The most dramatic evidence of efficacy was shown in the treatment of Lyme carditis (41); however, that study was carried out without antimicrobial therapy, and it is now suggested that steroids are indicated only if patients with severe cardiac involvement do not respond quickly to antimicrobial therapy (8).

Prognosis and Complications

Several complications of Lyme disease have been reported. However, what is lacking in the literature is an accurate estimate of development of complications in patients treated or untreated for Stage I disease (erythema migrans). In one series, 55 patients who did not receive antibiotic therapy for ECM were followed for a mean duration of 6 years (42); 11 (20%) had no subsequent manifestations of Lyme disease. Another 10 patients (18%) had brief episodes of joint or musculoskeletal pain for up to 6 years, without objective abnormalities of the joints ever developing. Twenty-eight (51%) had at least one episode or intermittent attacks of frank arthritis, usually enlarged joints; the number of these patients continuing to have recurrences decreased by 10% to 20% each year. Chronic synovitis developed in six patients (11%); two had radiographic evidence of erosive disease; and 1 had permanent limitation of motion. Of these six, three had spontaneous resolution of chronic joint involvement 1.5 to 3 years later, whereas the other three were treated successfully with parenteral antibiotic therapy.

The chronic or tertiary arthritic stage of Lyme disease is likely to come to the attention of rheumatologists and orthopedists (43). Following the migratory polyarthritis seen early in the disease, chronic arthritis generally begins months later. Recurrent episodes of synovitis with significant effusion may persist for weeks; swelling produced by the large waxing and waning effusion is often out of proportion to the pain patients frequently experience. Examination may show swelling and edema of the periarticular soft tissues, with a diminished range of motion of the involved joint. A boggy synovitis is frequently palpable but is often without redness or warmth. Radiographs of long-standing chronic Lyme disease may show destruction and erosion of bone and cartilage, calcifications of menisci, ossification of soft tissues, osteophytes, and subarticular cysts (Figures 19-2 and 19-3). Joint aspiration will usually produce cloudy yellow fluid with a white cell count ranging from 500 to 100,000 cells/cm^3, with a polymorphonuclear leukocyte predominance. Protein levels are elevated, and glucose levels are usually normal. As mentioned earlier, there is a predominance of DR4 and DR2 HLA types in individuals with chronic Lyme arthritis (21).

In one series, synovial specimens from 17 patients, of whom 14 had

A B C

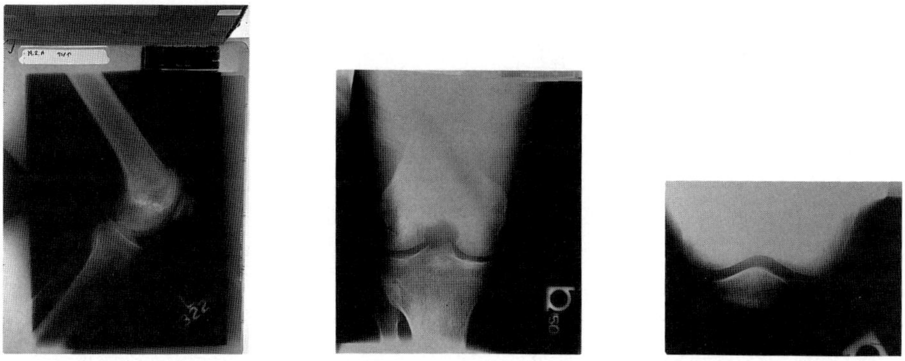

Figure 19-2. *A 30-year-old man with a total of 11 months of arthritis. (A) Radiograph of left knee, lateral. An erosion is noted in the posterosuperior margin of the tibia, and a soft-tissue mass is seen in the suprapatellar extension of the joint. (B) Radiograph of the left knee, posteroanterior. There is an erosion in the femoral condyle at the site of attachment of the lateral collateral ligament. Subarticular cysts are present in the medial tibial plateau. (C) Skyline radiograph of the patella. Calcification is present in the articular cartilage of the patella.* (Reproduced by permission from Lawson J, Steere A. Lyme arthritis: radiologic findings. Radiology 1985;154:37–43.)

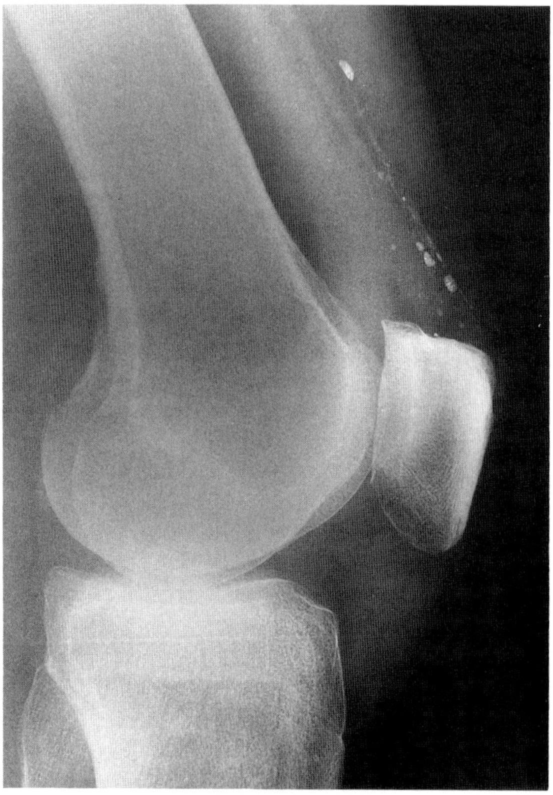

Figure 19-3. *A 39-year-old woman; arthritis has been present in the left knee for a total of 11 months. Multiple calcific densities are present in the insertion of the quadriceps femoris tendon.* (Reproduced by permission from Lawson J, Steere A. Lyme arthritis: radiologic findings. Radiology 1985;154:37–43.)

chronic (more than 6 months) arthritis in the knees, were studied (19). All had moderate to marked chronic cellular infiltrate; lymphocytes and plasma cells were the most numerous. Vascular abnormalities ranged from capillary arborization to vascular dilatation with congestion. Vascular microangiopathy was seen in 5 of 17 patients. There was striking villous hypertrophy and acidophilic proteinaceous material. In two patients, spirochetes were seen with Dieterle silver stains: the organisms were within edematous vascular beds and in one vessel wall. Organisms were present in only small numbers and were difficult to find. It was postulated that the scarcity of organisms and the difficulty of culturing is reminiscent of the lesions of tertiary syphilis or tuberculoid leprosy and that in Lyme arthritis, the stimulus for the chronic synovial lesions is small numbers of *B. burgdorferi* (17). This hypothesis is given support by the finding of spirochetes by histological staining in the tissues.

A second major complication of Lyme disease is carditis and reversible heart block. Carditis occurs in 4% to 10% of patients with Lyme disease, usually beginning 3 to 6 weeks after the initial illness (8,42,44). The average onset of carditis is 5 weeks (range, 4 days to 7 months) after the initial illness. The most common manifestation of carditis in Lyme disease is a varying degree of atrioventricular block; the majority reported had either complete or high-grade atrioventricular block and were almost always symptomatic.

Patients with atrioventricular block have an excellent prognosis; most infections resolved within 1 to 2 weeks and all but three resolved within 6 weeks (44). Of these three patients, two had persistent first-degree block for 4 to 5 months and the third had a transient Wenckebach atrioventricular block for 5 months before returning to normal. Perhaps most important, in no reported patient did complete atrioventricular block persist longer than 10 days. Most patients respond well to antimicrobial therapy, with a return to normal sinus rhythm. Recognizing Lyme carditis is important to avoid unnecessary permanent pacemaker implantation.

B. burgdorferi infection may produce involvement of both the central and peripheral nervous systems as late complications (>1 year) after initial onset of infection. The most clearly described central nervous system involvement is progressive encephalomyelitis, as described earlier (27). In one study, 36 patients with late Lyme disease, of whom 14 had prominent limb paresthesias, were described (45). All but one had neurophysiological evidence of peripheral neuropathy, whereas neurological examinations were normal in most. Antimicrobial treatment was associated with rapid improvement in 11 of the 12 treated patients. Resolution of symptoms occurred before any significant decrease in antibody titer, suggesting that the problem was a direct effect of infection with spirochetes and not an immune-mediated phenomenon (45).

Other complications of Lyme disease include septal panniculitis (46) and hepatitis (47). In both instances, complications occurred during recurrent episodes of Lyme disease. Both complications responded to antimicrobial therapy with tetracyclines. In the case of panniculitis, the histological appearance of the biopsy was consistent with the appearance of erythema nodosum and presumably represented a nonspecific response to infection. In contrast, in the patient with hepatitis, a liver biopsy identified spirochetal forms in the hepatic parenchyma.

The ultimate complication of any disease is death. A case of fatal adult respiratory distress syndrome in a patient with Lyme disease has been reported (48). Lyme disease developed in a 67-year-old woman following a trip to the Maryland shore. Approximately 1 month after the onset of her illness, she had abnormal liver function studies (both transaminase and alkaline phosphatase levels were elevated) and a negative chest radiograph. A course of intravenous penicillin was associated with initial improvement but gradual worsening. By the tenth day in the hospital, bibasilar rales were noted and a chest radiograph showed bilateral peripheral infiltrates. Her fever worsened, she became more hypoxic, and her chest radiograph showed diffuse bilateral patchy infiltrates consistent with acute respiratory distress syndrome (ARDS). She died of respiratory failure. At post-mortem, the cause of death was diffuse alveolar damage of the lungs consistent with ARDS. Lymph nodes showed spirochetes compatible with *B. burgdorferi*. This case was unusual for Lyme disease because respiratory symptoms are not generally described in human Lyme disease, although spirochetes have been demonstrated in the lungs of experimentally infected hamsters (48).

Unresolved Problems

The following problems remain unresolved and raise important questions in terms of diagnosis and management of this disease.

1. There is an urgent need for standardization of the serological testing for Lyme disease.
2. Definition of clinical syndromes is extremely important. There is a tendency to overdiagnose Lyme disease and to blame infection with *B. burgdorferi* for a variety of vague clinical complaints that may or may not have anything to do with infection with this organism. In particular, linking in the media of chronic fatigue syndrome and infection with the agent of Lyme disease is likely to lead to overdiagnosis and unnecessary treatment.
3. Optimal antimicrobial treatment for late complications of Lyme disease is also unclear. Currently, ceftriaxone appears to be the drug of choice, but treatment failures occur, and further investigation into other agents and other routes of administration should be examined.

References

1. Steere AC, Malawista SE, Snydman DR, et al. Lyme arthritis: an epidemic of oligoarticular arthritis in children and adults in three Connecticut communities. Arthritis Rheum 1977;20:7–17.
2. Steere AC, Broderick TF, Malawista SE. Erythema chronicum migrans and Lyme arthritis: epidemiologic evidence for a tick vector. Am J Epidemiol 1978;108:312–321.
3. Wallis RC, Brown SE, Kloter KO, Main AJ Jr. Erythema chronicum migrans and Lyme arthritis: field study of ticks. Am J Epidemiol 1978;108:322–327.
4. Steere AC, Malawista SE. Cases of Lyme disease in the United States: locations correlated with distribution of Ixodes dammini. Ann Intern Med 1979;91:730–733.
5. Lyme disease—Connecticut. MMWR 1988;37:1–3.
6. Kryger P, Hansen K, Vinterberg H, Pedersen F. Lyme borreliosis among Danish patients with arthritis. Scand J Rheum 1990;19:77–81.
7. Sigel L, Curran A. Lyme disease: A multifocal worldwide epidemic. Annu Rev Public Health 1991;12:85–109.
8. Steere AC. Lyme disease. N Engl J Med 1989;31:586–596.
9. Falco RC, Fish D. Potential for exposure to tick bites in recreational parks in a Lyme disease endemic area. Am J Public Health 1989;79:12–15.
10. Lastavica CC, Wilson ML, Berardi VP, Spielman A, Deblinger RD. Rapid emergence of a focal epidemic of Lyme disease in coastal Massachusetts. N Engl J Med 1989;320:133–137.
11. Costello C, Steere AC, Pinkerton RE, Feder HM Jr. A prospective study of tick bites in an endemic area for Lyme disease. J Infect Dis 1989;159: 136–138.
12. Paul H, Gerth H, Ackermann R. Infectiousness for humans of Ixodes ricinus containing Borrelia burgdorferi. Zentralbl Bakteriol Mikrobiol Hyg [A] 1986;263;473–476.
13. Shapiro E, Gerber M, Holabird N, et al. A controlled trial of antimicrobial prophylaxis for Lyme disease after deer-tick bites. N Engl J Med 1992;327: 1769–1773.
14. Berach J, Coleman J, Skinner R, Basler E. Adult Ixodes dammini on rabbits: a hypothesis for the development and transmission of Borrellia burgdorferi. J Infect Dis 1987;155:1300–1306.
15. Piesman J, Mather T, Sinsky R, Spielman A. Duration of tick attachment and Borrelia burgdorferi transmission. J Clin Microbiol 1987;25:557–558.
16. Piesman J, Maupin G, Campos E, Papp C. Duration of adult female Ixodes dammini attachment and transmission of Borrelia burgdorferi with description of a needle aspiration isolation method. J Infect Dis 1991;163: 895–897.
17. Steere A. Pathogenesis of Lyme arthritis. Implications for rheumatic disease. Ann NY Acad Sci 1988;39:87–92.

18. Duray P, Steere A. Clinical pathologic correlations of Lyme disease by stage. Ann NY Acad Sci 1988;39(Suppl):65–79.
19. Johnston Y, Duray P, Steere A, et al. Lyme arthritis. Spirochetes found in synovial microangiopathic lesions. Am J Pathol 1985;118:26–34.
20. Steere A, Gibofsky A, Patarroyo M, et al. Chronic Lyme arthritis: clinical and immunogenetic differentiation from rheumatoid arthritis. Ann Intern Med 1979;90:896–901.
21. Steere A, Dwyer E, Winchester R. Association of chronic Lyme arthritis with HLA-DR4 and HLA-DR2 alleles. N Engl J Med 1990;323:219–223.
22. Steere AC, Grodzicki RL, Kornblatt AN, et al. The spirochetal etiology of Lyme disease. N Engl J Med 1983;308:733–742.
23. Barbour AG, Hayes SF. Biology of Borrelia species. Microbiol Rev 1986; 50:381–400.
24. Asbrink E, Hovmark A. Early and late cutaneous manifestations of Ixodes-borne borreliosis (erythema migrans borreliosis, Lyme borreliosis). Ann NY Acad Sci 1988;539:4–15.
25. Snydman DR, Schenkein DP, Berardi VP, Lastavica CC, Pariser KM. Borrelia burgdorferi in joint fluid in chronic Lyme arthritis. Ann Intern Med 1986;104:798–800.
26. Schmidli J, Hunziker T, Moesli P, Schaad UB. Cultivation of Borrelia burgdorferi from joint fluid three months after treatment of facial palsy due to Lyme borreliosis. J Infect Dis 1988;158:905–906.
27. Ackerman R, Rehse-Kupper B, Gollmer E, Schmidt R. Chronic neurologic manifestations of erythema migrans borreliosis. Ann NY Acad Sci 1988; 539:16–23.
28. Asbrink E, Hovmark A. Successful cultivation of spirochetes from skin lesions of patients with erythema chronica migrans afzelius and acrodermatitis chronica atrophicans. Acta Pathol Microbiol Immunol Scand 1985;93: 161–163.
29. Duffy J, Mertz LE, Wobig GH, Katzmann JA. Diagnosing Lyme disease: the contribution of serologic testing. Mayo Clin Proc 1988;63:1116–1121.
30. Grodzicki RL, Steere AC. Comparison of immunoblotting and indirect enzyme-linked immunosorbent assay using different antigen preparations for diagnosing early Lyme disease. J Infect Dis 1988;157:790–797.
31. Hedberg C, Osterholm M. Serologic tests for antibody to Borrelia burgdorferi—another Pandora's box for medicine. Arch Intern Med 1990;150: 732–733.
32. Luger S, Krauss E. Serologic tests for Lyme disease. Interlaboratory variability. Arch Intern Med 1990;150:761–763.
33. Steere AC, Taylor E, Wilson ML, Levine JF, Spielman A. Longitudinal assessment of the clinical and epidemiological features of Lyme disease in a defined population. J Infect Dis 1986;154:295–300.
34. Dattwyler RJ, Volkman DJ, Luft BJ, Halperin JJ, Thomas J, Golightly MG. Seronegative Lyme disease. Dissociation of specific T- and B-lymphocyte responses to Borrelia burgdorferi. N Engl J Med 1988;22:1441–1446.

35. Steere AC, Malawista SE, Newman JH, Spieler PN, Bartenhagen NH. Antibiotic therapy in Lyme disease. Ann Intern Med 1980;93:1–8.
36. Steere AC, Hutchinson GJ, Rahn DW, et al. Treatment of the early manifestations of Lyme disease. Ann Intern Med 1983;99:22–26.
37. Steere AC, Green J, Schoen RT, et al. Successful parenteral penicillin therapy of established Lyme arthritis. N Engl J Med 1985;312:869–874.
38. Johnson RC, Kodner C, Russell M. In vitro and in vivo susceptibility of the Lyme disease spirochete, Borrelia burgdorferi, to four antimicrobial agents. Antimicrob Agents Chemother 1987;31:164–167.
39. Med Lett 1992;34:95–97.
40. Dattwyler RJ, Halperin JJ, Volkman DJ, Luft BJ. Treatment of late Lyme borreliosis—randomised comparison of ceftriaxone and penicillin. Lancet 1988;1:1191–1194.
41. Steere AC, Batsford WP, Weinberg M, et al. Lyme carditis: cardiac abnormalities of Lyme disease. Ann Intern Med 1980;93:8–16.
42. Steere AC, Schoen RT, Taylor E. The clinical evolution of Lyme arthritis. Ann Intern Med 1987;107:725–731.
43. McLaughlin TP, Zemel L, Fisher RL, Gossling HR. Chronic arthritis of the knee in Lyme Disease. J Bone Joint Surg [Am] 1986;68:1057–1062.
44. McAlister HF, Klementowicz PT, Andrews C, Fisher JD, Feld M, Furman S. Lyme carditis: an important cause of reversible heart block. Ann Intern Med 1989;110:339–345.
45. Halperin JJ, Little BW, Coyle PK, Dattwyler RJ. Lyme disease: cause of a treatable peripheral neuropathy. Neurology 1987;37:1700–1706.
46. Kramer N, Rickert RR, Brodkin RH, Rosenstein ED. Septal panniculitis as a manifestation of Lyme disease. Am J Med 1986;81:149–152.
47. Goellner MH, Agger WA, Burgess JH. Hepatitis due to recurrent Lyme disease. Ann Intern Med 1988;108:707–708.
48. Kirsch M, Ruben FL, Steere AC, Duray PH, Norden CW, Winkelstein AW. Fatal adult respiratory distress syndrome in a patient with Lyme disease. JAMA 1988;259:2737–2739.

CHAPTER 20

Soft-tissue Infections

Cellulitis

Cellulitis is an acute spreading bacterial infection of the skin and subcutaneous tissues that is sometimes difficult to distinguish from deeper infections, particularly septic arthritis and osteomyelitis, in sites such as the tibia or the ulna. A primary skin lesion can be identified in approximately 80% of patients (1) including traumatic wounds, ulcers, and fungal skin infections. Treatment is usually empiric, and the majority of patients are probably managed successfully in the community using oral antibiotics—although without antibiotics, and sometimes despite their use, it is a serious disease. The majority of infections are caused by Group A Streptococcus or *Staphylococcus aureus*. Other organisms isolated include other streptococci, *Hemophilus influenzae* type B, and occasionally gram-negative bacilli, such as *Escherichia coli, Pseudomonas aeruginosa,* and *Proteus* species. In immunocompromised individuals and in young children, cellulitis may result from bacteremia rather than as a consequence of skin trauma, and a wide variety of organisms, including atypical mycobacteria (2), may be involved.

Local features are tenderness, pain, erythema, swelling, and regional adenopathy. The edge of the infection is usually poorly demarcated. Skin bullae and occasional small subcutaneous abscesses may be found. Even with adequate antibiotic therapy, the natural history of cellulitis is often prolonged over many days, to the surprise and concern of both patients and physicians. Lymphangitis is an indicator of severity of infection but is no longer (as it was before antibiotics) an indication for surgical debridement or amputation. Initially, systemic signs (i.e., temperature, rigors, and malaise) may be prominent. An increased erythrocyte sedimentation rate (ESR) and polymorphonuclear leukocytosis are usually present. If discharge from a primary lesion is present, it can be examined by smear and culture; if not, aspiration or biopsy may occasionally be useful. Routine use of simple needle aspiration, either of the center of the lesion or of the leading edge, is not recommended because it will establish a bacteriological diagnosis in only approximately 10% of patients (1,3). The yield of positive culture is higher from skin biopsy (3,4), which may be justified in certain situations, including infections in compromised hosts or when unusual organisms are suspected.

Imaging techniques can demonstrate cellulitis and its complications. On radiographs and computerized tomography (CT), skin thickening and streaky increased density of the normal subcutaneous tissue layer are seen (5). Ultrasound also demonstrates these changes well and has the advantage of identifying any abscess deep to the cellulitis (6). The role of isotope imaging in cellulitis is controversial. Blood pool imaging may show a diffuse increase in activity involving both bones and soft tissues, whereas in osteomyelitis, areas of focal activity are present in bone (7,8). Comparison of ^{99m}Tc-MDP scanning with an indium-111 granulocyte study can aid differentiation of osteomyelitis and cellulitis (9).

Once swabs or aspirates, if indicated, have been taken, empiric antibiotic therapy should be started. Except in immunocompromised individuals, when a broad-spectrum agent should be used, or when there is a strong reason to suspect another organism, specific therapy effective against *S. aureus* and *S. pyogenes* should be chosen. If systemic signs are present, the intravenous route should be chosen until they are controlled, when oral therapy may be substituted and continued until local signs have resolved. Once an organism is identified in the laboratory, definitive antibiotic therapy should begin. Symptoms are eased by splintage and analgesics.

Cellulitis unduly slow to resolve suggests underlying abscess formation or necrotizing fasciitis and may indicate ultrasonography or biopsy. Dermal anesthesia and necrosis indicating thrombosis of skin vessels are findings that should raise suspicion of an underlying spreading fasciitis (10).

As resolution begins, the edema may resolve earlier than the skin erythema, giving rise to obvious wrinkling of the skin. However, many patients experience dependent skin capillary pooling for days or weeks after control of infection, continuing use of firm bandaging or stockings may be helpful.

Necrotizing Soft-tissue Infections

The literature describes a number of severe, spreading infections involving skin, fascia, and muscle to varying extent, which are characterized by failure, in general, to resolve with antibiotic treatment alone and a tendency to poor prognosis with significant mortality (10,11). They may be crepitant or noncrepitant. Bacterial synergy and involvement of fastidious strict anaerobes are common (12), but some severe infections involve single aerobic organisms of high virulence, particularly group A streptococci. Diabetes, malabsorption, malignancy, alcoholism, corticosteroid therapy, and immunosuppression are associated risk factors, but apparently healthy individuals may be involved. Some infections appear spontaneously, but a majority are associated with surgery or skin trauma, sometimes quite minor.

Classification of these conditions has been extremely confusing and clinical diagnosis is difficult. Terms used included *necrotizing fasciitis* (13), *streptococcal gangrene* (14), *Fournier's gangrene* (15), *anaerobic cellulitis* (16,17), and *synergistic gangrene* (18). In gas gangrene and nonclostridial anaerobic myonecrosis, muscle is also involved (16,17).

In the last decade, the trend has been to view these infections as a group of related conditions, initiated by a variety of organisms, the clinical course of which depends on the balance between host defenses and bacterial virulence factors (10–12). The problem in clinical practice is recognition of the context in which such infections may occur and the manner in which they present. Therefore, classification based on clinical appearance, particularly the patterns of tissue involvement (10,11) and rate of spread (12), are more helpful.

Ahrenholz (10) listed the features that should lead to the recognition of progressive necrotizing soft-tissue infection (Table 20-1) and thus to surgical exploration with biopsy and radical debridement, supplemented with antimicrobial therapy and, in some patients, hyperbaric oxygen. Some or most of these features are present in every necrotizing soft-tissue infection. In myonecrosis, pain and systemic signs are usually particularly marked.

Table 20-1. Features of Necrotizing Soft-tissue Infections

Systemic
Confusion
Tachycardia/tachypnea
Ketoacidosis/hyperglycemia
Local
Dermal gangrene
Cyanosis, blistering or bronzing of skin
Severe pain
Spreading cutaneous anesthesia
Thin, reddish drainage
Undermined wound edges
Progressive cellulitis
Severe edema around a wound
Crepitus or radiographic gas
Multiple cutaneous fistulae

Modified from Ahrenholz DH. Necrotizing soft tissue infections. Surg Clin North Am 1988;68:199–213.

Once an indication for surgical exploration has been established, appropriate fluid replacement and cardiovascular support must be ensured. Provisional antibiotic management should consist of penicillin, an aminoglycoside, and metronidazole (10). Culture of biopsy material will establish the definitive antibiotic program.

The key to optimal management of all these presentations is exploration and excision of all necrotic tissue, including skin. In severe fulminating infections, this approach may necessitate amputation; in others, thorough local debridement only is required. In the early stages of necrotizing fasciitis and when burrowing extensions of fat necrosis are absent, fascial necrosis may extend much further than skin necrosis, allowing partial preservation of skin flaps (19).

The role of hyperbaric oxygen therapy in necrotizing soft-tissue infections without myositis remains controversial (20–23). Overall, the mortality rate in this group of patients remains between 30% to 40% (10); it is higher in older patients (24), in patients with diabetes mellitus, and in immunocompromised individuals (25). Occasional cures of progressive bacterial synergistic gangrene have been reported using antibiotics alone (11).

Clostridial Myonecrosis (Gas Gangrene)

Although *Clostridia* may be cultured from 80% of war wounds and 10% to 30% of civilian open injuries (16), the incidence of gas gangrene is small. Rapid evacuation and early, competent wound management reduced its incidence from 1.8% of wounds in the Great War (1914–1918) to 0.016% among American casualties in the Vietnam conflict (26). Situations of increased risk include alcoholism (27), hip nailing in the elderly (28), vascular insufficiency (29), neoplasia (30), and previous splenectomy (31). High epidemic risk is associated with war and other disasters that temporarily overwhelm available medical services.

A collective review (32) suggests that approximately 50% of infections occur after trauma (including burns, bee stings, abortions, and injections), 35% are postoperative, and the remainder occur apparently spontaneously in such conditions as large bowel cancer, diabetes and peripheral vascular disease, burns, cholecystitis, and immunosuppression. Two thirds of infections in the extremities, and one third occur in the abdominal wall.

Approximately 80% of infections are caused by *Clostridium perfringens*. Two other toxin-elaborating species (*C. septicum* and *C. novyi*) and four species with proteolytic properties only (of which *C. bifermentans* is the most common) produce clinical gas gangrene. Although *Clostridia* are capable of survival for many hours in oxygen, growth and elaboration of toxin are favored by low oxygen tensions (33). Devitalized muscle greatly reduces the number of organisms required to produce experimental gas gangrene. The principal toxin is α-toxin, a lecithinase, but four major and four minor toxins are also described. *A*-toxin is responsible with other toxins for local necrosis and for intramuscular hemolysis. The gas in the tissues is believed to be mainly hydrogen (11). The combination of toxins, hemolysis, and local tissue breakdown produce widespread organ failure: brain dysfunction (34), cardiac failure, hypotension, and renal failure. Locally, once the infection is established, destruction of muscle spreads rapidly into adjacent healthy tissues. The process may proceed rapidly; death occurs as quickly as 12 hours from onset (32).

Following wounding or surgery, the incubation period may be as short as 6 hours or as long as 20 days (16), but most have occurred by 3 to 4 days. Pain of unexpected intensity is the most important early sign. Within hours, it is followed by systemic signs of tachycardia, tachypnea, confusion, irritability, and hypotension. The classic features of wound discoloration, hemorrhagic blistering, crepitation, odor, and discharge are late in onset, and diagnosis should be made before they become established.

The fundamental laboratory investigation is microscopic examination of the wound discharge. *Clostridia* are characteristically gram-positive, spore-forming, obligate anaerobic rods. However, *C. perfringens* may survive for many hours in oxygen, fail to demonstrate spores in clinical material, and occasionally even appear as gram-negative. The presence of gram-positive bacilli, even if there are other debatable signs, should be considered diagnostic of gas gangrene until proven otherwise (35). However, the clinical context is important, because the majority of isolates of clostridial species in hospital practice do not herald significant disease (36). Bacteremia occurs in 15% of patients with gas gangrene (37).

In early gas gangrene, the only radiological change is nonspecific soft-tissue swelling. Gas appears as a late sign and indeed may be sparse or absent. The typical streaky interfascicular pattern of gas (Figure 20-1) is highly suggestive of myonecrosis; in open wounds, anaerobic cellulitis, and cellulitis caused by gas-producing aerobes such as *E. coli,* the gas pattern is more discrete (38) (Figure 20-2).

The mortality in extremity gas gangrene after trauma has been reduced to approximately 5% by early recognition, meticulous surgical debridement, fluid replacement, cardiovascular support, and large doses of intravenous antibiotic (32). Penicillin (10–20 megaunits daily) or, in the presence of penicillin allergy, metronidazole, should be employed. Because tissue of marginal viability may survive, bacterial multiplication is inhibited, and capillary regrowth is stimulated after hyperbaric oxygen treatment (32,33), it is a valuable adjunct to the basic measures. Higher death rates in the spontaneous and postoperative group may reflect the age structure and the presence of underlying disease.

Pyomyositis

Pyomyositis, characterized by the formation of abscesses within striated muscles, is relatively common in tropical countries but unusual,

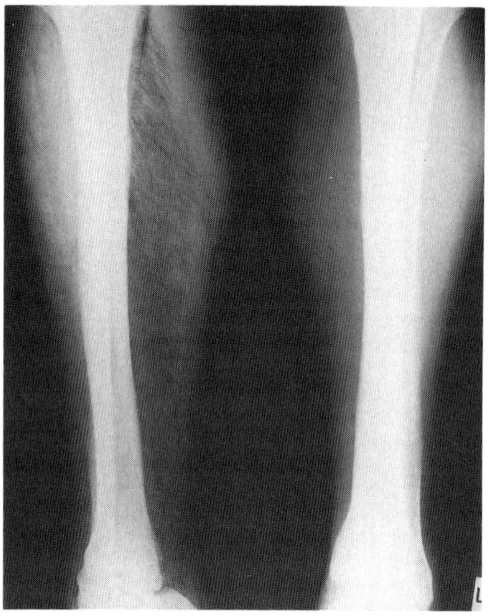

Figure 20-1. *The characteristic interfascicular gas pattern of clostridial myonecrosis.*

Figure 20-2. *In anaerobic cellulitis and postsurgical pocketing of air, the distribution of gas is more discrete.*

although increasingly reported, elsewhere. The high frequency in the tropics suggests predisposing environmental factors, although none have been authentically established (39,40). Diabetics may be predisposed to pyomyositis (41). Immunological deficits have been identified in nondiabetic patients with muscle abscesses; it is not clear whether these changes are primary or secondary (42).

Most infections occur in the first to fourth decades of life. The majority of abscesses occur in the lower limbs and trunk. Involvement of hands or feet is uncommon. Twenty to 40% of patients have multiple lesions. Suppuration is preceded by a clinically recognizable phase of inflammatory edema (43), during which aggressive antibiotic treatment may avert the formation of pus. Many patients, however, present with a fully developed intramuscular abscess. The route of bacterial spread is presumed to be hematogenous from skin or other lesions, although the yield from blood cultures is low. More than 90% of infections are caused by *S. aureus;* the remainder are caused mainly by *Streptococcus* species (43,44). A variety of other organisms, including *E. coli, Klebsiella,* and *Pseudomonas* species (45), have been isolated.

Anaerobic abscesses caused by *Clostridium* species also occur (27,46). Intermuscular abscesses are seen occasionally, associated with guinea worm (*Dracunculus medinensis*) infestation (47).

Trauma has been suggested as a predisposing factor (48), which is supported by early experimental work (49). Viral infections may be associated with pyomyositis (50,51). Pyomyositis has been reported in patients with human immunodeficiency virus infection (52,53).

In the typical subacute presentation, the history is of onset over some days. Local signs predominate: woody induration, local tenderness, and pain on stretching the muscle are characteristic. Erythema, skin warmth, and systemic signs are slight or absent. The second, less usual, presentation is dominated by systemic illness and pyemia (54). Most patients have a leukocytosis and an increased ESR. In tropical countries, eosinophilia is often present but is considered a nonspecific characteristic of coexisting parasitic infection. Serum levels of muscle enzymes generally remain normal (55). Overall, the yield from blood cultures is low, estimated at 5% to 25% (54,55).

Radiology is helpful but of secondary importance in a characteristic presentation. Plain films may show soft-tissue swelling and edema. Ultrasound (56), CT (57), and magnetic resonance imaging (58) provide precise localization and characterization, particularly within the pelvis (59) (Figures 20-3, 20-4).

Early lesions without suppuration respond to antibiotic therapy and rest (43). Aspiration may yield an organism even if pus has not formed. Once an abscess has developed, drainage is recommended. This may be achieved by surgery or using aspiration guided by CT or ultrasound. Because the great majority of patients are infected with *S. aureus*, provisional antibiotic therapy should be with a beta-lactamase–resistant penicillin, or with an agent such as clindamycin if penicillin allergy is suspected. The optimum duration of treatment has not been established. Mobilization may be initiated when systemic disease is controlled, local drainage has ceased, and pain allows. Significant loss of function is rare.

Rickettsial and Viral Myalgia and Myositis

Myalgia is prominent in the rickettsial diseases; the severity of the pain caused confusion between typhus and osteomyelitis in the nineteenth century.

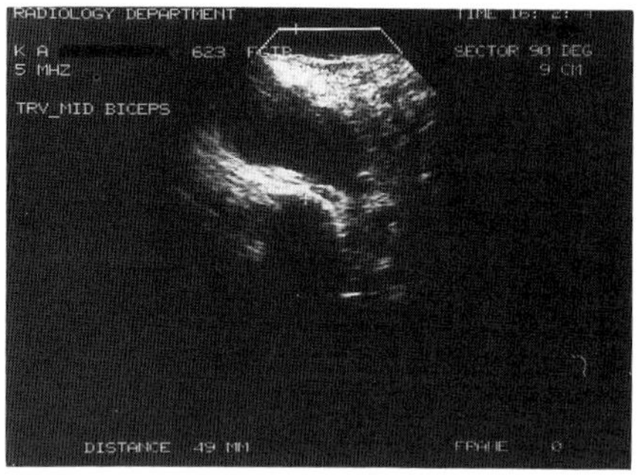

Figure 20-3. *Ultrasonic demonstration of pyomyositis in flexor aspect of left arm.*

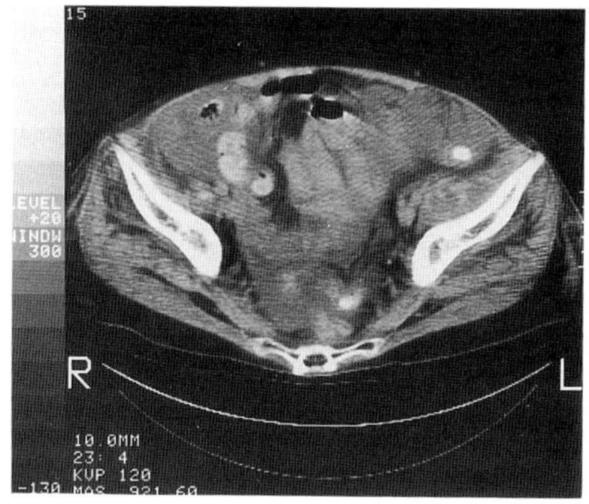

Figure 20-4. *Computerized tomography in a patient with rheumatoid arthritis and* Staphylococcus aureus *septicemia showing swelling of the iliacus muscle on the left side with a poorly defined abscess in its substance.*

Many viral infections are associated with muscle pain, and in some, such as influenza and dengue, this pain may be severe. Biopsy appearances in such circumstances are variable, showing either inflammatory reaction or muscle necrosis (60). Virus particles have been identified in muscle of some patients with scoliosis, in which their relevance is unknown (61), and in patients with polymyositis (62), in which a causative association might be more plausible.

Septic Bursitis

Septic bursitis, particularly on the extensor aspect of the knee and the elbow, is a well-recognized clinical entity (63–65). In a referral population, nonseptic bursitis (i.e., gout, rheumatoid arthritis, and idiopathic cases) exceeded septic infections by a ratio of 2:1 (64).

S. aureus is responsible for more than 90% of infections; other isolates include hemolytic streptococci and anaerobes (66). There is an association with overlying skin lesions in 50% of patients. Peribursal tenderness, edema, and cellulitis are usually present; fever, in contrast, is often absent. A sympathetic effusion may occur in the neighboring joint but is usually small. Associated septic arthritis has been described in patients with rheumatoid disease presenting with septic olecranon bursitis (67). Diabetes, alcoholism, chronic organ failure, and neoplasia are often associated in adults (65) but not in children (68).

Diagnosis is readily made by aspiration, gram-stain, and culture of the bursal fluid. Other features of the bursal fluid have been compared in septic and nonseptic patients (65). Although distinguishing features, such as cell count and fluid-to-serum glucose ratio are relatively consistent, they are not usually required for diagnosis. Treatment is bursal aspiration and administration of an appropriate antibiotic. Surgical drainage is not recommended unless the infection fails to respond to this program.

Chronic bursal infection is seen in patients with tuberculosis (69), atypical mycobacterial infection (70), brucellosis (71), fungal infections (72), and tertiary syphilis and yaws, in whom firm periarticular nodules, resembling those in rheumatoid arthritis, may occur (73). These chronic lesions are usually amenable to appropriate chemotherapy.

Infective Tenosynovitis

Infection of synovial tendon sheaths may arise from a penetrating injury, direct extension of a contiguous infection, or by hematogenous spread. In view of the serious consequences for function, attention has focussed particularly on infections in the hand (74). Tenosynovitis in the foot, particularly in diabetes mellitus or in leprosy, often arises from direct spread from other infected areas.

The majority of cases of acute suppurative tenosynovitis are confined to one sheath or bursa and are caused by *S. aureus* or *S. pyogenes* (74), but other organisms may be isolated, particularly *N. gonorrhoeae* (75,76). A history of penetrating injury is present in approximately 60% of patients (77). Clinical features are localized tenderness along the line of the tendon sheath, with limitation of passive and active movement. Fever and leukocytosis are usual but may be obscured by antibiotic treatment. This acute, closed-space infection, carrying a risk of tendon infarction and slough, requires surgical drainage. Ultrasonography is useful in confirming the clinical diagnosis and may also demonstrate the presence of radiolucent foreign bodies (78). A limited approach, with exposure of both ends of the infected sheath and irrigation (74,79,80), has been widely accepted. Empiric antibiotic treatment with a beta-lactamase–resistant penicillin and drainage of the sheath should be followed by definitive chemotherapy on identification of the organism.

Granulomatous tenosynovitis of infective origin is relatively rare, but it is seen increasingly in immunosuppressed individuals, often caused by nontuberculous mycobacterial infection, usually in the flexor synovium of the wrist and the hand (81). Possible explanations for this localization include the relative abundance of synovium in this area and the high risk of inoculation through minor penetrating injuries. The classic compound palmar ganglion of tuberculosis is now relatively rare (82). Other reported isolates include *Brucella* species (83), *H. influenzae* type B (84), *N. meningitidis* (85), fungi (86,87), and *Toxoplasma gondii* (88). Diagnosis requires a biopsy with a microbiological and a histological study of the chronic synovitis. Although surgical synovectomy is sometimes recommended (88,89), appropriate chemotherapy alone will often suffice once the diagnosis has been made (81).

Although the presence of multiple sites of tenosynovitis is also due most commonly to rheumatoid arthritis, there are clear associations with a number of infectious agents. Disseminated gonorrheal infection and meningococcemia, although occasionally a cause of an acute suppurative tenosynovitis, are more often associated with a polytenosynovitis, typically affecting the extensor aspects of the hand or the foot (see Chapter 18). Similar lesions are seen occasionally in infection with *H. influenzae* type B and in acquired syphilis and yaws (see Chapter 21). Appropriate chemotherapy results in resolution of these lesions.

References

1. Newell PM, Norden CW. Value of needle aspiration in bacteriologic diagnosis of cellulitis in adults. J Clin Microbiol 1988;26:401–404.
2. Sanderson TL. Disseminated Mycobacterium avium-intracellulare infection appearing as a panniculitis. Arch Pathol Lab Med 1982;106:112–114.
3. Hook EW, Hooton TM, Horton CA, Coyle MB, Ramsey PG, Turck M. Microbiologic evaluation of cutaneous cellulitis in adults. Arch Intern Med 1986;146:295–297.

4. Lee PC, Turnidge J, McDonald PJ. Fine needle aspiration biopsy in diagnosis of soft tissue infections. J Clin Microbiol 1985;22:80–83.
5. Magid D, Fishman EK. Musculoskeletal infections in patients with AIDS: CT findings. AJR 1992;158:603–607.
6. Greenberg RN, Poepsel PR, Reynaud SP, et al. Staphylococcal infection of fascial space diagnosed by ultrasonography. South Med J 1983;76:814.
7. Gilday DL, Paul DJ, Paterson J. Diagnosis of osteomyelitis in children by combined blood pool and bone imaging. Radiology 1975;117:331–335.
8. Gandsman EJ, McCullough RW. Dynamic bone imaging in the differential diagnosis of skeletal lesions. Int J Rad Appl Instrum [B] 1990;17:533–541.
9. Schauwecker DS, Park HM, Mock BH, et al. Evaluation of complicating osteomyelitis with Tc-99m MDP, In-111 granulocytes and Ga-67 citrate. J Nucl Med 1984;25:849–853.
10. Ahrenholz DH. Necrotizing soft tissue infections. Surg Clin North Am 1988;68:199–213.
11. Feingold DS. Gangrenous and crepitant cellulitis. J Am Acad Dermatol 1982;6:289–299.
12. Kingston D, Seal DV. Current hypotheses on synergistic microbial gangrene. Br J Surg 1990;77:260–264.
13. Sudarsky LA, Laschinger JC, Coppa GF, Spencer FC. Improved results from a standardized approach in treating patients with necrotizing fasciitis. Ann Surg 1987;206:661–665.
14. Meleney FL. Hemolytic streptococcus gangrene. Arch Surg 1924;9:317–364.
15. Nickel JC, Morales A. Necrotizing fasciitis of the male genitalia (Fournier's gangrene). Can Med Assoc J 1983;129:445–448.
16. Maclennan JD. The histotoxic clostridial infections of man. Bacteriol Rev 1962;26:177–276.
17. Bessman AN, Wagner W. Non-clostridial gas gangrene. Report of 48 cases and review of the literature. JAMA 1975;223:958–963.
18. Meleney FL. Bacterial synergism in disease processes. Ann Surg 1931;94: 961–981.
19. Baxter CR. Surgical management of soft tissue infections. Surg Clin North Am 1972;52:1483–1487.
20. Barzilai A, Zaaroor M, Toledano C. Necrotizing fasciitis: early awareness and principles of treatment. Isr J Med Sci 1985;21:127–132.
21. Pessa ME, Howard RJ. Necrotizing fasciitis. Surg Gynecol Obstet 1985; 161:357–361.
22. Riseman JA, Zamboni WA, Curtis A, Graham DR, Konrad HR, Ross DS. Hyperbaric oxygen therapy for necrotizing fasciitis reduces mortality and the need for debridements. Surgery 1990;108:847–850.
23. Kindwall EP, Gottlieb LJ, Larson DL. Hyperbaric oxygen therapy in plastic surgery: a review article. Plast Reconstr Surg 1991;88:898–908.
24. Rea WJ, Wyrick WJ. Necrotizing fasciitis. Ann Surg 1970;172:957–964.
25. Rouse TM, Malangoni MA, Schulte WJ. Necrotizing fascitis—a preventable disaster. Surgery 1982;92:765–770.

26. Brown PW, Kinman PB. Gas gangrene in a metropolitan community. J Bone Joint Surg [Am] 1974;56;1445–1451.
27. Gorbach SL, Thadepalli H. Isolation of clostridium in human infections: evaluation of 114 cases. J Infect Dis 1975;131(suppl):S81–S85.
28. Dykes RG. Gas gangrene after hip nailing. J Bone Joint Surg [Br] 1976; 58:263.
29. Parker MT. Post-operative clostridial infections in Britain. Br Med J 1969; 3:676–681.
30. Alpern RJ, Dowell VR. Clostridium septicum infections and malignancy. JAMA 1969;209:385–388.
31. Schwartz PE, Sterioff S, Mucha P, et al. Postsplenectomy sepsis and mortality in adults. JAMA 1982;248:2279–2283.
32. Hart GB, Lamb RC, Strauss MB. Gas gangrene. J Trauma 1983;23: 991–1000.
33. Kindwall EP. Uses of hyperbaric oxygen therapy in the 1990s. Cleve Clin J Med 1992;59:517–528.
34. Nora PF, Mousavirpur M, Mittelpunkt A, Rosenberg M, Laufman H. Brain as target organ in Clostridium perfringens exotoxin toxicity. Arch Surg 1966;92:243–246.
35. Altemeier WA, Fullen WD. Prevention and treatment of gas gangrene. JAMA 1971;209:806–813.
36. Lewis JF, Mullins N, Johnson P. Isolation and evaluation of clostridia from clinical sources. South Med J 1980;73:427–432.
37. Caplan ES, Kluge RM. Gas gangrene: review of 34 cases. Arch Intern Med 1976;136:788–791.
38. Nichols RL, Smith JW. Gas in the wound: what does it mean? Surg Clin North Am 1975;55:1289–1293.
39. Burkitt RT. Tropical pyomyositis. J Trop Med Hyg 1947;50:71–75.
40. Engel D. Tropical pyomyositis: a thiamine deficiency disease. Med Hypotheses 1981;7:345–352.
41. Walling DM, Kaelin WG. Pyomyositis in patients with diabetes mellitus. Rev Infect Dis 1991;13:797–802.
42. Giasuddin ASM, Idoko JA, Lawande RV. Tropical pyomyositis: is it an immunodeficiency disease? Am J Trop Med Hyg 1986;35:1231–1234.
43. Duvie SOA. Bacterial myositis and pyomyositis. J Coll Surg Edinb 1984; 29:237–241.
44. Foster WD. The bacteriology of tropical pyomyositis in Uganda. J Hyg (Camb) 1965;63:517–524.
45. Ajao OG, Ajao AO. Tropical pyomyositis. Int Surg 1982;67:414–416.
46. Kolbeinsson ME, Holder WDJ, Aziz S. Recognition, management, and prevention of Clostridium septicum abscess in immunosuppressed patients. Arch Surg 1991;126:642–645.
47. Anand SV, Evans KT. Pyomyositis. Br J Surg 1964;51:917–920.
48. Ashken MH, Cotton RE. Tropical skeletal muscle abscesses (Pyomyositis Tropicans). Br J Surg 1963;50:846–852.

49. Miyake H. Beitrage zur kenntnis der sogenannten myositis infectiosa. MH Grenzgib Med Chir 1904;13:155–198.
50. Taylor JF, Fluck D. Tropical myositis: ultrastructural studies. J Clin Pathol 1976;29:1081–1084.
51. Egelmeijer F, Markusse HM, Stolk B, Bloem JL. Pyomyositis associated with Epstein-Barr virus infection. Br J Rheumatol 1988;27:409–411.
52. Watts RA, Hoffbrand BI, Paton DF, Davis JC. Pyomyositis associated with human immunodeficiency virus infection. Br Med J 1987;294:1524–1525.
53. Victor G, Branley J, Opal SM, Mayer KH. Pyomyositis in a patient with the acquired immunodeficiency syndrome. Arch Intern Med 1989;149:705–709.
54. Traquair RN. Pyomyositis. J Trop Med Hyg 1957;50:81–89.
55. Levin MJ, Gardener P, Waldvogel FA. Tropical pyomyositis. N Engl J Med 1971;184:196–198.
56. Datz FL, Lewis SE, Conrad MR, Maravilla A, Parkey RW. Pyomyositis diagnosed by radionuclide imaging and ultrasonography. South Med J 1980;73:649–651.
57. Yousefzadeh DK, Schumann EM, Mulligan GM, Bosworth DE, Young CS, Pringle KC. The role of imaging modalities in diagnosis and management of pyomyositis. Skeletal Radiol 1982;8:285–289.
58. Yuh WTC, Schreiber AE, Montgomery WJ, Ehara S. Magnetic resonance imaging of pyomyositis. Skeletal Radiol 1988;17:190–193.
59. Broadfoot E, Chaitow J. Primary suppurative myositis. Aust Radiol 1981; 25:175–176.
60. Swartz MN. Myositis. In: Mandel GL, Douglas RG, Bennet JC, eds. Principles and practice of infectious diseases. Toronto: Wiley and Sons, 1979.
61. Webb JN, Gillespie WJ. Virus-like particles in paraspinal muscle in scoliosis. Br Med J 1976;2:912–913.
62. Gyorkey F, Cabral GA, Gyorkey PK. Coxsackievirus aggregates in muscle cells of a polymyositis patient. Inter-virology 1978;10:69–77.
63. Ho G, Tice AD, Kaplan SR. Septic bursitis in the prepatellar and olecranon bursae: an analysis of 25 cases. Ann Intern Med 1978;89:21–27.
64. Ho G, Tice AD. Comparison of non-septic and septic bursitis. Arch Intern Med 1979;139:1269–1273.
65. Thompson GR, Manshady BM, Weiss JJ. Septic bursitis. JAMA 1978;240: 2280–2281.
66. Tollerud DL, Albano L, Bia FJ. Anaerobic septic bursitis. Ann Intern Med 1979;91:494.
67. Viggiano DA, Garrett JC, Clayton ML. Septic arthritis presenting as olecranon bursitis in patients with rheumatoid arthritis. J Bone Joint Surg [Am] 1980;62:1011–1012.
68. Paisley JW. Septic bursitis in childhood. J Pediatr Orthop 1982;2:57–61.
69. Rehm-Graves S, Weinstein AJ, Calabrese LH, Cook SA, Boumphrey SR. Tuberculosis of the greater trochanteric bursa. Arthritis Rheum 1983;26:77–81.
70. Winter FE, Runyon EH. Prepatellar bursitis caused by Mycobacterium marinum. J Bone Joint Surg [Am] 1965;47:375–379.

71. Rotes-Querol J. Manifestationes osteoarticulares en 174 casos consecutives de brucellosis. Rev Esp Rheum 1957;7:59–62.
72. Torstrick RF, Harrison K, Heckman JD, Johnson JE. Chronic bursitis caused by Philaphora richardsiae. J Bone Joint Surg [Am] 1979;61:772–774.
73. King AJ, Nicol C. Venereal diseases. London: Bailliere Tindall, 1975.
74. Pollen AG. Acute infections of the tendon sheaths. Hand 1974;6:21–25.
75. Ogiela DM, Peimer CA. Acute gonococcal flexor tenosynovitis—case report and literature review. J Hand Surg 1981;6:470–472.
76. Balcomb T. Acute gonococcal flexor tenosynovitis in a woman with asymptomatic gonorrhoea. J Hand Surg 1982;7:521–522.
77. Flynn JE. Grave infections of the hand. N Engl J Med 1943;229:898–905.
78. Groleau S, Chem RK, Younge D, Basora J. Ultrasonography of foreign-body tenosynovitis. Can Assoc Radiol J 1992;43:454–456.
79. Nevaiaser RJ. Closed tendon sheath irrigation for pyogenic flexor tenosynovitis. J Hand Surg 1978;3:462–466.
80. Juliano PJ, Eglseder WA. Limited open–tendon-sheath irrigation in the treatment of pyogenic flexor tenosynovitis. Orthop Rev 1991;20:1065–1069.
81. Jones MW, Wahid IA. Mycobacterium marinum infections of the hand and wrist. Results of conservative treatment in 24 cases. J Bone Joint Surg [Am] 1988;70:631–632.
82. Klofkorn RW, Steigerwald JC. Carpal tunnel syndrome as the initial manifestation of tuberculosis. Am J Med 1976;60:583–586.
83. Mousa AR, Muhtaseb SA, Almudallal DS, Khodeir SM, Marafie AA. Osteoarticular complications of brucellosis: a study of 169 cases. Rev Infect Dis 1987;9:531–543.
84. Mustafa MM, Lebel MH, McCracken GHJ. Tenosynovitis and transient arthritis associated with Haemophilus influenzae type b bacteremia. Pediatr Infect Dis J 1988;7:517–519.
85. Pollet SM, Leek JC. Tenosynovitis in meningococcemia. Arthritis Rheum 1987;30:232–233.
86. Stratton CW, Lichtenstein KA, Lowenstein SR, Phelps DB, Reller LB. Granulomatous tenosynovitis and carpal tunnel syndrome caused by Sporothrix schenckii. Am J Med 1981;71:161–164.
87. Eglseder WA. Carpal tunnel syndrome associated with histoplasmosis: a case report and literature review. Milit Med 1992;157:557–559.
88. Vass M, Kullman L, Csoka R, Magyar E. Polytenosynovitis caused by Toxoplasma gondii. J Bone Joint Surg [Br] 1977;59:229–232.
89. Dixon JH. Non-tuberculous mycobacterial infection of the tendon sheaths in the hand. J Bone Joint Surg [Br] 1981;63:542–544.

CHAPTER 21

Other Pathogens Producing Bone Infection

Many different organisms have been reported to produce infection in the musculoskeletal system, and the list continues to increase. A number of these organisms are discussed in this chapter, including infections due to viruses, fungi, mycoplasma, *Brucella,* spirochaetes, actinomyces, protozoa, and helminths.

Viral Osteitis and Arthritis

Although viral infection may predispose to bacterial osteomyelitis by altering host defenses (1) or by allowing secondary bacterial infection of viral skin lesions, as in varicella (2), viral infections of the musculoskeletal system have not been regarded as an important clinical problem. Currently, the possible association of Paget's disease of bone (osteitis deformans) and viruses of the paramyxovirus group remains unproven (3).

Reported isolations from joints with synovitis include vaccinia (4), mumps (5), and varicella (6). Varicella may be manifest as an acute arthritis even in the absence of the typical exanthem (7). In rubella, synovitis may be associated with the multiplication of virus particles (8,9). Some rubella strains appear to grow in joint-derived tissue culture more readily than others; the pattern conforms to clinical experience of the incidence of joint involvement with different wild and vaccine strains (9). Immune complexes are seen in the arthritis associated with viral hepatitis (10). Involvement of the small joints of the hand has been described in the convalescent phase of lymphocytic choriomeningitis (11). Peripheral polyarthritis is also a feature of human parvovirus arthropathy associated with erythema infectiosum (12,13), and, occasionally, of infectious mononucleosis, Coxsackie virus infection, and Ross River fever (14–16). Small parvo-like viruses have been isolated from synovium in some patients with rheumatoid arthritis (17). Retrovirus-like particles may have a part in psoriatic arthropathy (18).

Osteomyelitis variolosa was the best recognized viral osteitis (19). Prior to the suppression of smallpox, 2% to 5% of affected children suffered bilateral symmetrical joint swelling 10 to 28 days after onset of the disease (20). The radiological appearances were of nonspecific lytic metaphyseal lesions, which often crossed the growth plate. Vaccinial osteomyelitis had a similar appearance (21). It occurred 10 to 14 days after vaccination of infants and sometimes presented as swelling or pseudoparalysis. Areas of metaphyseal lucency (Figure 21-1) are seen in congenital rubella. These areas have been considered to represent osteitis (22), although it may be that only osteoporosis is

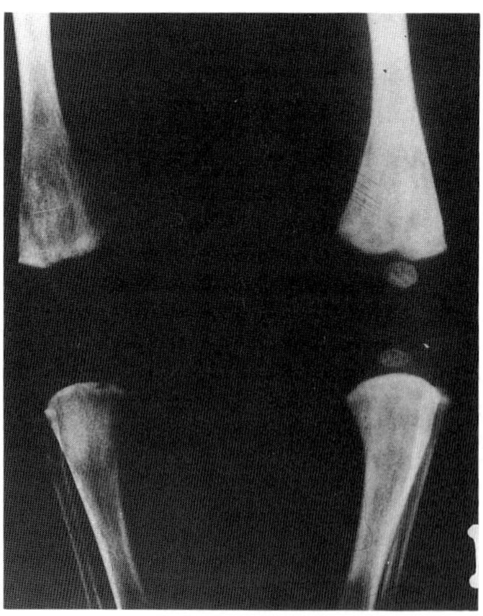

Figure 21-1. *Congenital rubella. Metaphyseal lucency involves both femur and tibia on the right side.*

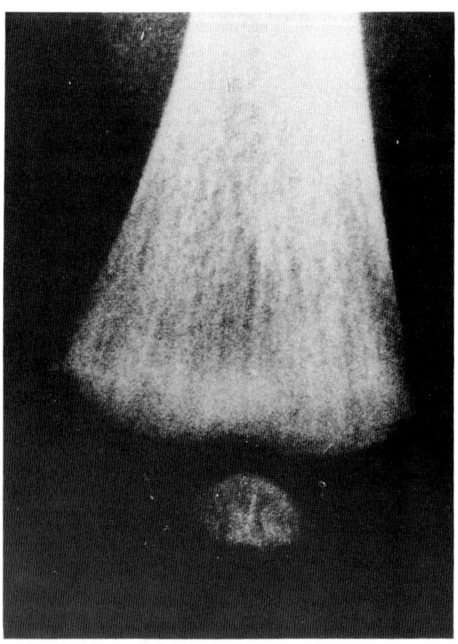

Figure 21-2. *Congenital rubella, showing a striate pattern of metaphyseal lucency.*

present (23). Occasionally, the lucency has a striking striated appearance (Figure 21-2). These lesions may be due to disturbance of endochondral ossification rather than true bone infection. Similar changes are seen in congenital cytomegalic inclusion disease (24; Figure 21-3) and occasionally in other viral illnesses in young children. Cytomegalovirus osteomyelitis has been described in association with human immunodeficiency virus infection (25). Periostitis has been noted in patients infected with the Epstein-Barr virus (26).

Fungal Infections

Fungal infections of bone may be divided into two groups according to the type of host in which they usually produce disease. Organisms such as *Histoplasma, Coccidioidomyces,* and *Blastomyces* generally attack "normal" hosts. Others, such as *Candida, Cryptococcus,*

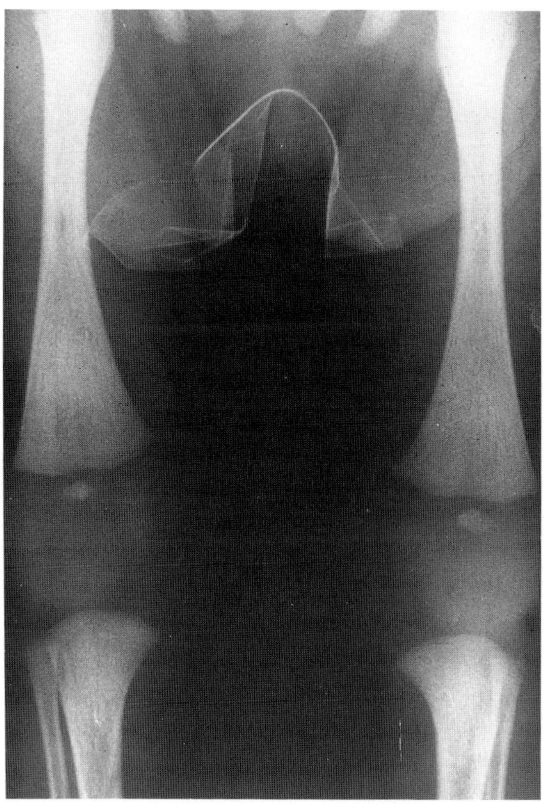

Figure 21-3.
Cytomegalovirus infection. Subtle metaphyseal lucency is present, particularly in the right femur.

Aspergillus, and *Sporotrichosis* generally infect immunocompromised hosts but may also attack "normal" hosts. Other fungi, such as penicillium, *Chrysosporium,* and *Fusarium,* tend almost exclusively to attack immunocompromised hosts or to occur following trauma and direct inoculation.

Infection Caused by *Candida* and *Torulopsis*

Candida and *Torulopsis* species are being recognized with increasing frequency as etiological agents of significant human infections. A review (27) of the 32 adult patients with *Candida* osteomyelitis reported in the literature up to 1987, with a description of five new patients, reported that the risk factors for *Candida* osteomyelitis include disseminated candidiasis, multiple antibiotic use, surgery, diabetes mellitus, and drug abuse. In the majority of patients, the pathogenesis appears to be seeding of bone as a sequela to disseminated candidiasis. The delay between positive blood culture results and the onset of symptoms of bone infection ranges from 2 to 15 months. Contiguous osteomyelitis may develop in an area of recent infection, sometimes surgically induced. Osteomyelitis may develop despite amphotericin B therapy at the time of diagnosis of disseminated candidiasis, and patients may be thought to be cured of disseminated candidiasis before bone infection is recognized.

In the majority of patients, the presentation of osteomyelitis is nonspecific, with relatively few systemic symptoms. The most frequent initial symptom is local pain. The majority of patients had involvement of either a single long bone or two adjacent vertebral bodies; the sternum was the most common site in patients with contiguous osteomyelitis. Laboratory findings were nonspecific and included elevated sedimentation rates in some patients, as well as elevated white blood cell counts in a few. Radiographic lesions were present, but there were no characteristic radiographic findings that helped to differentiate *Candida* osteomyelitis from other etiological agents (Figure 21-4). The diagnosis is established in the majority of patients by either needle biopsy or open procedure; closed needle biopsy frequently yields positive microbiological diagnoses. The majority of species isolated are *Candida albicans,* but several other species, including *C. stellatoidea, C. guillermondi, C. parapsilopsis,* and *C. tropicalis,* have been recovered.

Treatment regimens vary but primarily include amphotericin B or

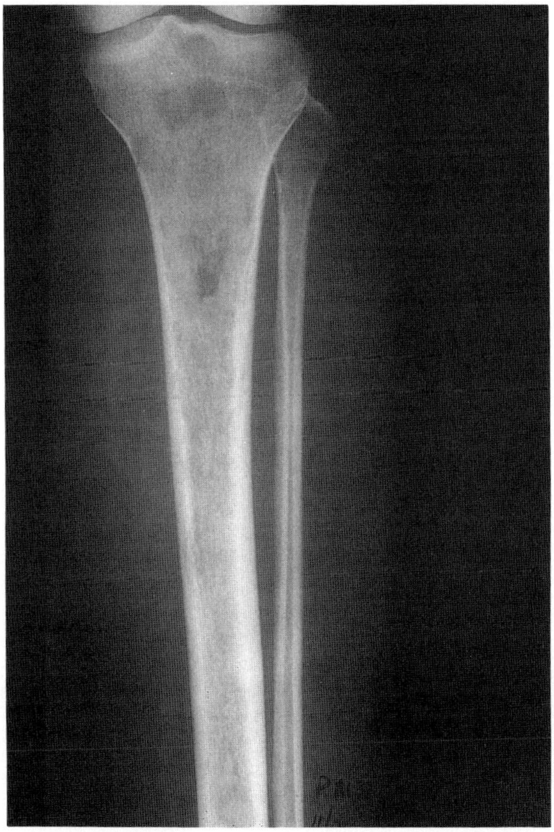

Figure 21-4. *Osteomyelitis due to* Candida albicans *in a woman with ulcerative colitis receiving chronic corticosteroid therapy.* (Provided by Dr. Alex Norman.)

ketoconazole. A combination of surgical debridement and antifungal therapy has been associated with marked clinical improvement or a completely healed radiograph on follow-up evaluation. Both ketoconazole and amphotericin B appear to be effective. There are no reports of chronic osteomyelitis due to *Candida* developing after adequate treatment of the initial bone lesions. Fluconazole, a new, orally administered triazole derivative, has been reported to treat osteomyelitis due to *Candida* (28,29) successfully. Patients who received the drug for approximately 1 year were apparently cured of infection.

In summarizing an approach to therapy, we suggest the following: (a) The decision whether to debride should be individualized; in patients with vertebral osteomyelitis, it does not appear to be critical, whereas it appears to be necessary in infection of the sternum. (b)

Although there are rare reports of spontaneous remission, treatment should be instituted with amphotericin B. Whether ketoconazole or fluconazole can replace amphotericin will require further studies. The target dose of amphotericin B for the treatment of osteomyelitis is not clear, but a suggested range would be up to 1,500 mg.

Torulopsis appears to produce disease in the same group of patients as *Candida* and generally manifests itself in the same way; however, the number of reported infections due to this species is much lower. In general, the same guidelines for diagnosis and management of *Candida* osteomyelitis apply to bone infections caused by *Torulopsis* (30,31).

Cryptococcus

The most common organ systems involved in cryptococcal infection are the lungs and the central nervous system. It is postulated that cryptococcal osteomyelitis is usually due to silent dissemination from a pulmonary source. However, many of the cases reported in the literature appear to be isolated bone lesions without any other focus of cryptococcal infection. It is estimated that bone infection develops in approximately 10% of patients with disseminated cryptococcosis.

In one review of 61 patients with osseous cryptococcosis, 29 infections were confined to bone (32). Nineteen patients had single lesions and the rest had multiple lesions. The most commonly involved bones were vertebrae, pelvis, ribs, and skull. Lesions are osteolytic, with minimal periosteal reaction (Figure 21-5); these findings are nonspecific and are also found in tuberculosis, histoplasmosis, coccidioidomycosis, and Ewing's sarcoma (33,34). The diagnosis is made by biopsy and demonstration of organisms. Culture of the organism is confirmatory.

Thirty-nine patients with skeletal cryptococcal infection reported in the literature since the development of chemotherapy for fungi were reviewed (35). In three fourths of patients, a single bone was involved; when more than one bone was involved, the process usually occurred in contiguous areas. The vertebrae were the most frequent site of involvement. Diagnosis was made either by aspiration or, in the majority of patients, at surgery. Data were available for 29 patients who were followed for periods ranging from 2 months to 15 years. During that time, none were reported to have recurrence of disease; three failed to show radiological improvement.

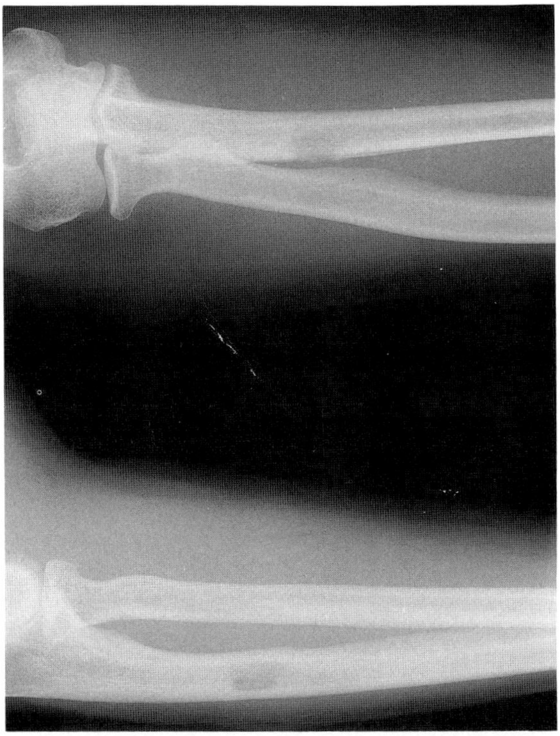

Figure 21-5. *A poorly defined lytic lesion in the ulna of a 40-year-old woman with extensive bilateral nodular pulmonary shadowing.* Cryptococcus neoformans *was identified at biopsy. Radiological appearances are nonspecific.*

If osseous cryptococcosis is found, a search for disease elsewhere in the body is critical. In particular, central nervous system involvement must be evaluated by lumbar puncture. One series noted that 16 of 19 reported lumbar punctures were negative for cryptococci; however, three were positive, indicating disseminated disease (35).

Although some have argued that surgical curettage is sufficient to treat osseous cryptococcosis, we believe that addition of antifungal agents is necessary, especially because the distinction between localized and disseminated disease is not always apparent. The optimal duration of therapy is unknown. A combination of amphotericin and 5-flucytosine and surgical debridement appears appropriate (35). The role of newer imidazole agents, such as fluconazole, is not yet clear in the management of this disease.

Coccidioidomycosis

Bony involvement is second only to skin as a manifestation of extrapulmonary spread; osteomyelitis occurs in 10% to 50% of all cases of coccidioidal dissemination (7). Virtually any bone may be involved, but lesions are particularly prominent at the sites of ligament or tendon insertion (i.e., malleoli, patella, and ankles). It was noted that in a series of 112 cases of coccidioidal osteomyelitis, 59% involved one bone with up to as many as eight different sites (36). Vertebrae were most frequently involved, followed by tibia, skull, metatarsals, and metacarpals. Blacks were more likely to have bone involvement than individuals of other racial origins.

Radiological appearances are nonspecific. Lesions in the long bones usually occur in the metaphysis and present with findings of rarefaction and periosteal proliferation. Punched out cystic areas in long or flat bones may be seen. Later, bone destruction, sequestrum, and sinus formation can occur (37).

Because infection of vertebrae is particularly common, it is worth noting radiographic differences from tuberculosis. In coccidioidomycosis, there is relative sparing of the disks, but there is also involvement of all portions of the vertebrae, including the arches and the processes, and there is absence of gibbus deformity; however, vertebral collapse may occur.

In the skull, lesions are either circular or irregular destructive lesions involving the outer table or both tables. Both skull and vertebral lesions pose a significant threat to life because direct spread to the meninges may occur in the absence of aggressive therapeutic intervention.

Antifungal chemotherapy is frequently not satisfactory in patients with coccidioidomycosis because of the lack of host immunity. Anergy, as defined by negative skin test to coccidioidin antigen, is a poor prognostic sign. However, the same basic principles of treatment, as have been described for other forms of fungal osteomyelitis, apply to coccidioidomycosis. Thus, the current recommendation for treatment is amphotericin B and surgical debridement where indicated. However, in patients with multiple bone lesions, surgical debridement is more difficult to perform and less likely to be useful.

Blastomycosis

As with many other fungi, *Blastomyces dermatitidis* (the agent of North American balstomycosis) primarily infects the lung and sets up a focus that either remains localized or may spread to involve other organs. Infection with this agent is prevalent in the mid-Atlantic areas and in the south central United States. However, with increasingly frequent and widespread travel, the pattern of geographic distribution is of limited help. Soil appears to be the ultimate source of infection.

Diagnosis is made by examination of histological tissue, and the histological appearance is usually sufficient to establish the diagnosis.

The incidence of bone involvement is reported to be between 14% and 60% in disseminated disease. Vertebrae are most commonly involved, followed by skull, ribs, and tibia. With long bone involvement, the infection may be located at the epiphysis or at the subarticular region, from which the infection may spread to the joint (38).

The radiographic appearance is not characteristic; generally, bone destruction predominates and periosteal proliferation is rare. If vertebrae are involved, there is usually massive destruction of the vertebral body, and the disk spaces are not spared (unlike coccidioidomycosis). Therefore, differentiation between tuberculosis and blastomycosis may be very difficult. Sequestrum formation is rare in blastomycosis.

Treatment involves appropriate orthopedic therapy and administration of amphotericin. Precise duration and dosage of therapy is not known. More recently, ketoconazole has been reported to be effective in treatment of bone infections due to *Blastomyces* (39). The organism is quite sensitive in vitro and the usual dose of 200 mg/day should provide adequate serum levels for treatment.

Aspergillus

The true incidence of osteomyelitis due to *Aspergillus* is unknown. In sino-orbital aspergillosis, contiguous bone involvement is probably relatively common but is often not reported.

Fifteen cases of *Aspergillus* osteomyelitis from the medical literature were reviewed (40). The most striking feature was that most patients had gross defects in immunocompetence. In children, chronic granulomatous disease is a significant risk factor. In adults, the most important predisposing condition was immunosuppressive drug therapy. In children, vertebrae and ribs were the most common sites; contiguous spread from a pulmonary infection was the most frequent mechanism postulated. Vertebrae were also the most common location of osteomyelitis in adults, but in half the patients (unlike children), the infections were spread hematogenously. *Aspergillus fumigatus* was responsible for two thirds of the infections. Surgery and antifungal chemotherapy, usually with amphotericin B, allowed survival of 10 patients; all deaths were directly related to *Aspergillus* infection. Patients who were immunosuppressed had a very high mortality rate. One series noted that when *Aspergillus* osteomyelitis is resistant to treatment with amphotericin, the presence of necrotic tissue or pus should be suspected and excised and drained in immunosuppressed patients (41).

Subsequent reports have identified vertebral osteomyelitis following laminectomy and several patients in whom infection extended to the vertebrae from infected aortic grafts with mycotic pseudoaneurysm (42). In the latter patients, a period of approximately 2 years elapsed between placement of the vascular graft and diagnosis of the adjacent osteomyelitis.

Two cases of hematogenously acquired *Aspergillus* vertebral osteomyelitis in drug addicts who appeared to be immunocompetent were reported (43). Both patients recovered with treatment consisting of debridement and administration of a total of 2 g amphotericin B. Patients with normal immune function appear to survive *Aspergillus* osteomyelitis in contrast to immunosuppressed individuals with similar infections (40,43).

Histoplasmosis

Reports of radiological evidence of lesions of bone due to *Histoplasma capsulatum* are rare; when reported, the lesion is usually a punched out lytic lesion. The clinical setting is usually that of disseminated histoplasmosis (44). In contrast, in disseminated histoplasmosis due to the African strain, *H. duboisii,* punched out lytic lesions are common (45). With vertebral involvement due to *H. duboisii,* the entire vertebral body is usually destroyed and undergoes liquefactive necrosis. The disks are initially preserved but subsequently are destroyed. Epidural extension of necrotic pus is common with spinal cord compression resulting.

Given the relative infrequency with which histoplasmosis of bone is reported, it is difficult to comment about efficacy of therapy. Treatment with amphotericin B appears to be the method of choice.

Miscellaneous Fungal Bone Infection

Sporotrichosis

Osteomyelitis has been reported as a complication of the localized cutaneous form of sporotrichosis, and arthritis may be seen with systemic sporotrichosis. However, osteomyelitis without arthritic involvement due to sporotrichosis is uncommon (46). In the localized cutaneous form, a skin lesion may involve underlying bone, producing an eccentric erosive lesion that may excite periosteal reaction. In the systemic form, a purulent arthritis develops, with multiple joints involved. In these instances, soft-tissue swelling, osteoporosis, bony erosion, and joint space narrowing may be noted. Usually, sporotrichosis seems primarily to involve the joint and to affect adjacent bone only secondarily.

An extensive review of the literature (47) of sporotrichosis found 22 patients with bone involvement. In almost 70%, local swelling developed over the site of bone destruction; approximately 40% had sinuses draining from bone to skin. Patients had disseminated disease with distant skin lesions. The combination of local areas of bone destruction and the appearance of distant skin lesions should suggest the possibility of sporotrichosis (47). In almost all patients, the bone lesions were osteolytic, with little reactive changes. Radiographic findings were not specific and may be seen in other fungal infections, tuberculosis of bone, and in tumors (Figure 21-6).

Although oral potassium iodide treatment of the skin lesions of sporotrichosis is frequently sufficient, osteomyelitis and arthritis may also require amphotericin B alone or with surgical debridement. However, successful treatment of osteomyelitis due to *S. schenckii* with potassium iodide and debridement has been reported (48).

Pseudallescheria boydii

P. boydii is a natural saprophyte that has been associated with mycetoma. A patient has been described with mycetoma of the scalp and osteomyelitis of the skull after blunt injury to the calvarium from a tree limb (49). The presumed mechanism was direct inoculation by vegetative material; surgical trauma and therapy with antibiotics and steroids probably facilitated subsequent development of infection. Wide resection of involved bone, without antifungal therapy, may achieve cure of cranial osteomyelitis due to this organism.

In another report, five patients with osteomyelitis due to *P. boydii* are described (50). All were previously healthy men, lived in rural areas, sustained traumatic injuries that caused contamination with soil or vegetative material, and required surgical debridement or amputation. The continuation of antifungal therapy in the management

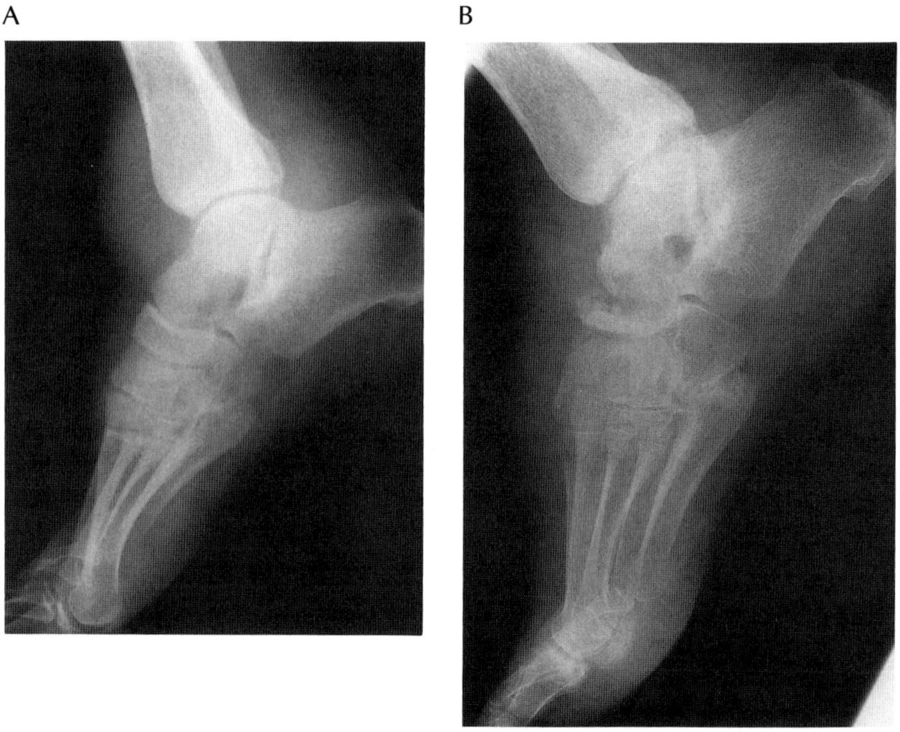

Figure 21-6. *Disseminated sporotrichosis. (A) Soft-tissue swelling and joint effusion are present. Joint spaces are maintained and no erosions are seen. (B) Four years later, there is narrowing of the tibia-talar joint and destruction of the talonavicular joint. Both the talus and the navicular bone are infected. The cuboid-fifth metatarsal is also involved.* (Provided by Dr. Robert Klein.)

of this form of osteomyelitis is difficult to assess, but may be useful as an adjunct in selected cases.

Alternaria

Alternaria has traditionally been considered harmless to humans, but there are now four cases of osteomyelitis due to this ubiquitous soil fungus in the literature (51). All four patients had normal immune systems and each experienced protracted infections, for which several courses of antifungal chemotherapy were required. It has been suggested that environmental factors peculiar to the nasal cavity and the paranasal sinuses favor growth of the organism at these sites; infection of bony structures in sites distant from sinuses are not reported (50). The reasons for the refractory nature of the infection are unclear, but aggressive surgical debridement and prolonged therapy with amphotericin B seems necessary.

Mucormycosis

The zygomycetes are a group of filamentous fungi that are ubiquitous in nature. They are most commonly seen in immunocompromised patients and may cause rhinocerebral, pulmonary, or disseminated zygomycoses. Osteomyelitis is an infrequent complication of these syndromes, although it has been reported secondary to contiguous spread of these organisms (52). It has also been reported to cause osteomyelitis with concomitant avascular necrosis (53). Although *Mucor* and *Rhizopus* are the organisms reported most frequently, *Saksenaea vasiformis* has been recently reported to cause significant osteomyelitis following trauma (54). Treatment of these infections requires vigorous surgical debridement as well as amphotericin B therapy.

Scedosporium Inflatum

Scedosporium inflatum is a relatively newly described species that differs from the clinically more well known *Scedosporium apiospermum* (55,56). Infections with this organism are primarily focally invasive and frequently involve musculoskeletal tissue. The great majority of infections follow penetrating trauma or surgery. There is a clear predilection for cartilage and joint areas, a striking lack of noncontiguous spread, and no real association with immunodeficiency. The organism was frequently difficult to identify and management was frequently protracted. The organisms frequently appeared to be resistant in vitro to amphotericin B, ketoconazole, miconazole, and fluconazole. No single mode of therapy appeared optimal. Currently, recommendations for treatment include local debridement or drainage, with intra-articular amphotericin B therapy if the response to systemic antifungal therapy is not adequate.

Other Fungi

Penicillium marneffei is a dimorphic fungus and an unusual pathogen in humans. A case of systemic infection with this organism was reported in a patient who presented with multiple osteolytic lesions as well as a chronic facial ulcer (57). A correct etiological diagnosis was made and treatment with amphotericin and oral 5-fluorocytosine was effective in curing the infection. The radiological appearance is similar to that seen in osteomyelitis caused by such organisms as African histoplasmosis, blastomycosis, and coccidioidomycosis. This infection is also frequently misdiagnosed as tuberculosis; such misdiagnoses are unfortunate because antifungal treatment may produce a rapid and gratifying response.

Isolated cases of osteomyelitis caused by fungi usually considered to be saprophytes have been reported. These cases include infection with *Chrysosparium* (58), *Fusarium solani* (59), and *Acremarium kiliense* (60). In most instances, infection of bone resulted from direct inoculation secondary to trauma. In general, these infections responded, albeit slowly, to surgical resection and antifungal chemotherapy (primarily amphotericin B).

Mycoplasma Species

Infections with mycoplasma species have rarely been reported to involve bone or joints. One case of wound infection with *Mycoplasma hominis* occurred following mandibular fracture in two patients (61) and was associated with osteomyelitis in one. Infections of sternotomy incisions have also been reported (62).

Infections with *Mycoplasma* species have been well described in patients who are immunocompromised, particularly those with hypogammaglobulinemia. In an interesting report, a 22-year-old man with known hypogammaglobulinemia for 18 years presented with osteomyelitis involving the femoral head and hip joint (63). Prior cultures of bone biopsy had been negative. Repeat exploration of the hip joint allowed the growth of colonies of *U. urealyticum,* and the patient responded appropriately to tetracycline and streptomycin. The need to consider infection with *Mycoplasma* species in patients with antibody deficiency who present with infection at extrapulmonary sites is underscored by this case report and another (64). Many patients also had genitourinary manipulation preceding infection with *M. hominis.* The ability of *M. hominis* to infect surgical wounds or trauma following a presumed mycoplasmemia is documented (60). The optimum treatment is not known, but we recommend surgical debridement and therapy with clindamycin and doxycycline (65).

Brucellosis

Brucellosis is currently comparatively rare in the developed world. Much of the recent literature has come from areas such as North Africa and the Middle East, where the disease remains endemic in cattle and goats. Human cases arise from ingestion of infected milk. Twenty to 85% of patients with brucellosis experience osteoarticular symptoms (66). The incidence of organism-positive skeletal infection, however, is much lower, and in some reports has been as low as 1% (67). Sacroiliac (68), hip, and knee joints are commonly affected, but involvement of most joints has been reported (69–72). Spondylodiskitis characteristically affects the lumbar rather than the thoracic spine (73).

Histologically, infection with *Brucella* species (*B. abortus, B. melitensis, B. suis*) characteristically shows multiple minute granulomata that closely resemble tuberculosis. Caseation may occur but is unusual. Sometimes the granulomatous nature of the chronic inflammatory lesion may not be obvious (74). At a macroscopic level, and on radiological examination, appearances are nonspecific, although calcification may occasionally be seen, giving rise to confusion with tuberculosis (75).

Potential exposure to infected animals or milk should alert clinicians. Acute brucellosis is a systemic disease, characterized by malaise, fatigability, fever, and an increased erythrocyte sedimentation rate. Signs may include splenomegaly, lymphadenopathy, and hepatomegaly. Many of these patients have arthralgia. However, individuals with localized osteoarticular brucellosis may lack significant systemic signs; indeed, up to one third may be free of fever (66). The local signs are those of a subacute bone, joint, or bursal infection. Although organisms may be isolated from blood culture, aspirate, or biopsy material, they grow poorly on ordinary media, and special notification of potential cases is advised. Only 20% of bone and joint infections give a positive culture. The most sensitive laboratory assay in contemporary practice appears to be the *Brucella* enzyme-linked immunosorbent assay (76).

In an appropriate clinical context, antimicrobial therapy should be begun on the basis of positive serology. A recent randomized study compared doxycycline plus rifampin with doxycycline plus streptomycin (77) and indicated that these regimens were equally effective for most patients with brucellosis, but that the classic regimen of doxycycline and streptomycin may be more effective in spondylodiskitis.

The role of surgery is in biopsy, drainage of significant abscesses, and, if necessary, late reconstruction.

Syphilis and Yaws

A number of osteoarticular manifestations are recognized in acquired, congenital, and endemic (nonvenereal) syphilis (*Treponema pallidum*), and yaws (*Treponema pertenue*). Acquired syphilis, in decline in the 1970s (78), has become more common in the late 1980s in North America, with a consequent increase in congenital syphilis (79). Nonvenereal syphilis has been, for the most part, eradicated (80). Yaws, largely controlled in the 1950s and 1960s by mass treatment campaigns, has also undergone a resurgence in the last decade in some tropical areas (81,82). Early antibiotic treatment has reduced the incidence of late manifestations in both diseases (82,83).

Acquired Syphilis and Yaws

The primary infection in both venereal syphilis and yaws is mucocutaneous. Osteoarticular involvement, similar in each disease, first occurs in the early or secondary stage, some weeks or months after the primary lesion (84). Three processes may become apparent: synovitis, osteomyelitis, and periostitis (85). Synovitis is relatively uncommon: it may be a blood-borne hematogenous infection, represent spread from an adjacent focus of bone infection, or be a sterile reactive effusion sympathetic to a nearby bone lesion. When multiple joints are involved, syphilis may present as a polyarthritis, resembling rheumatoid arthritis or systemic lupus erythematosus (86,87). This presentation may occur in association with human immunodeficiency virus infection (87,88).

Periostitis, osteomyelitis, arthritis, bursitis, or tenosynovitis occur in up to 20% of patients during the secondary stage of acquired syphilis; the reported incidence varies widely (89,90). Bone lesions present with swelling, tenderness, and pain that is often described as deep-seated, boring, and worse at night (91). Periostitis is the most common finding on radiological examination (92). It is typically laminar but may occasionally have a fluffy, radial appearance (93).

Osteomyelitis is less common and is most frequently found in the skull, but can occur in any situation (94).

In late (tertiary) syphilis and yaws, presenting years or decades after the early stages, periostitis and osteomyelitis are found. Periostitis in the tibia typically affects the subcutaneous surface in the middle third, producing the "saber tibia" deformity (Figure 21-7; 78). In yaws, hypertrophic periostitis of the maxilla may produce a characteristic thickening of the base of the nose (Figure 21-8) (95). Dactylitis (Figure 21-9), tenosynovitis and arthritis may also occur (96). In yaws, the hands may be the site of a deforming destructive osteoarthropathy producing a clinical appearance like psoriatic arthritis mutilans (97).

The characteristic bone lesion of tertiary syphilis is the gumma, which appears on radiography as a lytic lesion with a densely sclerotic

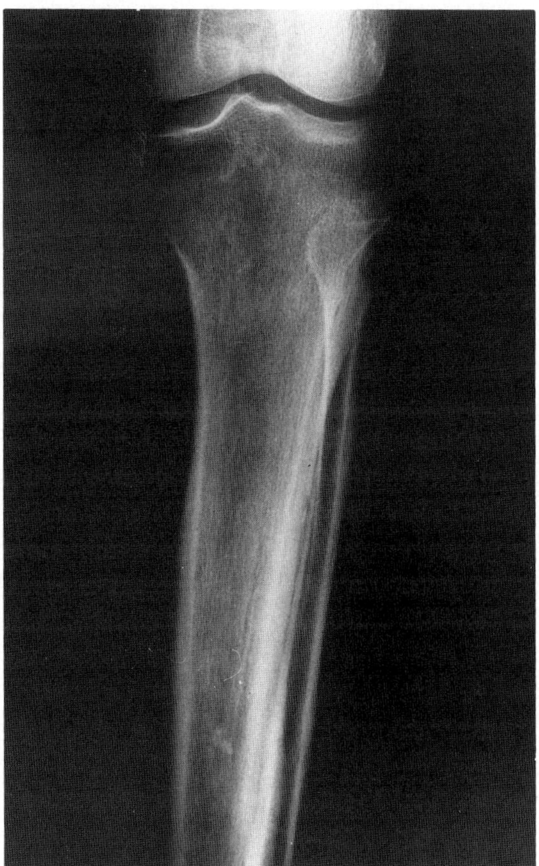

Figure 21-7. *Periostitis of the tibia particularly affecting the medial border (male, aged 45 years, tertiary syphilis).*

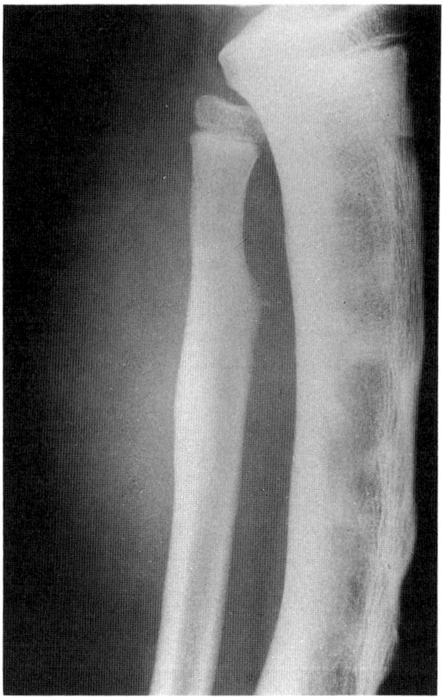

Figure 21-8. *Yaws osteoperiostitis of the tibia.*

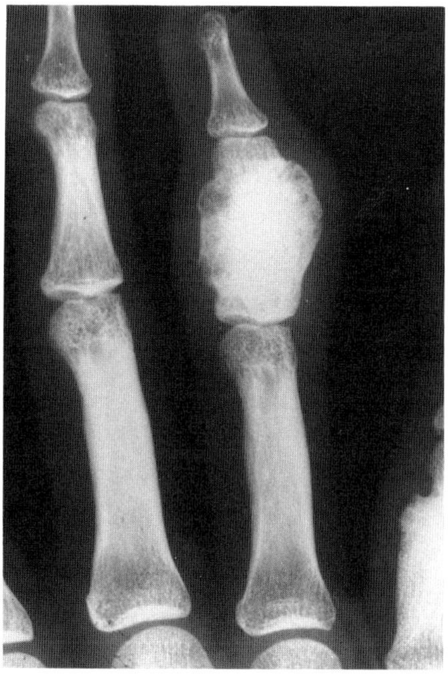

Figure 21-9. *Yaws dactylitis.*

bone reaction (78). Gummata, which may occur in any organ or tissue, differ from treponemal osteomyelitis in having histopathological characteristics of a hypersensitivity reaction, showing a central necrotic area surrounded by lymphocytes, plasma cells, epithelioid cells, and fibrosis with obliterative endarteritis (98). Persisting viable organisms may sometimes be identified.

Radiology, taken in conjunction with serological tests, is usually diagnostic (99). Characteristic scintigraphic appearances of periostitis and osteomyelitis have been described, but they add no new information if good quality radiographs are available (100,101).

Congenital Syphilis

Bone involvement in congenital syphilis presents in a manner similar to secondary acquired syphilis, usually within the first 4 months of life. Approximately 10% present with painful swollen joints resembling rickets or with pseudoparalysis (101). On radiological examination, disturbance of endochondral ossification with widening of the zone of provisional calcification (osteochondritis) is manifest as narrow horizontal bands of radiolucency, which may proceed to confluent areas of metaphyseal erosion if allowed to progress (85). In the medial aspect of the proximal tibia, this appearance is called Wimberger's sign. Metaphyseal changes are seen in 20% to 30% of seropositive infants (102,103). The incidence of focal destructive lesions and periostitis varies in the contemporary literature (103,104) and may depend on the stage of presentation. Pathological fractures occasionally occur (102). In treated children, these signs disappear during the first year of life, leading usually to normal growth and development (102).

Late Congenital Syphilis

Late congenital syphilis is characterized by lesions appearing for the first time 2 or more years after birth. In the musculoskeletal system, these lesions include chronic diaphyseal osteomyelitis and periostitis leading in the tibia to a characteristic saber deformity, and in the hands or feet to dactylitis (85). Destructive bone lesions also occur, particularly in the skull and the facial bones. A painless symmetrical chronic arthritis, thought to be a hypersensitivity phenomenon, generally affecting the knees (Clutton's joints) occurs occasionally, typically between the ages of 10 and 20 years (105,106).

Management

For clinicians in the 1990s, tertiary musculoskeletal manifestations of treponemal infections are relatively rare, even in the developing world, due to antibiotic treatment in the primary and secondary stages. Awareness of typical presentations and willingness to biopsy destructive lesions of uncertain etiology (107–109) are the important elements in diagnosis.

Management of syphilis and yaws is antibiotic chemotherapy. In the presence of penicillin allergy, erythromycin and tetracycline are probably effective; in its absence, penicillin is the antibiotic of choice for both diseases.

Actinomycosis

Actinomycosis is an uncommon chronic infection characterized by its ability to cross tissue planes; thus, for example, lesions in the facial bones may spread widely in the cervicofacial area, and pulmonary lesions may involve the chest wall. Thirty percent of infections are cervicofacial, less than 5% involve the extremities (110), and infections in the spine (111) are uncommon.

The actinomycotic lesion is a rather hard mass with edema, induration, sinus formation, and repeated episodes of surrounding cellulitis. Most are subacute, but occasionally the presentation is acute and rapidly progressive. The sinus discharge is particularly characteristic, containing distinctive yellow-orange clumps of organisms approximately 2 mm in diameter, known as sulphur granules.

The most common isolate in human disease is *Actinomyces israeli.* An oral commensal, it is a gram-positive branching filamentous bacterium that grows best under anaerobic conditions. Microbiological diagnosis can be made by examination of histological material, but carefully prepared smears (112) and anaerobic culture of material from discharge or lesion are more likely to identify the infection.

Radiological features are nonspecific. In the facial bones (112), actinomycosis may cause periostitis by involvement of neighboring soft tissues, a sclerotic honeycomb pattern of osteomyelitis, or a rather poorly marginated lytic lesion (Figure 21-10). In the spine, a cystic "soap bubble" appearance involving the vertebral bodies, with sparing of the disk, may occur (112), but typical vertebral infections with disk destruction are also described (111,113). In long bones, radiologically typical cases of chronic sclerosing osteomyelitis have occasionally yielded *Actinomyces* species (114).

Penicillin is the antibiotic of choice in the management of actinomycosis. Erythromycin and tetracycline are satisfactory in the presence of penicillin sensitivity. In the absence of significant abscess or sequestrum formation, antibiotic therapy alone can produce a cure. Abscesses should be aspirated or drained surgically, and clearly devitalized bone should be resected according to the principles established for chronic osteomyelitis (see Chapter 15).

Protozoal and Helminthic Infections

Protozoa

Although myalgia is a feature of the systemic disease in malaria and kala-azar, protozoal infections of muscle, bone, and joints are rare.

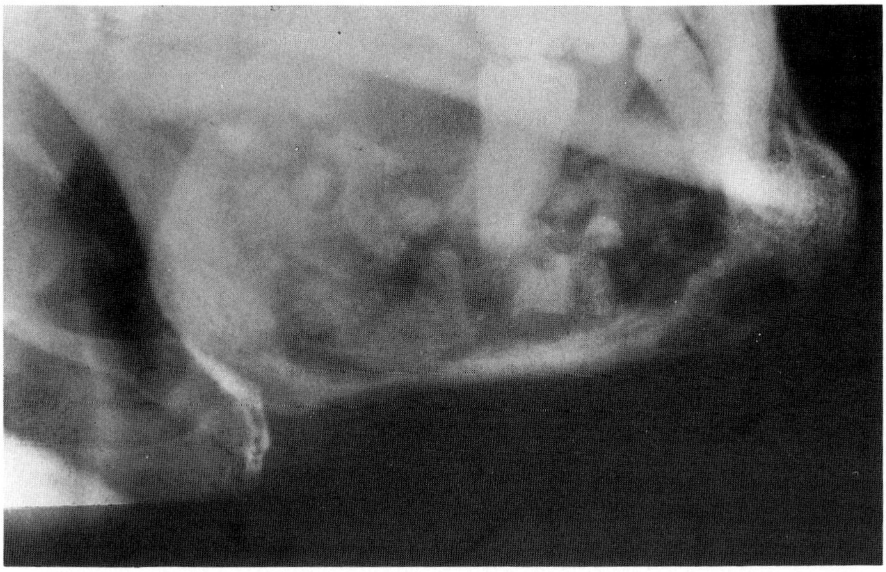

Figure 21-10. *Actinomycosis of the mandible. The lesion is predominantly destructive, with some foci of sclerosis.*

Bone and muscle lesions have been identified in congenital toxoplasmosis (115). Arthritis, myositis (116), and granulomatous tenosynovitis (117) occasionally occur in acquired toxoplasmosis.

Free-living amoebae have not been definitively described as producing infection in bone. In a prediabetic woman undergoing resection and autograft for a tumor of the mandible, acute suppurative osteomyelitis developed, from which gram-positive cocci, gram-positive bacilli, gram-negative bacilli, and *Acanthamoeba castellanii* were cultured (118). These amoebae may be oral commensals of transitory nature. The authors concluded that many factors, including use of broad-spectrum antibiotics and altered immune competence, contributed to the infection, which resolved after removal of the sequestrum without specific treatment for the amoebic infection.

It is also possible that some examples of slowly progressive postsurgical necrotizing cellulitis are caused by *Entamoeba hystolytica* (119).

Trichinosis

Myositis occurs in 90% of individuals with clinically manifest infection by the nematode *Trichinella spiralis*. The principal associated features are fever, malaise, periorbital edema, eosinophilia, and a history of ingestion of poorly cooked meat. Antibody titers are increased after 3 weeks. Diagnosis can be confirmed by biopsy of tender, swollen areas of muscle. Treatment is symptomatic and symptoms settle over 2 to 3 weeks (120).

Cysticercosis

Cysticercosis is also derived from the ingestion of poorly cooked, infected pork, due to infection with eggs of *Taenia solium*, the pork tapeworm. Cysts may form in any viscus. In muscle, the cysts, whose long axis is aligned with the muscle fasciculi, are palpable as small nodules that calcify after 3 to 5 years. The radiological appearances are characteristic (Figure 21-11).

Dracunculiasis (Guinea Worm Arthritis)

Dracunculus medinensis is widespread throughout the tropics, but osteoarticular involvement is uncommon. The female worm migrates

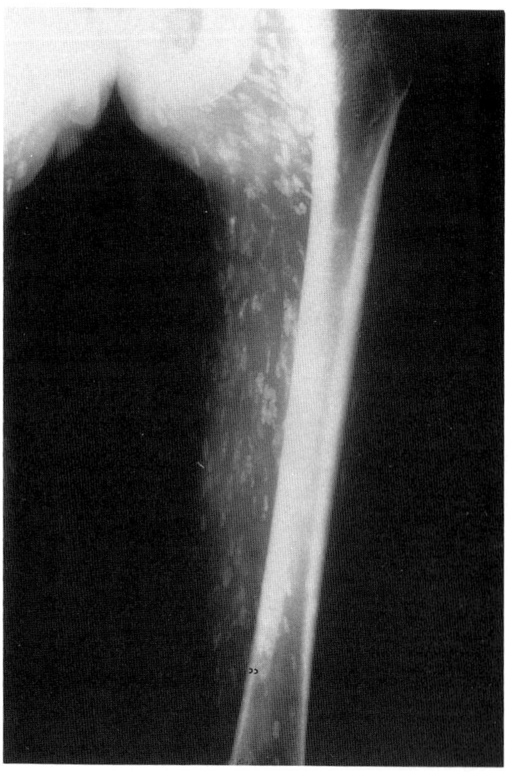

Figure 21-11. *Cysticercosis in muscles of the left thigh.*

to the subcutaneous tissues, usually of the limbs. Death of the worm results in an intense reaction, which produces ulceration and secondary involvement of bone or joint by bacterial infection. There are occasional reports of direct involvement of joints by migrating worms (121,122).

Hookworm

A hookworm (*Necator americanus*) has been identified from a lytic bone lesion in the hindfoot (123). Reactive arthritis has been diagnosed in a child with hookworm infestation, but the relationship is uncertain (124).

Hydatid Disease (Echinococcosis)

Of all human patients with echinococcosis, 1% to 4% have musculoskeletal disease (125,126). Reports of bone and joint hydatid have come mainly from South America (127), the Arabian peninsula (125,128), Australia and New Zealand (126), and East Africa (129).

Most cases are caused by *Echinococcus granulosus,* but human disease with two other species, *E. vogeli* and *E. multilocularis,* has also been reported (130,131). The dog is the principal host in which the adult worm parasitizes the small intestine, and complete control of the disease in dogs is essential to its eradication. Humans are occasional intermediate hosts. The ova, excreted by the dog, may be ingested. The oncosphere penetrates the gut mucosa and enters the portal circulation, lodging in the liver and hence spreading to many tissues, including bone, muscle, and synovium. Initially, the rigid structure of bone prevents the formation of typical cysts, but these cysts develop, and extensive destruction of bone occurs (132).

In musculoskeletal hydatid disease, it is usually the appearances on imaging that lead to diagnosis. In addition, there may be a history of exposure to dogs, particularly animals that may have ingested raw offal. Although the liver is the most common site of formation of a hydatid cyst in humans and should be examined in any case of hydatid, it may be spared. Eosinophilia is usual. If necessary, specific serological tests may also be employed (131). The radiological, computerized tomographic, and ultrasound appearances of hydatid cysts in soft tissue and in bone are usually characteristic, demonstrating large multilocular cysts (Figures 21-12 to 21-14), although early bone lesions may be less obvious. Established bone lesions may present

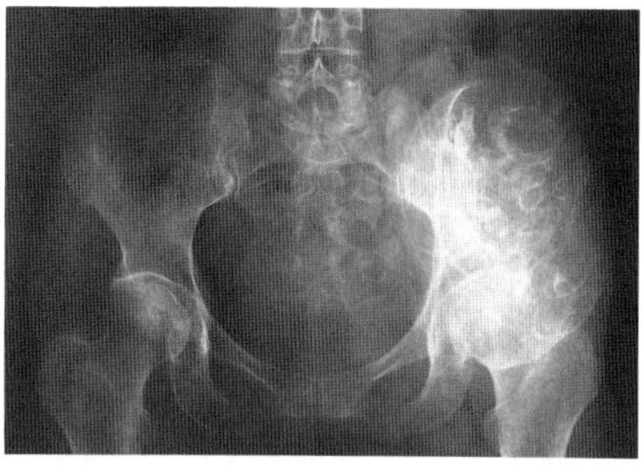

Figure 21-12. *Hydatid disease involving the left ilium.*

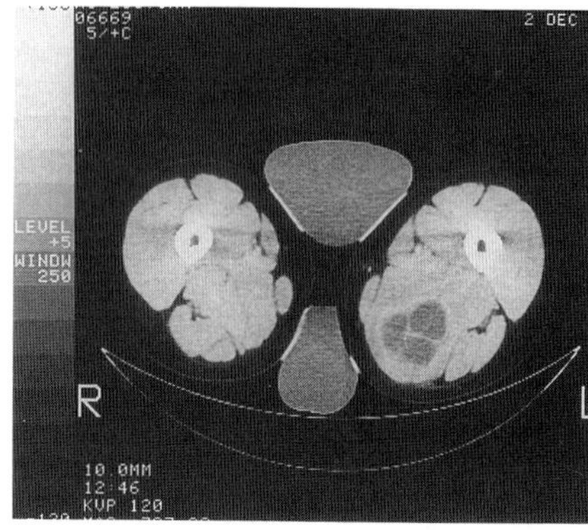

Figure 21-13. *Appearance of hydatid cysts in muscle on computerized tomography.*

with a fracture (Figure 21-15), or with bone pain or enlargement. Up to 50% of cases of osseous hydatid in some series have involved the spine; computerized tomography and magnetic resonance imaging may be of particular value in establishing the diagnosis (133). In muscle, the cyst presents as a slowly enlarging mass lesion with slight pain, although exacerbations of pain may occur and have been considered to be due to cyst rupture.

Diagnostic biopsy and aspiration are contraindicated in hydatid disease. When technically possible, management is radical surgical resection of the diseased area. Spillage from cysts during aspiration or surgery may cause spread of the disease, giving rise to chronic sinus formation with secondary bacterial infection. Should a cyst be accidentally punctured, the danger of spread may be reduced by application of cetyl-trimethyl ammonium bromide (Cetrimide) (134), 2% formalin, or 1% iodine (131), but this is no substitute for careful planning and meticulous surgery. Function following radical resection of bone may be restored by the use of allografts (135) or endoprosthetic surgery. In the past, surgical curettage, formalin swabbing, and bone grafting were recommended at sites where excision is difficult, such as the spine (125,128). Alternatively, if excision is impossible, chemotherapy with mebendazole or albendazole may be considered (129,136), but chemotherapy in the management of bone and joint hydatid has not been clearly established.

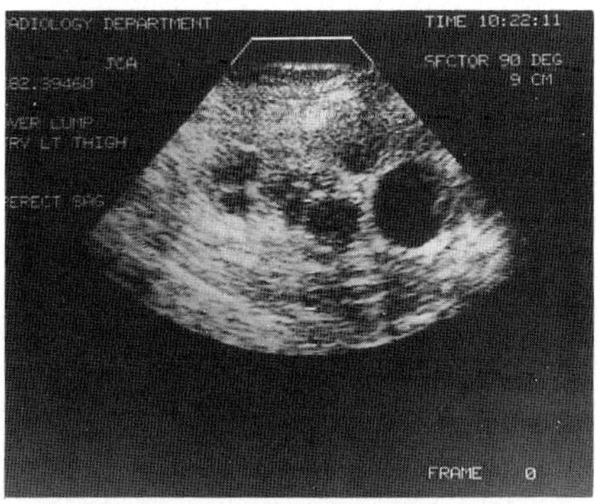

Figure 21-14. *Characteristic ultrasonic appearance of hydatid disease.*

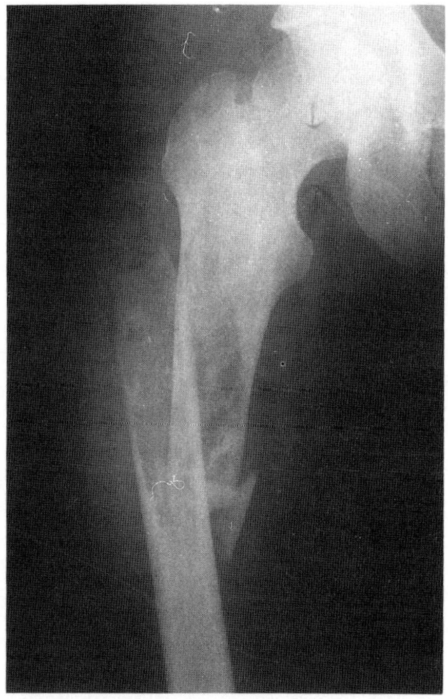

Figure 21-15. *Pathological fracture through hydatid disease of the femoral shaft.*

References

1. Larson HE, Blades R. Impairment of human polymorphonuclear leukocyte function by influenza virus infection. Lancet 1976;1:283.
2. Liebergall M, Porat S. Streptococcal osteomyelitis associated with varicella virus infection: a case report and review of the literature. J Pediatr Orthop 1984;4:756–758.
3. Ralston SH, Digiovine FS, Gallacher SJ, Boyle IT, Duff GW. Failure to detect paramyxovirus sequences in Paget's disease of bone using the polymerase chain reaction. J Bone Mineral Res 1991;6:1243–1248.
4. Sewell S. Vaccinia osteomyelitis: a report of a case with isolation of the vaccinia virus. Bull Hosp J Dis 1949;10:59–63.
5. Caranosos GJ, Gelker JR. Mumps arthritis. Arch Intern Med 1967;119: 394–398.
6. Ward JR, Bishop B. Varicella arthritis. JAMA 1970;212:1954–1956.

7. Fierman H. Varicella-associated arthritis occurring before the exanthem. Case report and literature. Clin Pediatr (Phila) 1990;29:188–190.
8. Grahame R, Armstrong R, Simmons N, et al. Chronic arthritis associated with the presence of intrasynovial rubella virus. Ann Rheum Dis 1983;42:2–13.
9. Miki NP, Chantler JK. Differential ability of wild-type and vaccine strains of rubella virus to replicate and persist in human joint tissue. Clin Exp Rheumatol 1992;10:3–12.
10. Alpert E, Isselbacher KJ, Schur PH. The pathogenesis of arthritis associated with viral hepatitis. Complement component studies. N Engl J Med 1971; 285:185–189.
11. Vanzee BE, Douglas RG, Betts RF, Bauman AW, Fraser DW, Hinman R. Lymphocytic choriomeningitis in university hospital personnel. Clinical features. Am J Med 1975;58:803–809.
12. White DG, Woolf AD, Mortimer PP. Human parvovirus arthropathy. Lancet 1985;1:419–421.
13. Reid DM, Reid TMS, Brown T, Rennie JA, Eastmond CJ. Human parvovirus associated arthritis: a clinical and laboratory description. Lancet 1985;1:422–425.
14. Sigal LH, Steere AC, Niederman JC. Symmetric polyarthritis associated with heterophile negative infectious mononucleosis. Arthritis Rheum 1982; 25:930–936.
15. Hurst NP, Martynoga AG, Nuki G, Sewell JR, Mitchell A, Hughes GR. Coxsackie B infection and arthritis. Br Med J 1983;286:605.
16. Bennett PH. Ross River virus infection. An acute polyarthritis caused by arborvirus. J Rheumatol 1983;10(suppl):34–36.
17. Simpson RW, McGinty L, Simon L, Smith CA, Godzeski CW, Boyd RJ. Association of parvoviruses with rheumatoid arthritis of humans. Science 1984;223:1425–1428.
18. Rsdahl E. Retroviruses and chronic arthritis. Possible significance of some recent observations. Scand J Rheumatol 1989;18:335–339.
19. Srivastava AN. Orthopaedic complications of smallpox. J Bone Joint Surg [Br] 1966;48:183.
20. Cockshott P, Macgregor M. Osteomyelitis variolosa. Q J Med 1958;27: 69–87.
21. Elliott WD. Vaccinial osteomyelitis. Lancet 1959;2:1053–1055.
22. Lindquist JM, Plotkin SA, Shaw L. Congenital rubella syndrome as a systemic infection: studies of affected infants born in Philadelphia. Br Med J 1965;2:1401–1406.
23. Reed BG. Rubella bone lesions. J Pediatr 1969;74:208–213.
24. McCandless AE, Davis C, Hall EG. Bone changes in congenital cytomegalic inclusion disease. Arch Dis Child 1975;50:160–162.
25. Berman S, Jensen J. Cytomegalovirus-induced osteomyelitis in a patient with the acquired immunodeficiency syndrome. South Med J 1990;83: 1231–1232.
26. Burrows FG. Transient periosteal reaction in an illness diagnosed as infectious mononucleosis. Radiology 1971;98:291–292.

27. Gathe JC, Harris RL, Garland B, Bradshaw MW, Williams TW. Candida osteomyelitis. Report of five cases and review of the literature. Am J Med 1987;82:927–937.
28. Sugar AM, Saunders C, Diamond RD. Successful treatment of candida osteomyelitis with fluconazole. A noncomparative study of two patients. Diagn Microbiol Infect Dis 1990;13:517–520.
29. Targ C. Successful treatment of Candida albicans osteomyelitis with fluconazole. J Infect 1993;26:89–92.
30. Imahori SC, Papademetriou T, Ogliela DM. Torulopsis glabrata osteomyelitis. A case report. Clin Orthop 1987;219:214–220.
31. Thurston AJ, Gillespie WJ. Torulopsis glabrata osteomyelitis of the spine: a case report and review of the literature. Aust NZ J Surg 1981;51:374–376.
32. Rolston KVI. Treatment of osseous cryptococcosis—report of a case and review of the literature. Orthopedics 1982;5:1610–1614.
33. Zach TL, Penn RG. Localized cryptococcal osteomyelitis in an immunocompetent host. Pediatr Infect Dis 1986;5:601–603.
34. Chleboun J, Nade S. Skeletal cryptococcosis. J Bone Joint Surg [Am] 1977;59:509–514.
35. Behrman RE, Masci JR, Nicholas P. Cryptococcal skeletal infections: case report and review. Rev Infect Dis 1990;12:181–190.
36. Durtz D, Catanzaro A. Coccidioidomycosis—part I. Am Rev Respir Dis 1978;117:559–585.
37. Moreno AJ. Nuclear imaging in coccidioidal osteomyelitis. Clin Nucl Med 1987;12:604–609.
38. Reigler HF, Goldstein LA, Betts RF. Blastomycosis osteomyelitis. Clin Orthop 1974;100:225–231.
39. Wagner DK, Varkey B, Head MD. Blastomycotic osteomyelitis of the mandible: successful treatment with ketoconazole. Oral Surg Oral Med Oral Pathol 1985;60:370–371.
40. Tack KJ, Rhame FS, Brown B, Thompson RC. Aspergillus osteomyelitis. Report of four cases and review of the literature. Am J Med 1982;73:295–300.
41. Bridwell KH, Campbell JW, Barenkamp SJ. Surgical treatment of hematogenous vertebral aspergillus osteomyelitis. Spine 1990;15:281–285.
42. Brandt SJ, Thompson RL, Wenzel RP. Mycotic pseudoaneurysm of an aortic bypass graft and contiguous vertebral osteomyelitis due to Aspergillus fumigatus. Am J Med 1985;79:259–262.
43. Brown DL, Musher DM, Taffet GE. Hematogenously acquired aspergillus vertebral osteomyelitis in seemingly immunocompetent drug addicts. West J Med 1987;147:84–85.
44. Jones RC, Goodwin RA. Histoplasmosis of bone. Am J Med 1981;70:864–866.
45. Williams AO, Lawson EA, Lucas AO. African histoplasmosis due to Histoplasma duboisii. Arch Pathol 1971;92:306–318.
46. Kumer R, van der Smissen E, Jorizzo J. Systemic sporotrichosis with osteomyelitis. J Can Assoc Radiol 1984;35:83–84.

47. Gladstone J, Littman M. Osseous sporotrichosis. Am J Med 1971;51: 121–133.
48. Govender S, Rasool MN, Ngcelwane M. Osseous sporotrichosis. J Infect 1989;19:273–276.
49. Fernandez-Guerrero ML, Ruiz Barns P, Ales JM. Postcraniotomy mycetoma of the scalp and osteomyelitis due to Pseudallescheria boydii. J Infect Dis 1987;156:855.
50. Travis LB, Roberts GD, Wilson WR. Clinical significance of Pseudallescheria boydii: a review of 10 years' experience. Mayo Clin Proc 1985;60:531–537.
51. Murtagh J, Smith JW, Mackowiak PA. Case report: alternaria osteomyelitis: eight years of recurring disease requiring cyclic courses of amphotericin B for cure. Am J Med Sci 1987;30:399–402.
52. Brown OE, Finn R. Mucormycosis of the mandible. J Oral Maxillofac Surg 1986;44:132–136.
53. Chaudhuri R, McKeown B, Harrington D. Mucormycosis osteomyelitis causing avascular necrosis of the cuboid bone: MR imaging findings. Am J Radiol 1992;159:1035–1037.
54. Pierce PF, Wood MB, Roberts GD, et al. Saksenaea vasiformis osteomyelitis. J Clin Microbiol 1987;25:933–935.
55. Wilson C, O'Rourke E, McGinnis M, Salkin I. Scedosporium inflatum: clinical spectrum of a newly recognized pathogen. J Infect Dis 1990;161: 102–107.
56. Salkin I, McGinnis M, Dykstra M, Rinaldi M. Scedosporium inflatum, an emerging pathogen. J Clin Microbiol 1988;26:498–503.
57. Chan YF, Woo KC. Penicillium marneffei osteomyelitis. J Bone Joint Surg [Am] 1990;72:500–503.
58. Stillwell WT, Rubin BD, Axelrod JL. Chrysosporium. A new causative agent in osteomyelitis. Clin Orthop 1984;184:190–192.
59. Nuovo MA. Fusarium solani osteomyelitis with probable nosocomial spread. Am J Clin Pathol 1988;90:738–741.
60. Brabender W. Acremonium kiliense osteomyelitis of the calvarium. Neurosurgery 1985;16:554–556.
61. Lee Y, Nersasian R, Lan M. Wound infections with Mycoplasma hominis. JAMA 1971;218:252–253.
62. Steffenson DO. Sternotomy infections with Mycoplasma hominia. Ann Intern Med 1987;106:204–208.
63. Mohiuddin AA. Ureaplasma urealyticum chronic osteomyelitis in a patient with hypogammaglobulinemia. J Allergy Clin Immunol 1991;87:104–107.
64. Forgacs P, Kundsin R, Margles S. A case of ureaplasma urealyticum septic arthritis in a patient with hypogammaglobulinemia. Clin Infect Dis 1993; 16:293–294.
65. McMahon D, Dummer J, Pasculle A, Cassell G. Extragenital Mycoplasma hominis infections in adults. Am J Med 1990;89:275–281.
66. Mikolich DJ, Boyce JM. Brucella species. In: Mandell GL, Douglas RG, Bennet JE, eds. Principles and practice of infectious diseases. New York: Churchill Livingstone, 1989:1735–1742.

67. Samra Y, Hertz M, Shaked Y, Zwas S, Altman G. Brucellosis of the spine. J Bone Joint Surg [Br] 1982;64:429–431.
68. Mousa AR, Muhtaseb SA, Almudallal DS, Khodeir SM, Marafie AA. Osteoarticular complications of brucellosis: a study of 169 cases. Rev Infect Dis 1987;9:531–543.
69. Mousa AM, Muhtaseb SA, Al Mudallal DS, Marafie AA, Habib FM. Brucellar sternoclavicular arthritis, the forgotten complication. Ann Trop Med Parasitol 1988;82:275–281.
70. Alarcon GS, Bocanegra TS, Gutuzzo E, Espinoza LR. Articular involvement in human brucellosis. J Rheumatol 1988;15:379–380.
71. Sharif HS, Clark DC, Aabed MY, et al. Granulomatous spinal infections: MR imaging. Radiology 1990;177:101–107.
72. Colmenero JD, Reguera JM, Cabrera FP, Cisneros JM, Orjuela DL, Fernandez Crehuet J. Serology, clinical manifestations and treatment of brucellosis in different age groups. Infection 1990;18:152–156.
73. Sharif HS, Aideyan OA, Clark DC, et al. Brucellar and tuberculous spondylitis: comparative imaging features. Radiology 1989;171:419–425.
74. Keenan MA, Gutmann GG. Brucella osteomyelitis of the distal part of the femur. J Bone Joint Surg [Am] 1982;64:142–144.
75. Lowbeer L. Experimental and spontaneous brucellotic osteomyelitis of the animal. Am J Pathol 1947;23:911–912.
76. Khateeb MI, Araj GF, Majeed SA, Lulu AR. Brucella arthritis: a study of 96 cases in Kuwait. Ann Rheum Dis 1990;49:994–998.
77. Ariza J, Gudiol F, Pallares R, et al. Treatment of human brucellosis with doxycycline plus rifampin or doxycycline plus streptomycin. A randomized, double-blind study. Ann Intern Med 1992;117:25–30.
78. Tramont EC. Treponema pallidum (syphilis). In: Mandell GL, Douglas RG, Bennet JE, eds. Principles and practice of infectious diseases. New York: Churchill Livingstone, 1979:1794–1807.
79. Holmes KK, Mardh P-A, Sparling PF, Wiesner PJ. Sexually transmitted diseases, ed 2. New York: McGraw-Hill, 1985.
80. Grin EI, Guthe T. Evaluation of a previous mass campaign against endemic syphilis in Bosnia and Herzegovina. Br J Venereal Dis 1973;49:1–19.
81. Noordhoek GT, Engelkens HJ, Judanarso J, et al. Yaws in West Sumatra, Indonesia: clinical manifestations, serological findings and characterization of new Treponema isolates by DNA probes. Eur J Clin Microbiol Infect Dis 1991;10:12–19.
82. Eason RJ, Tasman-Jones T. Resurgent yaws and other skin diseases in the western provinces of the Solomon Islands. Papua New Guinea Med J 1985;28:247–250.
83. Hopkins DR. Yaws in the Americas 1950–1975. J Infect Dis 1977;136: 548–554.
84. Csonka GW, Oates JK. Sexually transmitted diseases. A textbook of genitourinary medicine. London: Bailliere Tindall, 1990.
85. Resnick D, Niwayama G. Diagnosis of bone and joint disorders, ed 2. Philadelphia: WB Saunders, 1988.

86. Kazlow PG, Beyer B, Brandeis G. Polyarthritis as the initial symptom of secondary syphilis: case report and review. Mt Sinai J Med 1989;56:65–67.
87. Burgoyne M, Agudelo C, Pisko E. Chronic syphilitic polyarthritis mimicking systemic lupus erythematosus/rhematoid arthritis as the initial presentation of human immunodeficiency virus infection. J Rheumatol 1992;19: 313–315.
88. Radolf JD, Kaplan RP. Unusual manifestations of secondary syphilis and abnormal humoral immune response to Treponema pallidum antigens in a homosexual man with asymptomatic human immunodeficiency virus infection. J Am Acad Dermatol 1988;18:423–428.
89. Reynolds FW, Wasserman H. Destructive osseous lesions in early syphilis. Arch Intern Med 1942;69:263–276.
90. Bauer MF, Caravati CM. Osteolytic lesions in early syphilis. Br J Venereal Dis 1967;43:175–177.
91. Middleton S, Rowntree C, Rudge S. Bone pain as the presenting manifestation of secondary syphilis. Ann Rheum Dis 1990;49:641–642.
92. Wile UJ, Senear FE. A study of the involvement of the bones and joints in early syphilis. Am J Med Sci 1916;152:689–693.
93. Skapinker S, Minnaar D. Syphilitic diseases of the long bones in the Bantu. J Bone Joint Surg [Br] 1951;33:578–583.
94. Dismukes WE, Delgado DG, Mallernee SV, Myers TC. Destructive bone disease in early syphilis. JAMA 1976;236:2646–2648.
95. Whittet HB, Quiney RE. Nasal manifestations of yaws. J Laryngol Otol 1988;102:1147–1149.
96. King A, Nicol C. Venereal diseases. London: Bailliere Tindall, 1975.
97. Jones BS. Doigt en lorgnette and concentric bone atrophy associated with healed yaws osteitis. Report of two cases. J Bone Joint Surg [Br] 1972;54: 341–345.
98. Collins DH. Pathology of bone. London: Butterworths, 1966.
99. Antonio C, Davanzo R. Congenital syphilis in Mozambique: the diagnostic complementary role of laboratory and radiological investigations. Cent Arf J Med 1989;35:552–555.
100. du Cret RP, Aafedt BC, Griffiths HJ, Warner VT, Boudreau RJ, Kuni CC. Scintigraphic and radiologic manifestations of yaws. Clin Nucl Med 1990;15:580–581.
101. Cronin EB, Williams WH, Tow DE. Radionuclide imaging in a case of tertiary syphilis involving the liver and bones. J Nucl Med 1987;28: 1047–1051.
102. Rasool MN, Govender S. The skeletal manifestations of congenital syphilis. A review of 197 cases. J Bone Joint Surg [Br] 1989;71:752–755.
103. Brion LP, Manuli M, Rai B, Kresch MJ, Pavlov H, Glaser J. Long-bone radiographic abnormalities as a sign of active congenital syphilis in asymptomatic newborns. Pediatrics 1991;88:1037–1040.
104. Greenberg SB, Bernal DV. Are long bone radiographs necessary in neonates suspected of having congenital syphilis? Radiology 1992;182:637–639.

105. Clutton HH. Symmetrical synovitis of the knee in hereditary syphilis. Lancet 1886;1:391.
106. Kabuubi JB. Probable late congenital syphilis presenting as Clutton joints. J R Army Med Corps 1989;135:88–90.
107. Wallace AL, Ellis JM. Juxta-articular bone lesions in tertiary yaws. Med J Aust 1989;150:217–219.
108. Olle Goig JE, Barrio JL, Gurgui M, Mildvan D. Bone invasion in secondary syphilis: case reports. Genitourin Med 1988;64:198–201.
109. Rodriguez S, Teich DL, Weinman MD, Greene JM, Keroack MA, Apstein MD. Gummatous syphilis: a reminder. J Infect Dis 1988;157: 606–607.
110. Brown JR. Human actinomycosis: a study of 181 subjects. Hum Pathol 1973;4:319–330.
111. Conrad SE, Breivis J, Fried MA. Vertebral osteomyelitis caused by Arachnia propionica and resembling actinomycosis. J Bone Joint Surg [Br] 1951;33:204–214.
112. Cope VZ. Actinomycosis of bone with special reference to infection of the vertebral column. J Bone Joint Surg [Br] 1951;33:204–214.
113. Wilding K, Nade SML. Actinomycosis of bone. Aust NZ J Surg 1975;45: 61–65.
114. Kadish LJ, Muller CJB, Mezger H. Chronic sclerosing osteomyelitis in a long bone caused by actinomycosis. S Afr Med J 1982;62:658–659.
115. Millgram JW. Osseous changes in congenital toxoplasmosis. Arch Pathol 1974;97:150–151.
116. Chandar K, Mair HJ, Mair NS. Case of toxoplasma polymyositis. Br Med J 1968;1:158–159.
117. Vass M, Kullman L, Csoka R, Magyar E. Polytenosynovitis caused by Toxoplasma gondii. J Bone Joint Surg [Br] 1977;59:229–232.
118. Borochowitz D, Martinez AJ, Patterson GT. Osteomyelitis of a bone graft of the mandible with Acanthamoeba castellani infection. Hum Pathol 1981;12:573–576.
119. Davson J, Jones DM, Turner L. Diagnosis of Meleney's synergistic gangrene. Br J Surg 1988;75:267–271.
120. Corriden JP, Gray JJ. Trichinosis in South West Ireland. Br Med J 1969;2: 727–730.
121. Sivaramappa M, Reddy CR, Devi CS, Reddy AC, Reddy PK, Murthy DP. Acute guinea worm synovitis of the knee joint. J Bone Joint Surg [Am] 1969;51:1324–1330.
122. McLaughlin GE, Utsinger PD, Trackat WF, Resnick D, Moidel RA. Rheumatic syndromes secondary to guinea worm infestation. Arthritis Rheum 1984;27:694–697.
123. O'Connor RL, Luedke DC, Harkess JW. Hookworm lesion of bone. J Bone Joint Surg [Am] 1971;53:362–364.
124. Bissonette B, Beaudet F. Reactive arthritis with eosinophilic synovial infiltration. Ann Rheum Dis 1983;42:466–468.

125. Booz MK. The management of hydatid disease of bone and joint. J Bone Joint Surg [Br] 1972;54:698–709.
126. Alldred AJ, Nisbet NW. Hydatid disease of bone in Australasia. J Bone Joint Surg [Br] 1964;46:260–267.
127. Ivanessevich O. Hidatidosis osea. Buenos Aires: Amorrortu, 1934.
128. El Gazzar A, McCreadie DWA. Hydatid disease in Kuwait. Br Med J 1962;2:232–234.
129. Okela GBA. Albendazole in the treatment of inoperable hydatid disease in Kenya—a report of 12 cases. Trans R Soc Trop Med 1986;80:193–197.
130. D'Allessandro A, Rausch RL, Cuello C, Aristazabal N. Echinococcus vogeli in man with a review of polycystic hydatid disease in Colombia and neighboring countries. Am J Trop Med Hyg 1979;28:303–317.
131. Jones TC. Cestodes (Tapeworms). In: Mandell GL, Douglas RG, Bennet JE, eds. Principles and practice of infectious diseases. New York: Churchill Livingstone, 1989:2151–2156.
132. Braithwaite PA. Hydatid disease: epidemiology and pathology. Aust NZ J Surg 1983;53:203–209.
133. Hernigou P, Nabih A, Goutallier D. Vertebral hydatidosis. Complications and contribution of modern imaging. Rev Rhum Mal Osteoartic 1992;59: 131–135.
134. Frayha GJ, Bizhaki J, Kachachi TA. Treatment of hydatid cysts (Echinococcus granulosus) by Cetrimide (R). Trans R Soc Trop Med Hyg 1981; 75:447–450.
135. Ottolenghi EC. Massive osteoarticular bone grafts. J Bone Joint Surg [Br] 1966;48:646–659.
136. Levin MH, Weinstein RA, Axelrod JA, Schantz PM. Severe reversible neutropenia during high dose mebendazole therapy for echinococcosis. JAMA 1983;249:2929–2931.

Index